Age-related Macular Degeneration
Diagnosis and Treatment

Allen C. Ho • Carl D. Regillo

Editors

Age-related Macular Degeneration Diagnosis and Treatment

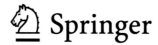 Springer

Editors
Allen C. Ho, MD, FACS
Wills Eye Institute
Thomas Jefferson University
Philadelphia, PA, USA
acho@att.net

Carl D. Regillo, MD, FACS
Wills Eye Institute
Thomas Jefferson University
Philadelphia, PA, USA
cregillo@aol.com

ISBN 978-1-4614-0124-7   e-ISBN 978-1-4614-0125-4
DOI 10.1007/978-1-4614-0125-4
Springer New York Dordrecht Heidelberg London

Library of Congress Control Number: 2011932176

Printed on acid-free paper

Springer is part of Springer Science+Business Media (www.springer.com)

Foreword

Few ocular diseases are so prevalent and devastating to daily life as age-related macular degeneration (AMD). Yet, very little is known about is pathogenesis and treatment. Given the expanding geriatric population, AMD is assuming epidemic proportion, prioritizing the disorder at the pinnacle of critical medical-retinal disease in need of better management.

Fortunately, considerable research has made notable advances in attempting to unravel the biochemical, immunologic, epidemiological and genetic complexities associated with this maculopathy. As a result, there is a wealth of burgeoning knowledge, led by discoveries in molecular biology, genetics, biochemical vasogenic and atrophic pathways, and imaging technology, which specifically displays the microabnormalities related to its pathogenesis. Many of these advances have also led to new opportunities for improved treatment modalities with a better visual prognosis than in the past. It is important to recall that knowledge in any field of medicine relates to a point in time, particularly for a complex disease such as AMD which is constantly under investigation which has led to converging lines of experimental and clinical evidence that modifies established ideas and new treatment concepts. Over the course of years, several comprehensive textbooks and atlases have been written to compile this encyclopedic changing and expanding knowledge related to AMD. The authors of this text have tried to provide a current comprehensive and systemic documentation of the practical and timely analysis of AMD for retinal specialists, comprehensive ophthalmologists, and patients alike. Given the wide range of related disciplines, the authors have engaged an elite corps of experts as contributing authors. They are all leaders in the field with specialized interest in one or more of the principal issues related to the diagnosis and treatment of the disorder. Each section of this text discusses the nature and visual expectations associated with treatment today, including the limitations and potential adverse effects and the anticipated benefits. A review of the ophthalmic literature leading to standards of care based on evidenced-based medicine, specifically the randomized clinical trial, is also incorporated into these discussions. In essence, all new information on retinal genetics, molecular biology, risk factors, and diagnostic testing and imaging have been compiled in this text in a comprehensive format not found in any previous publication.

Thanks to advances from anti-VEGF treatment and enhanced imaging, progress has been made in recent years in the management of neovascular AMD, but very little progress has been made to prevent, retard, and treat the mounting population of patients who suffer vision loss from apoptotic programmed cell loss or atrophy. Accordingly, they have also evaluated possibilities for future new forms of therapy for both the neovascular and non-neovascular forms of the disease. This text has examined all of the current concepts under investigation for management of this critical issue in AMD. It also presents a very erudite discussion on the economic impact of AMD to patients and our society realized by successful treatment. The authors do not fail to present an analysis of the complexities, and controversies and challenges in the study of AMD, assimilating information into logical explanations on the mechanisms of the related patho-physiological manifestations in the fundus, the array of future considerations for accelerating our understanding of the disease, and providing practical means for prevention and treatment.

Essentially, this new comprehensive text on AMD represents a labor of love by an elite corps of expert retinal specialists and clinical scientists. Their monumental efforts will be rewarded by the gratitude of clinicians and patients who will receive incalculable pleasure whether a casual or discerning reader.

Lawrence A. Yannuzzi, M.D.
Vice-Chairman, Dept. of Ophthalmology
and Director of Retinal Services
Manhattan Eye, Ear and Throat Hospital
Professor of Clinical Ophthalmology
College of Physicians and Surgeons
Columbia University, New York, USA

Preface

The field of ophthalmology has witnessed an unparalleled degree of progress over the last decade in the diagnosis and management of age-related macular degeneration (AMD). Before ten years ago, diagnostic techniques consisted of only fundus angiography and treatment was limited to laser photocoagulation for neovascular AMD. Unfortunately, many people suffered severe and irreversible loss of visual acuity from advanced AMD, both neovascular and atrophic or nonneovascular.

A new era began around 1990 with the introduction of photodynamic therapy, which effectively limited vision loss due to certain angiographic classes of neovascular AMD but generally did not afford significant visual gains. More recently, injectable vascular endothelial growth factor (VEGF) inhibiting pharmacotherapeutics have transformed the therapy of all types of neovascular AMD by giving patients a high likelihood of visual stability and a real chance of meaningful visual improvement Frequent intravitreal injections of anti-VEGF medicines remains the standard of care for neovascular AMD; however, there is still room for improvement since only the minority of patients experience significant visual gains and the treatment burden of frequent injections is high. The pace of finding even better therapies for neovascular AMD has quickened and new comparative information on anti-VEGF therapies will play a major role in treatment decision making.

Although the nutritional interventions established by the Age Related Eye Disease Study (AREDS) have incrementally improved the prognosis of patients with significant drusen and nonneovascular AMD, we have not yet witnessed a sea change event. This is about to change as our expanding understanding of the pathobiology of nonneovascular AMD points us toward new therapeutic strategies and targets. While all these therapeutic advances were emerging, our ability to diagnose AMD-related atrophy and exudation improved with the advent of fundus autofluorescence and optic coherence tomography (OCT). These invaluable tools have become essential for day-to-day patient care but also generate and measure important quantitative data in nearly all ongoing AMD clinical trials. Lastly, our understanding of disease has leaped forward with the discovery of various genetic factors and inflammatory mechanisms that are associated strongly with AMD.

This book aims to provide – for the retina specialist, general eye care professional, vision scientist, and those training in these areas – an update on the current understanding of AMD pathophysiology, the use of diagnostic tests, and the management of both nonneovascular and neovascular AMD. It also looks into the future with potential treatment options that are now under investigation in clinical trials. Finally, it covers the medical economics and societal impact of this major public health issue.

To cover this large array of topics in AMD, the editors are fortunate to have leading authorities in the field of retina to author the chapters of this book. We are grateful to the authors for all their time and efforts. We wish to acknowledge the ongoing support and inspiration of our associates at Mid Atlantic Retina and our ophthalmology colleagues, residents, and fellows at Wills Eye Institute. We also wish to thank our editors at Springer, Rebekah Amos, Shelley Reinhardt, Barbara Lopez-Lucio, and Catherine Paduani for their dedicated guidance and editorial expertise.

Philadelphia, PA   Allen C. Ho, MD
                                                                   Carl D. Regillo, MD

Contents

Contributors

Gary C. Brown, M.D., M.B.A. Department of Ophthalmology, Jefferson Medical College, Wyndmoore, PA, USA; Center for Value-Based Medicine, Flourtown, PA, USA

Kathryn Brown Center for Value-Based Medicine, Flourtown, PA, USA

Melissa M. Brown, M.D., M.B.A. Department of Ophthalmology, Jefferson Medical College, Wyndmoore, PA, USA; Center for Value-Based Medicine, Flourtown, PA, USA

Claudia Brue, M.D. URMNY, New York, NY, USA

Yuhong Chen, M.D., Ph.D. Department of Ophthalmology, University of California at San Diego, La Jolla, San Diego, CA, USA

Emily Y. Chew, M.D. Division of Epidemiology and Clinical Applications, National Eye Institute/National Institutes of Health, Bethesda, MD, USA

Allen Chiang, M.D. Retina Service, Wills Eye Institute/ Mid-Atlantic Retina, Philadelphia, PA, USA

Hanna R. Coleman, M.D. Department of Ophthalmology, New York Hospital Presbyterian-Columbia, New York, NY, USA

Jeffrey S. Heier, M.D. Ophthalmic Consultants of Boston, Boston, MA, USA

Allen C. Ho, M.D. Retina Service, Wills Eye Institute/Mid-Atlantic Retina, Philadelphia, PA, USA

Jonathan Jonisch, M.D. Barnes Retina Institute, MO, USA

Peter K. Kaiser, M.D. Cole Eye Institution, Cleveland Clinic, Cleveland, OH, USA

Daniel T. Kasuga, B.S. Department of Ophthalmology, University of California at San Diego, La Jolla, San Diego, CA, USA

Nupura Krishnadev, M.D., FRCSC Department of Epidemiology and Clinical Applications, National Eye Institute/National Institutes of Health, Bethesda, MD, USA

Ketan Laud, M.D. Vitreous-Retina-Macula Consultants of New York, Columbia University, New York, NY, USA

Heidi B. Lieske Center for Value-Based Medicine, Flourtown, PA, USA

Philip A. Lieske Center for Value-Based Medicine, Flourtown, PA, USA

Annal D. Meleth, M.D., M.S. Department of Epidemiology
and Clinical Applications, National Eye Institute/National Institutes
of Health, Bethesda, MD, USA

Sri Krishna Mukkamala, M.D. Department of Ophthalmology,
The New York Eye and Ear Infirmary, New York, NY, USA

Fernando M. Penha, M.D., Ph.D. Department of Ophthalmology,
Bascom Palmer Eye Institute, University of Miami, Miami, FL, USA

Veena R. Raiji, M.D., M.P.H. Department of Ophthalmology,
George Washington University, Washington, DC, USA

Carl D. Regillo, M.D., FACS Retina Service, Wills Eye Institute/
Mid-Atlantic Retina, Philadelphia, PA, USA

Philip J. Rosenfeld, M.D., Ph.D. Department of Ophthalmology,
Bascom Palmer Eye Institute, University of Miami, Miami, FL, USA

Chirag P. Shah, M.D., M.P.H. Ophthalmic Consultants of Boston,
Boston, MA, USA

Gaurav Shah, M.D. Barnes Retina Institute, MO, USA

Jason S. Slakter, M.D. Vitreous-Retina-Macula Consultants
of New York, New York, NY, USA

Nathan Steinle, M.D. Cole Eye Institute, Cleveland Clinic Foundation,
Cleveland, OH, USA

Andre J. Witkin, M.D. Retina Service, Wills Eye Institute/
Mid-Atlantic Retina, Philadelphia, PA, USA

Kang Zhang, M.D., Ph.D. Department of Ophthalmology,
Institute for Genomic Medicine, Shiley Eye Center,
University of California at San Diego, La Jolla, San Diego, CA, USA

Genetics of Age-Related Macular Degeneration

Daniel T. Kasuga, Yuhong Chen, and Kang Zhang

Key Points

- Age-related Macular Degeneration (AMD) is a multifactorial disease involving genetic and environmental influences.
- Complement Factor H (CFH) and HTRA1/ LOC387715 are the two main loci associated with AMD.
- A genetic understanding of AMD may allow for early diagnosis and treatment.

Introduction

Age-related macular degeneration (AMD) is the leading cause of irreversible blindness in the developed world. In the United States alone, over 10 million people are affected, with over 1.75 million people exhibiting advanced forms of the disease. By 2020, nearly 3 million people in the United States will suffer from advanced AMD [1]. AMD is a complex disease, with multiple genetic and environmental factors playing a role in its pathogenesis [2]. With an improved understanding of disease-causing genes, genetic testing of individuals has become increasingly commonplace for early diagnosis of various

D.T. Kasuga (✉)
Department of Ophthalmology, University of California at San Diego, Skaggs (SSPPS) Rm. 4186, 9500 Gilman Dr., La Jolla, San Diego, CA, USA
e-mail: dankasuga@gmail.com

diseases and conditions. Due to the increasing number of individuals affected by this disease, identification of genetic factors and early genetic screening will be needed to determine populations at risk and allow for early intervention. In this chapter, we will review our current understanding of the genetics associated with AMD.

Etiology

AMD can be classified into early and late phases. The early phase is characterized by large yellow subretinal deposits called drusen and retinal pigmented epithelium (RPE) changes (Fig. 1.1). The disease can progress to either choroidal neovascularization (CNV), a rapidly deteriorating late form of AMD characterized by new blood vessels that invade the macula (Fig. 1.1c), or to geographic atrophy (GA), a slower late form causing degeneration of the macula's retinal pigmented epithelium (Fig. 1.1d).

Although extensive research has investigated the underlying etiology of AMD, the exact mechanism remains unknown. Researchers have investigated inflammatory dysregulation, lipid metabolism defects, oxidative stress, and structural defects, to name a few. Many have looked for a genetic answer to the question. Coupled with an age-related time course and two distinct late-stage phenotypes, the possibility of a single genetic cause seems unlikely. However, researchers have identified unique polymorphisms, which harbor impressive associations to AMD.

A.C. Ho and C.D. Regillo (eds.), *Age-related Macular Degeneration Diagnosis and Treatment*,
DOI 10.1007/978-1-4614-0125-4_1, © Springer Science+Business Media, LLC 2011

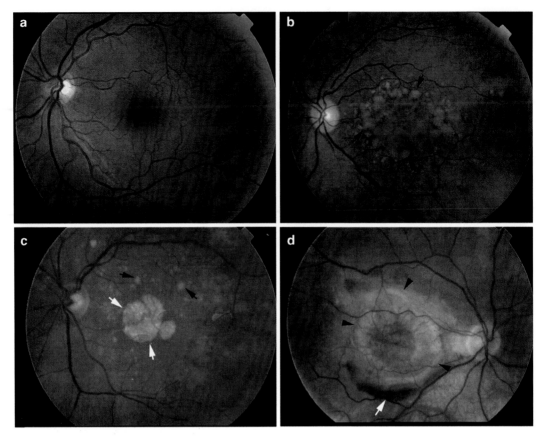

Fig. 1.1 Four fundus images showing a normal macula (**a**), confluent soft drusen (*black arrows*) covering the macula (**b**), geographic atrophy (*white arrows*) and soft drusen (*black arrows*) of the macula (**c**), and a choroidal neovascular membrane (*black arrow heads*) covering the macula with a concomitant subretinal hemorrhage (*white arrow*) (**d**) (Photographs were provided by Kang Zhang, MD, PhD, and James Gilman, CRA)

> **Pearl**
> Late AMD has two very different clinical manifestations.

> **Pearl**
> The etiology behind AMD is still unknown.

A Genetic Cause

Family Studies

The search for a genetic basis to AMD began with an understanding that family history is a significant risk factor. Over 20% of those with AMD have a family history of the disease [3, 4] and first-degree relatives of patients with late AMD have a fourfold increased risk of AMD. One case control study examining the frequency of AMD in siblings of affected patients found that 25% were also affected by the disease. In control patients, only 1% of the siblings exhibited signs of AMD [5]. Twin studies have also shown familial association [6, 7], with one study reporting a 19% concordance rate among dizygotic twins, and a 37% concordance rate among monozygotic twins [8]. Strong evidence for a familial component to AMD highlights a genetic predisposition to the disease.

Associations with Race

Research involving different populations has indicated that the risk of AMD varies by race. Across multiple studies, it has been shown that the prevalence of AMD is lower in blacks than in whites [9–13]. Friedman et al. found that the prevalence of AMD in a Baltimore population was higher in whites than blacks (1.91% versus 0.19%, respectively) [10]. More recently, the Salisbury Eye Evaluation (SEE) study showed black study participants had a significantly lower incidence of geographic atrophy when compared to white patients (0.3% versus 1.8%, respectively) [9]. Other studies have shown that Hispanics/Latinos have a lower prevalence than non-Latino whites [11, 13]. The Los Angeles Latino Eye Study determined that although early AMD findings were common in Latinos (9.7%, 95% Confidence Interval (CI) 8.7–10.2), late AMD findings were infrequent (0.52%, 95% CI 0.28–0.63) [13]. Regarding Asians, a recent meta-analysis showed similar prevalence rates to white populations for late AMD findings (0.56% versus 0.59%, respectively). However, early AMD findings were less common in Asians (6.8% versus 8.8%) [14]. Cumulatively, racial differences in disease prevalence point towards a genetic component to AMD.

After establishing that family history and race were risk factors, researchers turned to the task of elucidating those specific polymorphisms that confer an increased risk for AMD.

> **Pearl**
> Family history is a significant risk factor for AMD.

> **Pearl**
> Caucasians appear most susceptible to AMD, while black populations are least susceptible. Differences in race underline the importance of genetics in AMD pathogenesis.

Specific Genes Conferring AMD Risk

Although there is a clear genetic predisposition to AMD, finding specific genes has been difficult due to the late onset of the disease and its phenotypic heterogeneity. Even with these challenges, candidate genes have been identified, which confer considerable risk to the development of AMD. Along with family genetic studies, genome-wide linkage studies have aided in identifying key loci associated with AMD. Several of these studies found associations with chromosome 1q [15–21] and chromosome 10q [18, 20, 22, 23]. The most promising appear to be a loci found on chromosome 1, called ARMD1 (1q25–31), and one on chromosome 10 (10q26) [17, 24, 25]. Both likely account for more than 50% of all AMD cases.

Genetic Variants in Complement Factor Genes

An underlying inflammatory response has been postulated to be a cause of AMD [26, 27]. Specifically, researchers have hypothesized that dysfunction of the complement cascade may cause inflammatory changes in the retina, leading to the AMD phenotype [28]. This hypothesis has been strengthened by the findings of complement factors in drusen, an increase in activation of the alternative complement factor in the serum of AMD patients, and specific variants in complement factor genes that confer susceptibility to AMD [29–32]. The most significant of those variants was found in the gene for Complement Factor H (CFH).

Complement Factor H

CFH is a major inhibitor of the alternative complement pathway at multiple steps (Fig. 1.2). It inhibits the conversion of C3 to its C3a/C3b components and competes with Factor B to prevent activation of C3b to C3bB. CFH also binds heparin and C-reactive protein (CRP), which may help deter CRP-induced complement activation [33].

Investigation of the ARMD1 locus for unique AMD-associated polymorphisms identified the single nucleotide polymorphism (SNP) rs1061170 in exon 9 of the CFH gene as having a high concordance with AMD (p value: 4.95×10^{-10}) [28]. SNP rs1061170 encodes a tyrosine to histidine change at the 402 position of the gene (Y402H) [30]. The structural change caused by Y402H is found in the heparin and the C-reactive protein

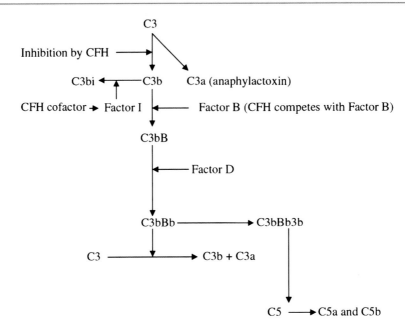

Fig. 1.2 The inhibitory role of CFH in the alternate complement pathway (Reprinted by permission from Macmillan Publishers Ltd: [33]. Copyright 2006)

binding site of CFH. Decreased binding to these factors may alter the ability of CFH to inhibit the alternative complement pathway, leading to over-activity of complement proteins [34]. Meta-analysis of eight studies showed that a single histidine allele (heterozygous for risk C allele, CT genotype) confers a 2.5-fold increased risk of AMD (95% CI 1.96–3.30), while individuals with two risk alleles (CC) were 6.35 times more likely to have AMD than those with the homozygous non-risk TT genotype (95% CI 4.25–9.48). This indicates a multiplicative model of the Y402H variant [35]. In a prospective study, additional risk alleles increased the risk of disease progression. Over a six-year period, 30% of those with the CC genotype, 18% with the CT genotype, and 10% with the TT genotype progressed to advanced disease [36]. Predicted population-attributable risk (PAR) for the risk genotype (CC or CT) ranges from 22% to 58.9%, indicating that persons homozygous or heterozygous for the CFH variant comprise roughly 20–60% of all AMD cases [35, 37]. Taken collectively, the association of Y402H to AMD has been firmly established.

Most CFH studies have investigated primarily Caucasian populations. Looking at the Y402H variant prevalence in multiple populations reveals large differences between ethnicities. Allele frequencies for Caucasian (34–39%) and African-American populations (30.7–35%) were higher than Hispanic (17%) and Asian populations (Japanese 8.1%, Chinese 6.8%) [38, 39]. These numbers do not correlate with the prevalence of AMD found among respective ethnicities, indicating that other genetic or environmental factors are at play [38].

Recently, a noncoding SNP rs1410996, found in an intron of CFH, has been significantly associated with AMD (p value: 2.65×10^{-61}) [40]. Its association was repeated in multiple studies, including recent studies of Chinese and Japanese populations [41–43]. Further research will hopefully find an associated coding SNP that confers a functional mechanism of action to the genetic variant.

C2-CFB Locus

Set in a locus on chromosome 6p21, variations in Complement Component 2 (C2, classic pathway) and Complement Factor B (BF, CFB, alternative pathway) genes have been associated with AMD. Gold et al. investigated haplotypes involving these two genes. Although one haplotype conferred risk for AMD, two haplotypes did not. A haplotype involving the nearly complete linkage disequilibrium (LD) set of the L9H variant of BF and the E318D variant of C2 was highly protective against AMD (p value: 2×10^{-4}, OR 0.37, 95% CI 0.18–0.60). A haplotype combining the nearly complete LD set of the R32Q variant of BF with the rs547154 variant of C2 intron 10, was highly protective as well (p value: 6.43×10^{-9}, OR 0.32, 95% CI 0.21–0.48). Further analysis showed a codominant model for these two haplotypes [44]. Another study investigating similar SNPs in a Caucasian family-based data set hypothesized that rs547154 is the same as R32Q due to their high LD. It purported that BF R32Q may be the most significant protective variant of the C2-BF locus, after controlling for age, common risk variants on chromosome 1 and 10, and smoking (OR 0.21, 95% CI 0.11–0.39) [45]. Functional studies of the R32Q variant supported this claim by showing a fourfold decreased affinity for C3b, and subsequent decreased formation of activated convertase [46]. Future functional studies will continue to elucidate the protective effects of C2 and BF variants.

Complement Component 3

Unlike C2-BF, variants in the complement component 3 (C3) gene confer susceptibility to AMD [47–50]. Two SNPs in high LD with each other have been implicated: rs2230199 (R102G) and rs1047286 (P314L). Yates et al. and Maller et al. [48, 50] examined the rs2230199 SNP in different cohorts of Caucasian patients. Odds ratios for being homozygous or heterozygous for the G risk allele were 1.7 (95% CI 1.3–2.1) and 2.6 (95% CI 1.6–4.1), respectively [50]. The rs2230199 SNP encodes an arginine to glycine switch in the third exon of C3 (R120G). The normal arginine provides a positive charge that may help stabilize a thioester binding motif. A switch to a neutral glycine residue at this position could weaken the thioester motif –a motif implicated in CFH binding [50]. Weakening of a CFH-binding site would prevent proper inhibition of C3. This variant also

results in two separate allotypes based upon their electrophoretic characteristics (slow, C3S; fast C3F). The fast allotype has been implicated in renal diseases much like variants of CFH [49].

Although multiple researchers have indicated that rs2230199 is a stronger risk variant for AMD [49, 50], others contend that both SNPs have a role in AMD risk [48]. No functional explanation has been assigned to SNP rs1047286. However, a recent meta-analysis showed a pooled susceptibility odds ratio of 1.50 for the P314L allele (95% CI 1.31–1.71) and 1.61 for the R102G allele (95% CI 1.46–1.78). Further studies will help refine these associations.

> **Pearl**
> The Y402H Complement Factor H genetic variant accounts for over 50% of the risk associated with AMD. Most variants in C2/BF are protective of AMD, while C3 variants confer AMD risk.

Other Inflammatory Factor Variants

Toll-Like Receptor

Some believe that underlying bacterial or viral infections instigate inflammatory ocular cascades that promote the propagation of AMD. Along this line of thinking, variant rs4986790 in the toll-like receptor (TLR) 4 gene (encodes a bacterial endotoxin receptor) was associated with AMD susceptibility [51]. Yang et al. investigated SNPs in both TLR3 and TLR4. Although they did not confirm the TLR4 variant associations, they showed that SNP rs3775291 of TLR3 conferred protection against geographic atrophy. Odds ratios for heterozygotes and homozygotes of this variant were 0.712 (95% CI 0.5–1.00) and 0.437 (95% CI 0.23–0.84), respectively [52].

VEGF-A

Vascular endothelial growth factor (VEGF) has been implicated in the pathogenesis of neovascular AMD (CNV) [53]. The VEGF-A protein can be alternatively spliced to create multiple isoforms.

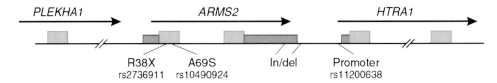

Fig. 1.3 Genetic variants within the chromosome 10q26 locus (Reprinted by permission from Macmillan Publishers Ltd: [56]. Copyright July 2008)

The VEGF-A 165 isoform is important in ocular angiogenic control and is elevated in AMD patients [54]. Genetic variations in the VEGF gene confer increased susceptibility to AMD. Churchill et al. found that those homozygous for the C risk allele of variant SNP rs1413711 were at an increased risk of AMD (OR 2.4, 95% CI 1.09–5.26) [55]. As more data becomes available, we may be able to predict how well AMD patients will respond to current anti-VEGF therapies based upon genetic modifiers.

Genetic Variants on Chromosome 10q26

Although ARMD1 was the first confirmed susceptibility locus, chromosome 10q26 harbors the locus most significantly associated with AMD [24]. This region contains three genes: a hypothetical gene LOC387715/ARMS2, and two known genes: PLEKHA1 and HTRA1 (Fig. 1.3).

LOC387715/ARMS2

The LOC387715/ Age-Related Maculopathy Susceptibility 2 (ARMS2) region lies between PLEKHA1 and HTRA1 on chromosome 10q26. In multiple association studies, this gene has been implicated in AMD susceptibility [57–59]. Using two separate German cohorts, researchers identified SNP rs10490924, which results in an alanine to serine (A69S) change, as a high-risk variant for AMD. Pooled data showed that cases heterozygous or homozygous for the T risk allele of rs10490924 had a 2.69-fold (95% CI 2.22–3.27) or 8.21-fold (95% CI 5.79–11.65) increased risk of AMD, respectively, compared with the homozygous non-risk genotype (GG) [59]. This association was independent of the Y402H

variant of CFH. A meta-analysis comprising five datasets showed similar results (TG heterozygous OR 2.48, 95% CI 1.67–3.70; TT homozygous OR 7.3, 95% CI 4.33–12.42) [58]. Phenotypically, the A69S variant was associated with a younger age of CNV onset [57, 60]. Although numbers vary by study, the population attributable risk for the A69S variant has been estimated between 34% and 57%, indicating that possibly over 50% of the AMD risk can be attributed to this variant [61–63].

Recently, an insertion-deletion (in/del) variant in LOC387715 was found that exists in perfect LD with the researched A69S variant. This in-del variant specifically removes the mRNA's polyadenylated tail, leading to rapid mRNA turnover and a decreased LOC387715 mRNA expression. The in/del variant was highly correlated with AMD risk (p value: 4.1×10^{-29}, OR 2.85, 95% CI 2.37–3.43) [64]. In contrast to the loss of function role of the in/del in *LOC387715,* the T allele of SNP rs2736911, a nonsynonymous coding SNP leading to a predicted premature stop (R38X) in *LOC387715,* is associated with a protective haplotype. These findings present a paradox. The in/del causes destabilization of *LOC387715,* suggesting that loss of function at that locus might confer risk to AMD. However, the introduction of the R38X mutation, which is also predicted to give rise to loss of the *LOC387715* message, is protective [65]. Yang et al. showed that both the R38X and in/del have the same mode of action, which decreases expression of LOC387715. Therefore, the loss of *LOC387715* is insufficient to explain AMD susceptibility.

Another criticism of the LOC387715/ ARMS2 gene is that it encodes a hypothetical gene with an unknown function. Present only in some primate lineages, it may encode a protein expressed mainly in placenta, but only weakly in the retina [59]. Using human retinal RNA, Kanda et al. expressed the purported LOC387715 protein in COS-1 cells. The expressed protein localized to the outer wall of mitochondria [66]. In comparison, Wang et al. used immunofluorescence and immunoblot analysis to show that the LOC387715 protein localized to the cytosol, not the mitochondria [67]. Further research will hopefully elucidate a possible functional mechanism by which this genetic variant confers risk for AMD.

HTRA1

The HTRA1 gene (also known as PRSS11) lies approximately 6.1 kb downstream of the LOC387715 gene. Its association to AMD has been established in a number of independent cohorts [68–75]. The SNP rs11200638 is found in the promoter region of HTRA1 and tagged a major disease haplotype. This variant's A risk allele (G625A) alters a conserved binding element, AP2/SRF [70]. In a cohort of 581 AMD patients and 309 normal controls, it was found that those heterozygous or homozygous for the A allele were at a significantly increased risk for AMD (OR 1.83, 95% CI 1.25–2.68; OR 7.29, 95% CI 3.18–16.74, respectively) [74]. Similar numbers were obtained in a meta-analysis of 14 studies (OR 2.13, 95% CI 1.9–2.39; OR 6.92, 95% CI 5.74–8.34, respectively) [76]. The population-attributable risk for HTRA1 ranges between 22% and 53% across studies [37].

The HTRA1 gene's protein, HtrA serine protease 1, is an inhibitor of the angiogenesis regulator transforming growth factor-β (TGF-β). It also appears to increase the degradation of extracellular matrix (ECM) proteins by modifying the activity of matrix metalloproteinase enzymes [77]. It could be possible that overexpression of HTRA1 weakens Bruch's membrane and promotes angiogenesis, creating the phenotypic CNV picture in advanced AMD. This hypothesis is strengthened by a study indicating its association specifically with CNV in a Chinese population [70] and data showing an increased

association with large CNV (≥4 disc areas, OR 3.4, 95% CI 1.2–9.5) [57]. Researchers implicating HTRA1 in GA have shown a threefold increased expression of HTRA1 in the retinal pigmented epithelium of patients with the rs11200638 risk variant [74] and evidence of the HTRA1 protein in the drusen of AMD patients [70, 74]. Together, these studies add weight to the claim that HTRA1 has a significant role in AMD risk.

Although research disagrees about transcript expression levels of HTRA1 and LOC387715 in AMD patients, haplotype analysis has linked both genes. Yang et al. showed a synergistic relationship between the reported in/del variant of LOC387715 [64] and the A risk allele of rs11200638 in HTRA1. In-vitro experiments showed either was insufficient to generate increased expression of HTRA1. However, a two-fold increase in expression was exhibited when a disease haplotype was used, which included both risk variants (Fig. 1.4). Animal invivo experiments and mRNA expression levels in human placentas with risk haplotypes confirmed this association [65]. The relationship between LOC387715 and HTRA1 highlights the importance of haplotype examination in complex diseases such as AMD.

> **Pearl**
> HTRA1 is the most significant AMD susceptibility gene on chromosome 10q26.

Other Genetic Variants

Apolipoprotein E

Apolipoprotein E (ApoE) is a glycoprotein involved in lipid transport and lipid homeostasis in the central nervous system [79]. In the eye, it is found in the RPE, outer segments of photoreceptors, Bruch's membrane, and drusen. Of the different isoforms of ApoE, the E4 allele appears to confer a protective effect, providing a two- to threefold decrease in AMD, while the E2 allele may be associated with AMD risk [80–84].

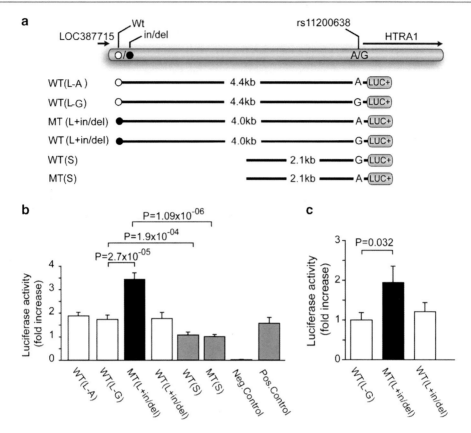

Fig. 1.4 Effects of the in/del variants and rs11200638 on HTRA1 expression in cultured human RPE cells and mouse RPE in vivo using luciferase activity. (**a**) Schematic diagram of constructs for luciferase reporter assays. *L* = long promoter construct. *S* = short promoter construct. A/G represents the allele at rs11200638. *Black dot* indicates in/del variant. (**b**) Luciferase activity in human cultured RPE of different HTRA1 promoter sequences corresponding to risk (MT) and wild-type (*WT*) alleles of in/del and rs11200638 (WT(L-A), WT(L-G), (MT(L + in/del), (WT(L + in/del), WT(S) and MT(S)) (**c**) Luciferase activities in mouse RPE in vivo corresponding to different HTRA1 promoter reporter constructs. *Error bars* represent the mean (6 SEM) (Reprinted from [78])

Although subsequent papers do not share similar results [85, 86], one meta -analysis found that having one E4 allele provided up to a 38% reduction in the risk of AMD [87].

Fibulin 5

Fibulin 5 is an extracellular matrix protein found in Bruch's membrane. Patients with AMD have a faster degradation of Bruch's membrane as they age, possibly increasing the risk for extension of blood vessels across this membrane and progression of CNV [88]. In a case-control Iowa cohort, Stone et al. found that missense variations in the gene encoding Fibulin 5 were statistically associated with AMD [89]. Lotery et al. showed that reduced Fibulin 5 secretion was associated with AMD [90]. Together, this data points towards the hypothesis that variations in the Fibulin 5 protein may weaken Bruch's membrane, thus contributing to the AMD phenotype. However, this association has not been consistently replicated in further research.

Hemicentin-1

Hemicentin 1 is another fibulin protein found in Bruch's membrane. Family-association studies identified the gene encoding Hemicentin 1 as a candidate gene for AMD [25]. However, further studies in larger populations have not found this association [91, 92].

Genetic Associations Between AMD and Heritable Macular Dystrophies

The clinical picture of many heritable macular dystrophies mirrors certain aspects of AMD. However, studies are inconclusive regarding the association between the inherited genetic variants and AMD risk. Genetic variants of CX3CR1, PON1, ERCC, LRP6, MMP9, ABCA4, and ELOVL4 proteins cause a variety of known heritable macular dystrophies. Although some studies have shown that they may also play a role in AMD, this data has been less consistently replicated.

Elongation of very long chain fatty acids-like 4 (ELOVL4) is highly expressed in human photo-receptors [93]. Genetic variants of ELOVL4 encoding premature stop codons result in an autosomal dominant form of Startgardt-like macular dystrophy (STGD3) [94]. Genetic studies involving AMD patients found that a M299V variant of ELOVL4 may have a role in CNV [95]. However, other studies failed to repeat this association with ELOVL4 and AMD [96]. Future studies will help confirm associations between AMD and genetic variants of heritable macular dystrophies.

Interactions of Multiple Genetic Variants

LOC387715/HTRA1 and CFH

Conley et al. showed that CFH and LOC387715 have a synergistic effect on disease susceptibility [58]. Individuals with one risk allele had a significantly higher risk for AMD than those with no risk alleles. Odds ratios for a Y402H T allele or A69S T allele were 2.8 (95% CI 1.6–5.0) and 3.2 (95% CI 1.7–6.0), respectively. Those heterozygous for both variants had a greater-than-twofold increase in risk (OR 7.2, 95% CI 3.8–13.5). In a combined cohort analysis of a German population, it was found that there was a high concordance of LOC387715 A69S risk (T) alleles and CFH Y402H risk (C) alleles. The odds ratio for the double homozygous (CCTT) haplotype was 57.28

(95%CI 37.24–89.00) [59]. In a study involving AREDS patients, the population attributable risk (PAR) of AMD progression for carrying both CFH Y402H and LOC387715 A69S variants was calculated to be 71.8% [36]. In summary, CFH and LOC387715 have an independent, yet multiplicative effect on the risk for AMD [58].

Cameron et al. examined the influence of both the HTRA1 rs11200638 variant and the CFH rs1061170 variant (Y402H) on AMD risk. Their results showed that an individual homozygous for both risk variants had a significantly increased risk of late AMD [29]. Together, the variants confer a PAR of 75% [29]. Yang et al. complemented these findings, stating that CFH and HTRA1 variants together confer an additive effect on AMD risk (Fig. 1.5). The estimated PAR for a haplotype with a risk allele at either locus was 71.4% [74].

> **Pearl**
> HTRA1 and LOC387715 variants, when combined with CFH variants, confer an increased susceptibility to AMD.

Genetic Predisposition to a Specific Late Phenotype

Due to the phenotypic heterogeneity of late AMD, researchers have investigated whether specific genetic variants confer more risk to geographic atrophy or choroidal neovascularization.

Magnusson et al. found that the Y402H variant confers similar risk to GA (OR 2.05, 95% CI 1.40–3.00), CNV (OR 2.17, 95% CI 1.66–2.84), and soft drusen formation (OR 2.10, 95% CI 1.5–2.95) [39]. Francis et al. confirmed the finding that SNPs around the CFH gene, including the Y402H variant, do not preferentially direct progression of disease towards one late phenotype [98]. Seddon et al. found that the A69S variant of LOC387715 conferred a stronger risk for progression to CNV (OR 6.1, 95% CI 3.3–11.2) than to GA (OR 3.0, 95% CI 1.4–6.5) [36]. Although Cameron et al. concluded that HTRA1 had an

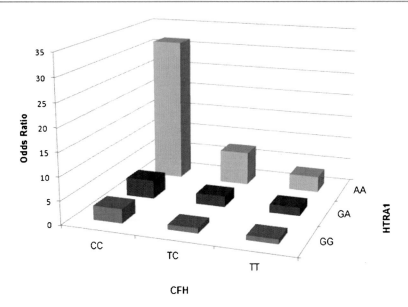

Fig. 1.5 AMD risk odds ratios for haplotypes involving the Y402H CFH variant (C risk allele) and the rs11200638 HTRA1 variant (A risk allele) (Adapted from [97])

equal contribution to both CNV and GA [68], a recent meta- analysis indicated that HTRA1 conferred a higher risk of CNV than GA [76]. Still, the differing results from multiple studies on CFH, LOC387715, and HTRA1 prevent us from making a definitive conclusion.

The rs3775291 variant of toll-like receptor 3 (TLR-3) was associated with a protective effect against geographic atrophy. No association was found between the variant and CNV [52]. Although later studies placed these results into question, rs3775291 is the closest current literature has come to a late phenotype-specific causal genetic variant.

Interactions Between Genetic Variants and Environmental Factors

Age-related Macular Degeneration is a true multi-factorial disease. It is well established that both genetic variants and environmental factors confer disease susceptibility [62, 63, 99–104]. The most significant environmental risk factor, after age, may be cigarette smoking. Of 17 studies investigated, 13 found a statistically significant link between smoking and AMD [104]. Smokers were at a two- to three-fold increased risk of AMD

compared to nonsmokers. Research investigating the link between smoking and genetic variants has shown that the effects of the Y402H variant and A69S variant are stronger among patients who smoke [63, 100]. However, statistically significant data is lacking. Although Francis et al. were able to show the A69S LOC387715 variant and current cigarette smoking as risk factors for AMD, no statistical interaction between the genetic and environmental factors was found [101]. Seddon et al. showed that the CC genotype (OR 7.4, 95% CI 4.7–11.8) of Y402H and current smoking (OR 5.1) conferred independent risks of AMD. However, their joint interaction odds ratio of 10.2 was less than the odds ratio generated from an additive model of each risk factor (7.4+5.1=12.5) [102]. Although no statistically significant multiplicative interactions were found, one study indicated that the incidence of AMD in those homozygous for the CFH Y402H risk allele was fivefold higher than a control population. If these patients were obese or current smokers, there was an estimated 12-fold and 9-fold increased risk of AMD, respectively [62]. In summary, both genetic and environmental factors surely play a role in the complex pathophysiology of AMD, even if the interaction between genetic and environmental factors has not been fully defined.

Conclusion

With the advent of improved genomic technology, there has been an increasing shift towards research addressing the interplay between genetics and common medical diseases. Age-related Macular Degeneration is a perfect example. There has been an exponential growth in research investigating genetic associations to AMD. Perturbations in the complement system, including the Y402H variant of Complement Factor H, have been repeatedly linked to AMD susceptibility. The 10q26 locus has yielded multiple genetic variants with strong associations to AMD, including HTRA1 and LOC387715. Beyond these two major loci, myriad variants with varying disease mechanisms have been implicated in AMD risk or protection. Future research will undoubtedly discover new variants in known or novel loci. With a mixture of environmental and genetic factors playing a role in its pathogenesis, construction of strong risk haplotypes may provide the best correlations with this multifaceted disease. Moving forward, these genetic profiles will be invaluable in helping to develop screening tools, diagnose AMD earlier and more accurately, and direct genetically-specific treatments to the appropriate patients.

References

1. Friedman DS, O'Colmain BJ, Munoz B, et al. Prevalence of age-related macular degeneration in the United States. Arch Ophthalmol. 2004;122(4):564–72.
2. Seddon JM, Ajani UA, Mitchell BD. Familial aggregation of age-related maculopathy. Am J Ophthalmol. 1997;123(2):199–206.
3. De Jong PT, Klaver CC, Wolfs RC, Assink JJ, Hofman A. Familial aggregation of age-related maculopathy. Am J Ophthalmol. 1997;124(6):862–3.
4. Klaver CC, Wolfs RC, Assink JJ, van Duijn CM, Hofman A, de Jong PT. Genetic risk of age-related maculopathy. Population-based familial aggregation study. Arch Ophthalmol. 1998;116(12):1646–51.
5. Silvestri G, Johnston PB, Hughes AE. Is genetic predisposition an important risk factor in age-related macular degeneration? Eye (Lond). 1994;8(Pt 5):564–8.
6. Klein ML, Mauldin WM, Stoumbos VD. Heredity and age-related macular degeneration. Observations in monozygotic twins. Arch Ophthalmol. 1994;112(7):932–7.
7. Meyers SM, Greene T, Gutman FA. A twin study of age-related macular degeneration. Am J Ophthalmol. 1995;120(6):757–66.
8. Hammond CJ, Webster AR, Snieder H, Bird AC, Gilbert CE, Spector TD. Genetic influence on early age-related maculopathy: a twin study. Ophthalmology. 2002;109(4):730–6.
9. Bressler SB, Munoz B, Solomon SD, West SK. Racial differences in the prevalence of age-related macular degeneration: the Salisbury Eye Evaluation (SEE) Project. Arch Ophthalmol. 2008;126(2):241–5.
10. Friedman DS, Katz J, Bressler NM, Rahmani B, Tielsch JM. Racial differences in the prevalence of age-related macular degeneration: the Baltimore eye survey. Ophthalmology. 1999;106(6):1049–55.
11. Klein R, Klein BE, Jensen SC, Mares-Perlman JA, Cruickshanks KJ, Palta M. Age-related maculopathy in a multiracial United States population: the national health and nutrition examination survey III. Ophthalmology. 1999;106(6):1056–65.
12. Klein R, Klein BE, Knudtson MD, et al. Prevalence of age-related macular degeneration in 4 racial/ethnic groups in the multi-ethnic study of atherosclerosis. Ophthalmology. 2006;113(3):373–80.
13. Varma R, Fraser-Bell S, Tan S, Klein R, Azen SP. Prevalence of age-related macular degeneration in Latinos: the Los Angeles Latino eye study. Ophthalmology. 2004;111(7):1288–97.
14. Kawasaki R, Yasuda M, Song SJ, et al. The prevalence of age-related macular degeneration in Asians: a systematic review and meta-analysis. Ophthalmology. 2010;117:921–7.
15. Abecasis GR, Yashar BM, Zhao Y, et al. Age-related macular degeneration: a high-resolution genome scan for susceptibility loci in a population enriched for late-stage disease. Am J Hum Genet. 2004;74(3):482–94.
16. Iyengar SK, Song D, Klein BE, et al. Dissection of genomewide-scan data in extended families reveals a major locus and oligogenic susceptibility for age-related macular degeneration. Am J Hum Genet. 2004;74(1):20–39.
17. Klein ML, Schultz DW, Edwards A, et al. Age-related macular degeneration. Clinical features in a large family and linkage to chromosome 1q. Arch Ophthalmol. 1998;116(8):1082–8.
18. Majewski J, Schultz DW, Weleber RG, et al. Age-related macular degeneration – a genome scan in extended families. Am J Hum Genet. 2003;73(3):540–50.
19. Schmidt S, Scott WK, Postel EA, et al. Ordered subset linkage analysis supports a susceptibility locus for age-related macular degeneration on chromosome 16p12. BMC Genet. 2004;5:18.
20. Seddon JM, Santangelo SL, Book K, Chong S, Cote J. A genomewide scan for age-related macular degeneration provides evidence for linkage to several chromosomal regions. Am J Hum Genet. 2003;73(4):780–90.
21. Weeks DE, Conley YP, Tsai HJ, et al. Age-related maculopathy: an expanded genome-wide scan with

evidence of susceptibility loci within the 1q31 and 17q25 regions. Am J Ophthalmol. 2001;132(5): 682–92.

22. Weeks DE, Conley YP, Mah TS, et al. A full genome scan for age-related maculopathy. Hum Mol Genet. 2000;9(9):1329–49.

23. Weeks DE, Conley YP, Tsai HJ, et al. Age-related maculopathy: a genomewide scan with continued evidence of susceptibility loci within the 1q31, 10q26, and 17q25 regions. Am J Hum Genet. 2004;75(2): 174–89.

24. Fisher SA, Abecasis GR, Yashar BM, et al. Meta-analysis of genome scans of age-related macular degeneration. Hum Mol Genet. 2005;14(15): 2257–64.

25. Schultz DW, Klein ML, Humpert AJ, et al. Analysis of the ARMD1 locus: evidence that a mutation in HEMICENTIN-1 is associated with age-related macular degeneration in a large family. Hum Mol Genet. 2003;12(24):3315–23.

26. Anderson DH, Mullins RF, Hageman GS, Johnson LV. A role for local inflammation in the formation of drusen in the aging eye. Am J Ophthalmol. 2002; 134(3):411–31.

27. Donoso LA, Kim D, Frost A, Callahan A, Hageman G. The role of inflammation in the pathogenesis of age-related macular degeneration. Surv Ophthalmol. 2006;51(2):137–52.

28. Edwards AO, Ritter 3rd R, Abel KJ, Manning A, Panhuysen C, Farrer LA. Complement factor H polymorphism and age-related macular degeneration. Science. 2005;308(5720):421–4.

29. Johnson LV, Leitner WP, Staples MK, Anderson DH. Complement activation and inflammatory processes in Drusen formation and age related macular degeneration. Exp Eye Res. 2001;73(6):887–96.

30. Klein RJ, Zeiss C, Chew EY, et al. Complement factor H polymorphism in age-related macular degeneration. Science. 2005;308(5720):385–9.

31. Mullins RF, Russell SR, Anderson DH, Hageman GS. Drusen associated with aging and age-related macular degeneration contain proteins common to extracellular deposits associated with atherosclerosis, elastosis, amyloidosis, and dense deposit disease. FASEB J. 2000;14(7):835–46.

32. Scholl HP, Charbel Issa P, Walier M, et al. Systemic complement activation in age-related macular degeneration. PLoS ONE. 2008;3(7):e2593.

33. Sivaprasad S, Chong NV. The complement system and age-related macular degeneration. Eye (Lond). 2006;20(8):867–72.

34. Giannakis E, Jokiranta TS, Male DA, et al. A common site within factor H SCR 7 responsible for binding heparin, C-reactive protein and streptococcal M protein. Eur J Immunol. 2003;33(4):962–9.

35. Thakkinstian A, Han P, McEvoy M, et al. Systematic review and meta-analysis of the association between complement factor H Y402H polymorphisms and age-related macular degeneration. Hum Mol Genet. 2006;15(18):2784–90.

36. Seddon JM, Francis PJ, George S, Schultz DW, Rosner B, Klein ML. Association of CFH Y402H and LOC387715 A69S with progression of age-related macular degeneration. JAMA. 2007;297(16): 1793–800.

37. Ting AY, Lee TK, MacDonald IM. Genetics of age-related macular degeneration. Curr Opin Ophthalmol. 2009;20(5):369–76.

38. Grassi MA, Fingert JH, Scheetz TE. Ethnic variation in AMD-associated complement factor H polymorphism p.Tyr402His. Hum Mutat. 2006;27(9):921–5.

39. Magnusson KP, Duan S, Sigurdsson H, et al. CFH Y402H confers similar risk of soft drusen and both forms of advanced AMD. PLoS Med. 2006;3(1):e5.

40. Maller J, George S, Purcell S, et al. Common variation in three genes, including a noncoding variant in CFH, strongly influences risk of age-related macular degeneration. Nat Genet. 2006;38(9):1055–9.

41. Cui L, Zhou H, Yu J, et al. Noncoding variant in the complement factor H gene and risk of exudative age-related macular degeneration in a Chinese population. Invest Ophthalmol Vis Sci. 2010;51(2):1116–20.

42. Li M, Atmaca-Sonmez P, Othman M, et al. CFH haplotypes without the Y402H coding variant show strong association with susceptibility to age-related macular degeneration. Nat Genet. 2006;38(9):1049–54.

43. Mori K, Gehlbach PL, Kabasawa S, et al. Coding and noncoding variants in the CFH gene and cigarette smoking influence the risk of age-related macular degeneration in a Japanese population. Invest Ophthalmol Vis Sci. 2007;48(11):5315–9.

44. Gold B, Merriam JE, Zernant J, et al. Variation in factor B (BF) and complement component 2 (C2) genes is associated with age-related macular degeneration. Nat Genet. 2006;38(4):458–62.

45. Spencer KL, Hauser MA, Olson LM, et al. Protective effect of complement factor B and complement component 2 variants in age-related macular degeneration. Hum Mol Genet. 2007;16(16):1986–92.

46. Montes T, Tortajada A, Morgan BP, Rodriguez de Cordoba S, Harris CL. Functional basis of protection against age-related macular degeneration conferred by a common polymorphism in complement factor B. Proc Natl Acad Sci USA. 2009;106(11): 4366–71.

47. Despriet DD, van Duijn CM, Oostra BA, et al. Complement component C3 and risk of age-related macular degeneration. Ophthalmology. 2009;116(3): 474–80. e472.

48. Maller JB, Fagerness JA, Reynolds RC, Neale BM, Daly MJ, Seddon JM. Variation in complement factor 3 is associated with risk of age-related macular degeneration. Nat Genet. 2007;39(10):1200–1.

49. Spencer KL, Olson LM, Anderson BM, et al. C3 R102G polymorphism increases risk of age-related macular degeneration. Hum Mol Genet. 2008; 17(12):1821–4.

50. Yates JR, Sepp T, Matharu BK, et al. Complement C3 variant and the risk of age-related macular degeneration. N Engl J Med. 2007;357(6):553–61.

51. Zareparsi S, Buraczynska M, Branham KE, et al. Toll-like receptor 4 variant D299G is associated with susceptibility to age-related macular degeneration. Hum Mol Genet. 2005;14(11):1449–55.
52. Yang Z, Stratton C, Francis PJ, et al. Toll-like receptor 3 and geographic atrophy in age-related macular degeneration. N Engl J Med. 2008;359(14):1456–63.
53. Lip PL, Blann AD, Hope-Ross M, Gibson JM, Lip GY. Age-related macular degeneration is associated with increased vascular endothelial growth factor, hemorheology and endothelial dysfunction. Ophthalmology. 2001;108(4):705–10.
54. Kliffen M, Sharma HS, Mooy CM, Kerkvliet S, de Jong PT. Increased expression of angiogenic growth factors in age-related maculopathy. Br J Ophthalmol. 1997;81(2):154–62.
55. Churchill AJ, Carter JG, Lovell HC, et al. VEGF polymorphisms are associated with neovascular age-related macular degeneration. Hum Mol Genet. 2006;15(19):2955–61.
56. Allikmets R, Dean M. Bringing age-related macular degeneration into focus. Nat. Genet. 2008;40(7):820–821.
57. Andreoli MT, Morrison MA, Kim BJ, et al. Comprehensive analysis of complement factor H and LOC387715/ARMS2/HTRA1 variants with respect to phenotype in advanced age-related macular degeneration. Am J Ophthalmol. 2009;148(6):869–74.
58. Conley YP, Jakobsdottir J, Mah T, et al. CFH, ELOVL4, PLEKHA1 and LOC387715 genes and susceptibility to age-related maculopathy: AREDS and CHS cohorts and meta-analyses. Hum Mol Genet. 2006;15(21):3206–18.
59. Rivera A, Fisher SA, Fritsche LG, et al. Hypothetical LOC387715 is a second major susceptibility gene for age-related macular degeneration, contributing independently of complement factor H to disease risk. Hum Mol Genet. 2005;14(21):3227–36.
60. Shuler Jr RK, Schmidt S, Gallins P, et al. Phenotype analysis of patients with the risk variant LOC387715 (A69S) in age-related macular degeneration. Am J Ophthalmol. 2008;145(2):303–7.
61. Jakobsdottir J, Conley YP, Weeks DE, Mah TS, Ferrell RE, Gorin MB. Susceptibility genes for age-related maculopathy on chromosome 10q26. Am J Hum Genet. 2005;77(3):389–407.
62. Schaumberg DA, Hankinson SE, Guo Q, Rimm E, Hunter DJ. A prospective study of 2 major age-related macular degeneration susceptibility alleles and interactions with modifiable risk factors. Arch Ophthalmol. 2007;125(1):55–62.
63. Schmidt S, Hauser MA, Scott WK, et al. Cigarette smoking strongly modifies the association of LOC387715 and age-related macular degeneration. Am J Hum Genet. 2006;78(5):852–64.
64. Fritsche LG, Loenhardt T, Janssen A, et al. Age-related macular degeneration is associated with an unstable ARMS2 (LOC387715) mRNA. Nat Genet. 2008;40(7):892–6.
65. Yang Z, Tong Z, Chen Y, et al. Genetic and functional dissection of HTRA1 and LOC387715 in age-related macular degeneration. PLoS Genet. 2010;6(2):e1000836.
66. Kanda A, Chen W, Othman M, et al. A variant of mitochondrial protein LOC387715/ARMS2, not HTRA1, is strongly associated with age-related macular degeneration. Proc Natl Acad Sci USA. 2007;104(41):16227–32.
67. Wang G, Spencer KL, Court BL, et al. Localization of age-related macular degeneration-associated ARMS2 in cytosol, not mitochondria. Invest Ophthalmol Vis Sci. 2009;50(7):3084–90.
68. Cameron DJ, Yang Z, Gibbs D, et al. HTRA1 variant confers similar risks to geographic atrophy and neovascular age-related macular degeneration. Cell Cycle. 2007;6(9):1122–5.
69. Chen H, Yang Z, Gibbs D, et al. Association of HTRA1 polymorphism and bilaterality in advanced age-related macular degeneration. Vision Res. 2008;48(5):690–4.
70. Dewan A, Liu M, Hartman S, et al. HTRA1 promoter polymorphism in wet age-related macular degeneration. Science. 2006;314(5801):989–92.
71. Gibbs D, Yang Z, Constantine R, et al. Further mapping of 10q26 supports strong association of HTRA1 polymorphisms with age-related macular degeneration. Vision Res. 2008;48(5):685–9.
72. Lu F, Hu J, Zhao P, et al. HTRA1 variant increases risk to neovascular age-related macular degeneration in Chinese population. Vision Res. 2007;47(24):3120–3.
73. Mori K, Horie-Inoue K, Kohda M, et al. Association of the HTRA1 gene variant with age-related macular degeneration in the Japanese population. J Hum Genet. 2007;52(7):636–41.
74. Yang Z, Camp NJ, Sun H, et al. A variant of the HTRA1 gene increases susceptibility to age-related macular degeneration. Science. 2006;314(5801):992–3.
75. Yoshida T, DeWan A, Zhang H, et al. HTRA1 promoter polymorphism predisposes Japanese to age-related macular degeneration. Mol Vis. 2007;13:545–8.
76. Chen W, Xu W, Tao Q, et al. Meta-analysis of the association of the HTRA1 polymorphisms with the risk of age-related macular degeneration. Exp Eye Res. 2009;89(3):292–300.
77. Grau S, Richards PJ, Kerr B, et al. The role of human HtrA1 in arthritic disease. J Biol Chem. 2006;281(10):6124–9.
78. Yang Z et al. Genetic and functional dissection of HTRA1 and LOC387715 in age-related macular degeneration. PLoS Genet. 2010;6(2):e1000836.
79. Han X. The role of apolipoprotein E in lipid metabolism in the central nervous system. Cell Mol Life Sci. 2004;61(15):1896–906.
80. Baird PN, Guida E, Chu DT, Vu HT, Guymer RH. The epsilon2 and epsilon4 alleles of the apolipoprotein gene are associated with age-related macular degeneration. Invest Ophthalmol Vis Sci. 2004;45(5):1311–5.
81. Klaver CC, Kliffen M, van Duijn CM, et al. Genetic association of apolipoprotein E with age-related macular degeneration. Am J Hum Genet. 1998;63(1):200–6.

82. Schmidt S, Klaver C, Saunders A, et al. A pooled case-control study of the apolipoprotein E (APOE) gene in age-related maculopathy. Ophthalmic Genet. 2002;23(4):209–23.

83. Schmidt S, Saunders AM, De La Paz MA, et al. Association of the apolipoprotein E gene with age-related macular degeneration: possible effect modification by family history, age, and gender. Mol Vis. 2000;6:287–93.

84. Simonelli F, Margaglione M, Testa F, et al. Apolipoprotein E polymorphisms in age-related macular degeneration in an Italian population. Ophthalmic Res. 2001;33(6):325–8.

85. Pang CP, Baum L, Chan WM, Lau TC, Poon PM, Lam DS. The apolipoprotein E epsilon4 allele is unlikely to be a major risk factor of age-related macular degeneration in Chinese. Ophthalmologica. 2000;214(4):289–91.

86. Zareparsi S, Reddick AC, Branham KE, et al. Association of apolipoprotein E alleles with susceptibility to age-related macular degeneration in a large cohort from a single center. Invest Ophthalmol Vis Sci. 2004;45(5):1306–10.

87. Thakkinstian A, Bowe S, McEvoy M, Smith W, Attia J. Association between apolipoprotein E polymorphisms and age-related macular degeneration: a HuGE review and meta-analysis. Am J Epidemiol. 2006;164(9):813–22.

88. Fiotti N, Pedio M, Battaglia Parodi M, et al. MMP-9 microsatellite polymorphism and susceptibility to exudative form of age-related macular degeneration. Genet Med. 2005;7(4):272–7.

89. Stone EM, Braun TA, Russell SR, et al. Missense variations in the fibulin 5 gene and age-related macular degeneration. N Engl J Med. 2004;351(4):346–53.

90. Lotery AJ, Baas D, Ridley C, et al. Reduced secretion of fibulin 5 in age-related macular degeneration and cutis laxa. Hum Mutat. 2006;27(6):568–74.

91. Fisher SA, Rivera A, Fritsche LG, et al. Case-control genetic association study of fibulin-6 (FBLN6 or HMCN1) variants in age-related macular degeneration (AMD). Hum Mutat. 2007;28(4):406–13.

92. Hayashi M, Merriam JE, Klaver CC, et al. Evaluation of the ARMD1 locus on 1q25–31 in patients with age-related maculopathy: genetic variation in laminin genes and in exon 104 of HEMICENTIN-1. Ophthalmic Genet. 2004;25(2):111–9.

93. Zhang K, Kniazeva M, Han M, et al. A 5-bp deletion in ELOVL4 is associated with two related forms of autosomal dominant macular dystrophy. Nat Genet. 2001;27(1):89–93.

94. Agbaga MP, Brush RS, Mandal MN, Henry K, Elliott MH, Anderson RE. Role of Stargardt-3 macular dystrophy protein (ELOVL4) in the biosynthesis of very long chain fatty acids. Proc Natl Acad Sci USA. 2008;105(35):12843–8.

95. Conley YP, Thalamuthu A, Jakobsdottir J, et al. Candidate gene analysis suggests a role for fatty acid biosynthesis and regulation of the complement system in the etiology of age-related maculopathy. Hum Mol Genet. 2005;14(14):1991–2002.

96. Ayyagari R, Zhang K, Hutchinson A, et al. Evaluation of the ELOVL4 gene in patients with age-related macular degeneration. Ophthalmic Genet. 2001;22(4):233–9.

97. Yang Z et al. A variant of the HTRA1 gene increases susceptibility to age-related macular degeneration. Science. 2006;314(5801):992–3.

98. Francis PJ, Schultz DW, Hamon S, Ott J, Weleber RG, Klein ML. Haplotypes in the complement factor H (CFH) gene: associations with drusen and advanced age-related macular degeneration. PLoS ONE. 2007;2(11):e1197.

99. DeAngelis MM, Ji F, Kim IK, et al. Cigarette smoking, CFH, APOE, ELOVL4, and risk of neovascular age-related macular degeneration. Arch Ophthalmol. 2007;125(1):49–54.

100. Despriet DD, Klaver CC, Witteman JC, et al. Complement factor H polymorphism, complement activators, and risk of age-related macular degeneration. JAMA. 2006;296(3):301–9.

101. Francis PJ, George S, Schultz DW, et al. The LOC387715 gene, smoking, body mass index, environmental associations with advanced age-related macular degeneration. Hum Hered. 2007;63(3–4):212–8.

102. Seddon JM, George S, Rosner B, Klein ML. CFH gene variant, Y402H, and smoking, body mass index, environmental associations with advanced age-related macular degeneration. Hum Hered. 2006;61(3):157–65.

103. Seddon JM, Willett WC, Speizer FE, Hankinson SE. A prospective study of cigarette smoking and age-related macular degeneration in women. JAMA. 1996;276(14):1141–6.

104. Thornton J, Edwards R, Mitchell P, Harrison RA, Buchan I, Kelly SP. Smoking and age-related macular degeneration: a review of association. Eye (Lond). 2005;19(9):935–44.

Modifiable Risk Factors of Age-Related Macular Degeneration

2

Hanna R. Coleman

Key Points

- The causative factors for AMD have not been elucidated, but disease development is likely a combined result of gene vulnerability interacting with predisposing and often modifiable risk factors.
- Many studies have linked AMD to the effects of oxidative stress. Several of the risk factors discussed below are thought to further increase oxidative damage and/or limit the retina's ability to repair.
- While inferences can be made about the effect of many of these modifiable risk factors, additional studies are necessary before definitive recommendations are possible.

Pearl

Thornton's criteria for causal attribution when evaluating risk factors:
- Consistency of findings: between study types, settings, populations and time
- Strength of association
- Evidence of dose–response: greater intensity and/or duration of smoking associated with greater effect
- Evidence of reversibility: reduced risk with removal of exposure (i.e., among ex-smokers compared with current smokers)
- Temporal relationship: evidence that exposure preceded effect
- Biological plausibility: evidence of supporting biological evidence from animal and tissue models or other sources

H.R. Coleman (✉)
Department of Ophthalmology, New York Hospital
Presbyterian-Columbia, 635 W. 165th Street,
New York, NY 10032, USA
e-mail: hrcoleman@hotmail.com

A.C. Ho and C.D. Regillo (eds.), *Age-related Macular Degeneration Diagnosis and Treatment*,
DOI 10.1007/978-1-4614-0125-4_2, © Springer Science+Business Media, LLC 2011

Introduction

Age-related macular degeneration (AMD) is a chronic progressive disorder characterized by drusen in the early stages and atrophy and/or choroidal neovascularization in the late stages. It is a leading cause of blindness in the elderly white population and carries a large individual and social burden.

Risk factors for AMD are numerous and multiple studies have been designed to identify and assess them (Table 2.1) [1]. The most consistently significant, yet nonmodifiable, factors are genetic predisposition and age. Multiple chromosomal susceptibility loci are currently being studied and are discussed elsewhere in this book.

Table 2.1 Risk factors for age related maculopathy

Genetic predisposition
  Family history of ARM
  Complement factor H gene
  Apolipoprotein E gene
  LOC gene
Cardiovascular disease
  Clinical evidence of atherosclerosis
  Angina/heart attack/stroke
  Subclinical evidence of atherosclerosis
  Carotid atherosclerosis
  Aortic atherosclerosis
Cigarette smoking
Diabetes mellitus
Hypertension and associated disease
Ischemic cerebral white matter changes
Abnormalities of the retinal vasculature
Cholesterol
  Total cholesterol
  Low-density Lipoprotein (LDL) cholesterol
  High-density Lipoprotein (HDL) cholesterol
Obesity
Female sex hormones
  Endogenous estrogen exposure
  Age at menarche
  Age at menopause
  Number of pregnancies
  Exogenous estrogen exposure
  Oral contraceptives
  Hormone replacement therapy

Novel risk factors for atherosclerosis
Lipid-related factors
  Apolipoproteins
  Lipoproteins
Inflammatory markers
  C-reactive protein
  Interleukins
  Serum amyloid A
Vascular and cellular adhesion molecules
Homocysteine/folate/vitamin B12/vitamin B6
Infectious agents
  Cytomegalovirus
  Helicobacter pylori
  Chlamydia pneumoniae
Systemic diseases with inflammatory components
  Gout
  Emphysema
Anti-inflammatory medications
  NSAIDs
  Steroids
Markers of systemic inflammation
  White blood cell count
  Serum albumin
  Plasma fibrinogen
  C-reactive protein
  Complement factor H Y402H polymorphism
  CRP haplotype
  Interleukin-6
  Tumor necrosis factor-α
Markers of endothelial dysfunction
  Intercellular adhesion Molecule-1
  E-selectin
Indicators of oxidative stress
Anti-oxidants
  Vitamin C
  Vitamin E
  Vitamin A
  Carotenoids
  Lutein
  Zeaxanthin
  α- and β-carotene
  β-cryptoxanthin
  Lycopene
Enzymes
  Plasma glutathione peroxidase
  Superoxide dismutase
Trace elements
  Zinc
Pro-oxidant status

(continued)

Table 2.1 (continued)

Dietary fat intake
Total fat
Saturated fat
Polyunsaturated fat
Fish/fish oils
Visible light exposure
Sunlight/blue light
Ultraviolet-B
Ocular factors
Refractive error
Emmetropia
Myopia
Hypermetropia
Iris Color
Cataract
Nuclear sclerosis
Cortical lens opacities
Posterior subcapsular cataracts
Cataract surgery
Miscellaneous factors
Alcohol consumption
Beer
Wine
Spirits
Medication use
Estrogens
Lipid-lowering agents
CNS medications
Anti-hypertensive medications
Coffee consumption
Frailty
Physical activity

From Connell et al. [1], used with permission

Advancements are being made in locating others, but ultimately disease development is likely a combined result of gene vulnerability interacting with predisposing risk factors. As such the identification and management of modifiable risk factors is of particular epidemiological interest in the control of this disease.

Possible modifiable risk factors for AMD include smoking, body mass index (BMI), cumulative sunlight exposure, diet, alcohol consumption, and cardiovascular disease. Of these, diet and nutritional supplements have been the focus of many multi-center trials. The recommendations regarding the impact of micronutrients such as AREDS and AREDS-like supplements as well as carotenoids and omega fatty acids among others are covered in detail in this book in Chapter 5. Here, we will discuss the background and the emerging data that point toward some of the other modifiable risk factors.

Although still unproven, many studies have linked AMD to the effects of oxidative stress in the macula [2]. The naturally increased oxygen consumption from the photoreceptors combined with the lack of autoregulatory capacity of the choriocapillaris to increased metabolic demand and the decreased choroidal blood flow due to diminished vessel volume and density that occurs with age contributes to an increased formation of oxygen free-radicals and inflammatory response that promotes degenerative changes [3]. Several of the risk factors discussed below are thought to further increase oxidative damage and/or limit the retina's ability to repair [4].

Smoking

Smoking has been shown to be one of the strongest environmental risk factors for AMD. Current smokers tend to have a fourfold higher risk of 5-year incident advanced AMD than never smokers. Past smokers have a threefold higher risk of geographic atrophy [5]. Long-term longitudinal studies demonstrated that exposure to smoking precedes the development of AMD and that there is a dose–response: the risk of developing AMD increases as the intensity of smoking increases [6]. Smoking cessation was associated with a marked, nonlinear decrease of the risk of progression to AMD. This protective effect was independent of smoking intensity [7]. Recent studies have shown that the presence of certain gene polymorphisms, specifically complement factor H (CFH) gene, Y402H and LOC387715 A69S genes influence the effect of smoking on AMD development [8]. It is expected that other gene and smoking interactions will be discovered as the field progresses. Therefore, it is reasonable to advise all smokers of their increased prospect of AMD development.

Pearl

Smoking has been shown to be one of the strongest risk factors for AMD.

- Current smokers have a fourfold higher risk of late AMD than never smokers.
- Past smokers have a threefold higher risk for geographic atrophy.
- Ever smokers (past or present) have on average a 30% increased risk of either exudative or nonexudative AMD.
- Smoking cessation decreases the risk of AMD progression, albeit nonlinearly.

Alcohol

The epidemiologic data on the association of AMD with alcohol consumption is inconsistent [9]. In the Beaver Dam Eye Study, there was an association with retinal drusen in men and beer drinking (seven drinks per week), but none in women [10]. In the Blue Mountains Eye Study, there was no association found, and in the National Health and Nutrition Examination Survey I, wine consumption was reported to be protective leading to a 34% reduction in relative risk. The authors of that report speculated that antioxidant phenolic compounds found in high concentrations in red wine may explain their finding [8]. However, it similarly has been shown to increase oxidative stress or to modify the mechanisms that protect against oxidative stress, so it is hypothesized that alcohol may have a J-shaped effect on AMD risk: protective for AMD when consumed in moderate amounts and associated with an increased risk with heavier consumption. Further studies are necessary to allow for a recommendation, but results are hampered by the lack of a widely accepted definition of heavy or moderate alcohol use. Low-risk recommendations vary between less than 10–60 g/day among developed nations [9].

Increased Light Exposure

Macular pigments are thought to filter out damaging blue light and act as an antioxidant by quenching reactive oxygen species [11]. Light exposure, specifically blue light, bright sunlight, and ultraviolet (UV) radiation, has been implicated in photochemical oxidative damage and light-induced apoptosis of the RPE cells [5, 8]. Clinical studies have had difficulty quantifying light exposures. Some suggest that the use of hats and sunglasses from an early age may be slightly protective, but others show no statistically significant effect and no definite conclusion on the protective effect of modern filtering lenses can be made [12, 13]. On the other hand, it is known that the anterior structures of the eye, such as the cornea and the lens, filter UV light but allow visible blue light to reach the retina [11]. An association of cataract surgery and subsequent onset and progression AMD exists, but has not been statistically proven; a protective effect of cataracts has been postulated and attributed to additional filtering of blue light by the opaque lens [14]. Based on this, prophylactic 'yellow' intraocular lenses (IOLs) have been introduced and although indications for their use are not clear, theoretically they should be considered in patients at risk [15]. Additional clinical trials would be needed to prove this assumption.

Obesity

The relationship between obesity and AMD is also inconsistent. Most studies have examined AMD associations with weight parameters defined by the BMI (calculated as weight in kilograms divided by height in meters squared). Some have found no association while others found associations within specific population subgroups [16]. The waist to hip ratio (WHR), however, is a measure of central or abdominal obesity that is emerging as a better predictor of diabetes and cardiovascular diseases than the BMI. Early studies also suggest that a reduction in WHR in middle-aged persons may be associated with a decrease in the likelihood of prevalent AMD [17]. With increasing rates of obesity in developed countries, future studies are needed to assess the additional benefit of weight loss in patients at risk of AMD.

Pearl

Calculating WHR (Waist to Hip Ratio)
- Measure around the hips where at their widest, then measure the waist around the largest part of the belly.
- Divide the waist measurement by the hip measurement to get the WHR
- Normal values range from 0.7 to 0.85 for women and 0.9 to 1 for men

Calculating BMI (Body Mass Index)
- Divide the weight taken in kilograms by the square of the height taken in meters.
- Bellow 18.5 is considered underweight
- 18.5–24.9 is within normal
- 25–29.9 is considered overweight
- >30 is considered obese

Exercise

Studies show that higher doses of physical activity correlate to lower incidence of exudative AMD [18]. In the Beaver Dam Eye study, persons with an active lifestyle (defined as regular activity three or more times a week) were found 70% less likely to develop neovascular AMD; an increased number of blocks walked per day decreased the risk of exudative AMD by 30% [19]. This is consistent with findings from the Eye Disease Case Control Study in which neovascular AMD was associated with less physical activity. However, physical activity has not been related to the incidence of early AMD or geographic atrophy. The benefits on exudative

AMD may be the result of lowering systolic blood pressure, lowering white blood cell count, and decreasing BMI, factors found to be associated with neovascularization. Although at this time it is difficult to recommend specific activities, it seems that more general physical activity would be beneficial to patients at risk [8].

Dietary Fat Intake

Dietary fats can be divided into "bad" fats such as cholesterol, monounsaturated and polyunsaturated fats, and linoleic acid and "good" fats such as omega-3 and omega-6 monounsaturated fatty acids, the benefits of which are discussed in detail elsewhere in this book. There is a growing body of evidence suggesting that diets high in bad fats, rather than total fat intake, may contribute to the risk of intermediate and advanced AMD and that diets high in good fats may be protective [20, 21]. Proposed mechanisms for this increased risk include progressive accumulation of lipids in Bruch's membrane, atherosclerosis causing hemodynamic changes in the retinal and choroidal blood supply, and the depletion of omega-3 fatty acids and high serum levels of polyunsaturated fatty acids that cause oxidative damage to the retina. Given the overall health benefits found for a diet low in cholesterol and saturated fats, it is reasonable to consider it as well in this population [5].

Phytochemicals

Phytochemicals or phytonutrients are active plant compounds that are thought to have health-protecting qualities. While the antioxidant, immune-boosting, and other health-promoting properties of a number of compounds are being studied, the most publicized phytochemicals have been vitamin C, vitamin E, and beta-carotene (which the body converts into vitamin A); their antioxidant properties are covered in detail in the review of the AREDS studies elsewhere in this book. However, data has been

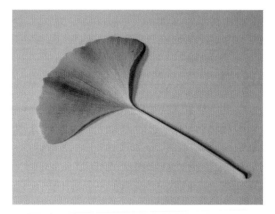

Fig. 2.1 Gingko biloba (From: http://upload.wikimedia.
org/wikipedia/commons/2/2a/Ginkgo_biloba_leaf_3.jpg)

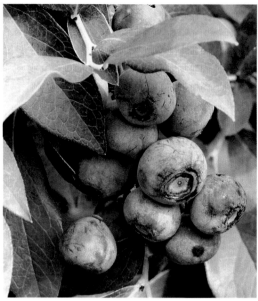

Fig. 2.2 Blueberries (From: http://upload.wikimedia.org/
wikipedia/commons/7/7e/Blueberries_on_branch.jpg)

generally inconsistent, particularly concerning their relationship to AMD, because it is difficult to control other influencing lifestyle choices [22]. A few of the more commonly known compounds are reviewed here.

Ginkgo Biloba

Ginkgo biloba is one of the oldest living tree species (Fig. 2.1). Its leaves contain flavonoid glycosides that have been studied for their role in reduction of platelet aggregation, increased vasodilatation, and quenching of free radicals – the latter of which has sparked interest for its use on AMD. To date, there are no studies that demonstrate a definite positive effect on AMD, but also there have been few reports of toxicity, although it can increase the risk of bleeding in anticoagulated patients. Clinical trials have used between 120 and 240 mg daily [23, 24]. Dietary supplements generally provide 40–80 mg in a single dose.

Anthocyanins

Anthocyanins, also known as berry extracts, are water-soluble flavonoid pigments found in fruit such as blueberries, cranberries, bilberries, blackberries, blackcurrants, red currants, cherries, and purple grapes among others (Fig. 2.2). They act as potent antioxidants and are thought to reduce inflammation, aging, neurological diseases, cancer, and diabetes. In the retina, they are thought to

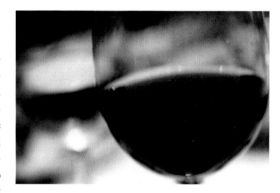

Fig. 2.3 Red wine (From: http://commons.wikimedia.
org/wiki/File:Red_wine_closeup_in_glass.jpg)

inhibit photo oxidation and membrane permeability changes that can lead to AMD [23].

Resveratrol

Resveratrol is a polyphenolic antioxidant found in red wine that appears to have antiinflammatory antioxidant and antiproliferative benefits (Fig. 2.3). Treatment with 50 and 100 µmol/L resveratrol has recently been shown to have significantly reduced in vitro the proliferation of retinal pigment epithelium cells by 10–25%, respectively, and as such is a compound of interest for ongoing studies [25].

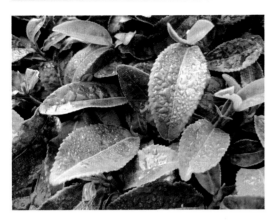

Fig. 2.4 Green tea (From: http://flickr.com/photos/barnkim/932910717/)

Epigallocatechin Gallate

Epigallocatechin gallate (EGCG) is the principal flavonoid present in green tea (Fig. 2.4). It has powerful antioxidant abilities and, in the eye is thought to confer neuroprotection of retinas injured by ischemia and reperfusion. It has also been shown to be an effective inhibitor of RPE cell migration and adhesion to fibronectin and its role in AMD prevention is being explored [26, 27].

Pearl

Phytochemicals are increasingly studied for the following possible effects:
- As antioxidants
- In enzyme stimulation
- Hormonal action
- Antibacterial properties

Mineral Supplements

Several metals and minerals play a significant role in the visual cycle and photoreceptor survival. Zinc and copper are cofactors and are major constituents in several important enzymes. The AREDS study showed a reduction in the development of advanced AMD as well as a decrease in the rate of progression of intermediate AMD to advance AMD [28]. Selenium activates the antioxidant enzyme glutathione peroxidase,

which protects cell membranes from oxidative damage [22].

Summary

The retina is the most metabolically active tissue of the body. Its high rate of oxygen consumption puts it at risk for increased oxidative damage, which is further aggravated by environmental and aging processes. In genetically susceptible individuals, this can lead to degenerative changes of the RPE and age-related macular degeneration. While current treatment modalities aim to stabilize vision and select patients do gain visual acuity, identification of preventable risk factors and behavior modification remain critical for best long-term visual prognosis.

References

1. Connell PP, Keane PA, O'Neill EC, et al. Risk factors for age-related maculopathy. J Ophthalmol. 2009; 2009:360764. Epub 2009 Sep 6.
2. Beatty S, Koh H, Phil M, Henson D, Boulton M. The role of oxidative stress in the pathogenesis of age-related macular degeneration. Surv Ophthalmol. 2000;45(2):115–34.
3. Neelam K, Nolan J, Chakravarthy U, et al. Psychophysical function in age-related maculopathy. Surv Ophthalmol. 2009;54(2):167–210.
4. Winkler BS, Boulton ME, Gottsch JD, Sternberg P. Oxidative damage and age-related macular degeneration. Mol Vis. 1999;5:32.
5. Feigl B. Age-related maculopathy – linking etiology and pathophysiological changes to the ischemia hypothesis. Prog Retin Eye Res. 2009;28(1):63–86.
6. Thornton J, Edwards R, Mitchell P, et al. Smoking and age-related macular degeneration: a review of association. Eye. 2005;19:935–44.
7. Neuner B, Komm A, Wellman J, et al. Smoking history and the incidence of age-related macular degeneration – results from the Muenster Aging and Retina Study (MARS) cohort and systematic review and meta-analysis of observational longitudinal studies. Addict Behav. 2009;34:938–47.
8. Klein EK, Klein R. Perspective: lifestyle exposures and eye diseases in adults. Am J Ophthalmol. 2007;144(6):961–9. Epub 2007 Oct 18.
9. Chong EW, Kreis AJ, Wong TY. Alcohol consumption and the risk of age-related macular degeneration: a systematic review and meta-analysis. Am J Ophthalmol. 2008;145(4):707–15.
10. Moss SE, Klein R, Klein BE, et al. Alcohol consumption and the 5-year incidence of age-related maculopathy:

the Beaver Dam eye study. Ophthalmology. 1998; 105(5):789–94.

11. Ahmed SS, Lott MN, Marcus DM. The macular xanthophylls. Surv Ophthalmol. 2005;50(2):183–93.

12. Ambati J, Ambati BK, Yoo SH, et al. Age-related macular degeneration: etiology, pathogenesis, and therapeutic strategies. Surv Ophthalmol. 2003;48(3): 257–93.

13. Johnson EJ. Obesity, lutein metabolism, and age-related macular degeneration: a web of connections. Nutr Rev. 2005;63(1):9–15.

14. Pollack A, Bukelman A, Zalish M, et al. The course of age-related macular degeneration following bilateral cataract surgery. Ophthalmic Surg Lasers. 1998;29(4): 286–94.

15. Algvere PV, Marshall J, Seregard S. Age-related maculopathy and the impact of blue light hazard. Acta Ophthalmol Scand. 2006;84(1):4–15.

16. Klein R, Knudtson MD, Lee KE, et al. Age–period–cohort effect on the incidence of age-related macular degeneration the Beaver Dam eye study. Ophthalmology. 2008;115(9):1460–7.

17. Peeters A, Magliano DJ, Stevens J, et al. Changes in abdominal obesity and age-related macular degeneration the atherosclerosis risk in communities study. Arch Ophthalmol. 2008;126(11):1554–60.

18. Williams PT. Prospective study of incident age-related macular degeneration in relation to vigorous physical activity during a 7-year follow-up. Invest Ophthalmol Vis Sci. 2009;50(1):101–6.

19. Knudtson MD, Klein R, Klein BE. Physical activity and the 15-year cumulative incidence of age-related macular degeneration: the Beaver Dam eye study. Br J Ophthalmol. 2006;90(12):1461–3.

20. CAREDS Research Study Group. Association between dietary fat intake and age-related macular degeneration in the Carotenoids in Age-Related Eye Disease Study (CAREDS): an ancillary study of the women's health initiative. Arch Ophthalmol. 2009;127 (11):1483–93.

21. Seddon JM, Rosner B, Sperduto RD, et al. Dietary fat and risk for advanced age-related macular degeneration. Arch Ophthalmol. 2001;119(8):1191–9.

22. Bartlett H, Eperjesi F. An ideal ocular nutritional supplement? Ophthalmic Physiol Opt. 2004;24: 339–49.

23. Rhone M, Basu A. Phytochemicals and age-related eye diseases. Nutr Rev. 2008;66(8):465–72.

24. Sierpina VS, Wollschlaeger B, Blumenthal M. Ginkgo biloba. Am Fam Physician. 2003;68(5):923–6.

25. King RE, Kent KD, Bomser JA. Resveratrol reduces oxidation and proliferation of human retinal pigment epithelial cells via extracellular signal-regulated kinase inhibition. Chem Biol Interact. 2005;151(2): 143–9.

26. Chan CM, Huang JH, Chiang HS, et al. Effects of (-)-epigallocatechin gallate on RPE cell migration and adhesion. Mol Vis. 2010;16:586–95.

27. Zhang B, Osborne NN. Oxidative-induced retinal degeneration is attenuated by epigallocatechin gallate. Brain Res. 2006;1124(1):176–87.

28. The Age-Related Eye Disease Research Group: A randomized, placebo-controlled, clinical trial of high-dose supplementation with vitamins C and E, beta carotene, and zinc for age-related macular degeneration and vision loss: AREDS report no. 8. Arch Ophthalmol. 2001;119(10):1417–36.

Literature Search References were identified through a systematic search of the Medline database using Pub Med Web site. Further articles, abstracts, and textbook references, generated from reviewing the bibliographies of the initial search, were retrieved and included.

Diagnosis of Age-Related Macular Degeneration

3

Jonathan Jonisch and Gaurav Shah

Key Points

- Classifying AMD helps physicians counsel patients, make treatment decisions, and standardize clinical trials.
- The presentation of AMD can vary widely and thus the differential diagnosis is large.
- Medical and ocular history, ophthalmoscopy, and ancillary testing can be used in combination to narrow the differential diagnosis.
- When the response to standard therapy is not typical, the diagnosis of AMD may need to be revisited.

Introduction

Age-related macular degeneration (AMD) is a heterogeneous group of disorders affecting the macula of elderly individuals. The classification scheme of this complex disorder continues to evolve as our understanding improves. The macula appearance of many other diseases can mimic AMD, thus the differential diagnosis is large. This chapter will focus on the classification schemes of AMD, the clinical presentations of AMD, and the differential diagnosis of AMD.

G. Shah (✉)
Barnes Retina Institute, 1600 S. Brentwood Blvd,
Ste. 800, St. Louis, MO 63144, USA
e-mail: gkshah1@gmail.com

Classification

The clinical appearance of age-related macular generation (AMD) includes drusen, retinal pigment epithelial (RPE) changes, atrophy of the RPE (geographic and nongeographic atrophy) and choroidal neovascularization (CNV). AMD can be classified in several ways. Classification is useful for multiple reasons, including counseling patients concerning prognosis, performing population-based incidence and natural history trials, and for evaluating new therapies. AMD is most commonly classified by the presence or absence of abnormal neovascularization; exudative versus nonexudative. In colloquial terms, it is referred to as dry or wet. Neovascular AMD is a term used commonly synonymously with exudative AMD. These terms will be used interchangeably for our purposes. AMD can also be classified based on the extent of visual impairment; early versus late. In this scheme, the advanced forms of non-neovascular AMD that can severely affect vision, such as geographic atrophy (GA) are combined with neovascular AMD to be classified as late AMD. All other findings are considered early AMD (Fig. 3.1).

Nonexudative (Non-neovascular or Dry) AMD

Dry AMD accounts for 80–90% of all cases of AMD [1]. The dry form of AMD is characterized

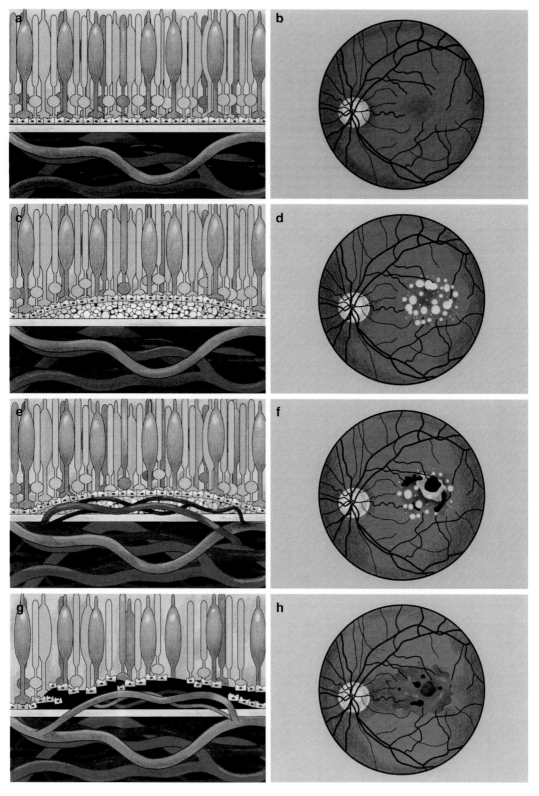

Fig. 3.1 Fundus illustrations with corresponding illustrations of the choriocapillaris, Bruch's membrane, RPE, and photoreceptor complex. (**a, b**) Normal fundus and complex. (**c, d**) Drusen due to nonexudative AMD with deposits between the RPE and Bruch's membrane. (**e, f**) Choroidal neovascularization due to exudative AMD with breaks through Bruch's membrane and vessels entering the subretinal space. (**g, h**) Advanced neovascular AMD highlighting chronic subretinal vasculature with subretinal fibrosis and atrophy of the RPE with photoreceptor loss

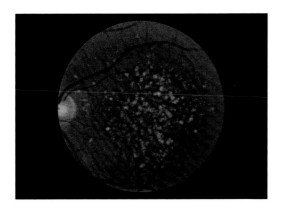

Fig. 3.2 Drusenoid fundus in young patient without macular degeneration

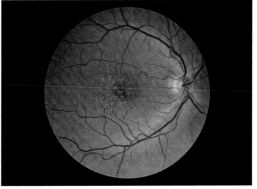

Fig. 3.4 Hard drusen in a patient with dry AMD

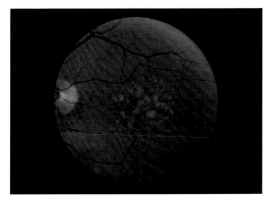

Fig. 3.3 Soft drusen in a patient dry AMD

by drusen, with or without RPE alterations. Drusen are discrete yellow lesions that can represent deposits within Bruch's membrane (basal linear deposits) or deposits between the plasma and basement membrane of the RPE (basal linear deposits) [2–4]. Drusen result in thickening of the Bruch's membrane and RPE degeneration. Vision loss may follow due to secondary photoreceptor loss [5] (Fig. 3.2). Different types of drusen include:

Soft drusen — yellow lesions with poorly defined edges. They are usually found in people over 55 years of age and represent shallow RPE detachments. These drusen lead to RPE atrophy, photoreceptor degeneration, and predispose to CNV [6–8]. Soft drusen may also calcify giving rise to refractile appearing lesions (Fig. 3.3).

Hard drusen — small (<50 μ(mu)m), round, yellow subRPE deposits. They are common in young people and do not result in AMD (Fig. 3.4) [9].

Cuticular drusen — histologically and anatomically similar to soft drusen, though they are found in younger patients (<50) and do not predispose to AMD. The angiographic feature of numerous small hyperfluorescent lesions have been described by Gass as "starry night" [10].

Drusen can be stable, can disappear, can progress to geographic atrophy, or progress to neovascular AMD. High-risk drusen characteristics for progression to neovascular AMD include drusen number (>5), size (>63 μ(mu)m), type (soft), confluence, and associated hyperpigmentation [11–14].

Geographic atrophy is an advanced form of nonexudative AMD. This form of dry AMD accounts for most of the severe loss among people with dry AMD, though it only accounts for 20% of legal blindness due to AMD overall [15]. GA appears as a well-demarcated area of retinal pigment epithelial and choroidal thinning allowing for increased visualization to the underlying choroidal circulation. There is marked choriocapillaris and RPE atrophy. Fluorescein angiography (FA) highlights the areas of atrophy that translate into hyperfluorescence due to transmission defects over the areas of atrophy. The natural history of GA is to enlarge at a median rate of 1.8 disc areas over a two-year period [16]. Eyes with GA are at risk of developing CNV and are at even

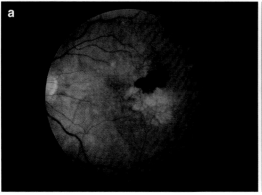 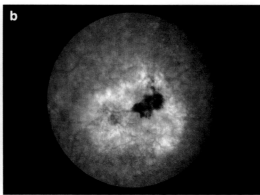

Fig. 3.5 (**a**) Color photo and (**b**) late angiogram of chor-oidal neovascularization in a patient with exudative AMD highlighted by an area of hemorrhage with adjacent atro-phy of the RPE with leakage in the late frames of the fluo-rescein angiogram

higher risk if the fellow eye has CNV with a risk as high as 45% over a five-year period [17].

Exudative (Neovascular or Wet) AMD

The neovascular form of AMD, although less common than the dry form, carries a more guarded prognosis for vision. In addition, unlike dry AMD, most patients with exudative AMD are symptomatic. Wet AMD includes pigment epi-thelial detachments (PED) sub-RPE neovascular-ization, and subretinal neovascularization. CNV can be classified by its location (subfoveal, juxta-foveal, extrafoveal) or by its FA findings (classic or occult) (Fig. 3.5). The spectrum of neovascular AMD has been expanded beyond the classic and occult CNV to include entities like idiopathic polypoidal choroidal neovascularization (IPCV) and retinal angiomatous proliferation (RAP). These entities should be distinguished from typi-cal neovascular AMD as their clinical course and response to treatment may be different than typi-cal neovascular AMD.

The Macular Photocoagulation Study (MPS) helped define a classification based on the dis-tance of CNV from the foveal avascular zone center [14]:
Subfoveal: 0 μ(mu)m
Juxtafoveal: 1 –199 μ(mu)m
Extrafoveal: 200 –2,500 μ(mu)m

This classification scheme remains important as treatment options vary depending on the loca-tion of the lesion.

CNV can also be classified as either classic or occult based on FA findings. Classic CNV has a bright, distinct, and lacy hyperfluorescence in the early transit phase with well-demarcated borders that become obscured in the late phases (Fig. 3.6). Occult CNV can be divided into two types (Fig. 3.7):

Fibrovascular PED — Hyperfluorescence best seen 90 s after dye injection with irregular RPE eleva-tions and either late staining or persistent leakage, though not as intense as in classic lesions.

Late leakage of undetermined source — There is poorly demarcated lesion boundary with late punctuated leakage best seen at 2–5 min. There is no early hyperfluorescence.

This classification is useful for describing var-ious lesions and has been useful in treatment tri-als and in providing patients with prognostic information based on natural history data. Occult CNV carries a better visual prognosis than clas-sic lesions [18]. This classification has been used less frequently in the age of anti-vascular endothe-lial growth factor (VEGF) therapies, as these agents are used for all CNV subtypes on FA.

There remains poor consensus as to the defini-tion of early nonexudative macular degeneration

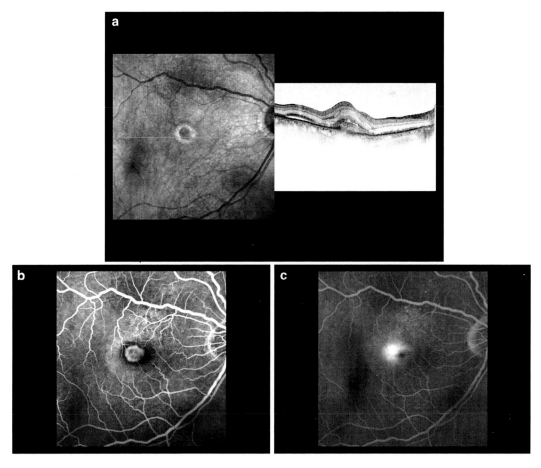

Fig. 3.6 (**a**) Red free photo and OCT and corresponding, (**b**) early, and (**c**) late frame fluorescein angiogram of classic subfoveal CNV due to exudative AMD

versus age-related maculopathy (ARM). Attempts have been made to classify age-related changes in the macula for purposes of clinical trials. Attempts of classifying non-neovascular changes have included diagnostic tools such as perimetry, contrast sensitivity, fundus photos (color or black and white), angiography, and histology. These have resulted in studies that are difficult to compare. An international epidemiologic study group classified soft drusen at least 63 μ(mu)m and RPE hyper- or hypopigmentation in patients ≥50 years of age as early age-related maculopathy (ARM). Geographic atrophy represented late ARM, which would be synonymous with dry AMD. Visual acuity was not taken into account. In this classification scheme, there is then the entity of neovascular AMD which includes RPE detachment, hemorrhages, and/or

scars [19]. Others have classified dry AMD as drusen with associated visual acuity loss due to overlying RPE atrophy [20].

In a more recent classification system, the Age-Related Eye Disease Study Group (AREDS) created a new classification without the use of the term ARM. This group classified AMD into four levels depending on the type and extent of drusen, as well as the presence of geographic atrophy and neovascular changes. In this scheme, AMD was divided into categories. Drusen were classified as <63 μ(mu)m, between 64 and 125 μ(mu)m, or >125 μ(mu)m. Early AMD was characterized by the presence of a few (<20) medium-size drusen or retinal pigmentary abnormalities; intermediate AMD was characterized by at least one large drusen, numerous medium-size drusen, or

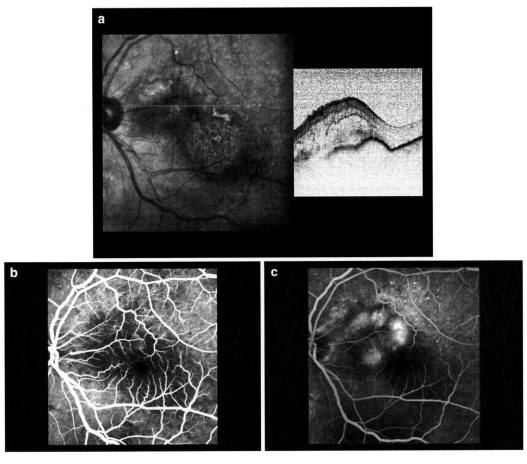

Fig. 3.7 (**a**) Red free photo and OCT and corresponding, (**b**) early, and (**c**) late frame fluorescein angiogram of occult CNV due to exudative AMD

geographic atrophy that does not extend to the center of the macula. Advanced or late AMD can be either non-neovascular (dry, atrophic, or non-exudative) or neovascular (wet or exudative). Advanced non-neovascular AMD is characterized by drusen and geographic atrophy extending to the center of the macula while advanced neovascular AMD is characterized by CNV and subsequent scar [21, 22].

Retinal Angiomatous Proliferation

Retinal angiomatous proliferation (RAP) is largely considered a subset of AMD with a different disease course, pathology, and response to treatment compared with typical neovascular AMD. In AMD, CNV originates below the RPE, in the choroidal circulation, and progresses into the retina. In advance neovascular AMD, there is then a communication between the choroidal circulation and the retinal circulation [23, 24]. RAP lesions are presumed to originate in the retinal circulation (as opposed to choroidal circulation) and ultimately form a retinal choroidal anastomosis in the late stages. RAP lesions may represent up to 15% of newly diagnosed wet AMD patients. Epidemiologic characteristics of patients with RAP include older age (81–82 years), Caucasian, female, and bilateral predilection. RAP lesions tend to be more aggressive with a worse clinical course than typical neovascular AMD and may be less responsive to anti-VEGF therapy (Fig. 3.8) [25–27].

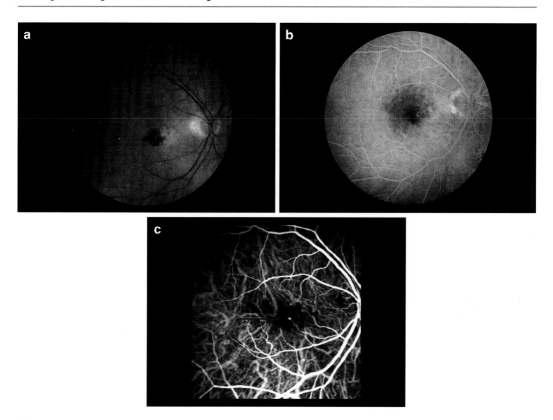

Fig. 3.8 (**a**) Color photo, (**b**) late phase fluorescein angiogram, and (**c**) ICG highlighting the hot spot in a patient with retinal angiomatous proliferation

A three-stage classification has been proposed to describe the progression of RAP lesions. Stage 1, intraretinal neovascularization (IRN) is usually slow-growing and asymptomatic. The location is usually extrafoveal and has not been described in the peripapillary area. IRN can result in intraretinal edema and multiple retinal hemorrhages. Fluorescein angiography usually reveals a focal area of intraretinal staining with indistinct borders corresponding to the IRN. This can be confused with idiopathic juxtafoveal telengectasia and classic AMD CNV lesions.

Stage II, subretinal neovascularization (SRN), is seen when the vessels proceed posteriorly beyond the photoreceptor level and into the subretinal space. At this stage, detachment of the neurosensory retina can ensue with further intraretinal edema. SRN may reach the RPE causing a PED.

Stage III, choroidal neovascularization (CNV), is diagnosed when vascularized PED are seen. At this stage, the neovascularization is being fed by the choroidal circulation.

ICG angiography is superior to FA in diagnosing RAP cases. A focal "hot spot" of intense hyperfluorescence corresponding to the area of activity can be seen in all stages. ICG angiography better images the presence of vascularized PED, because the serous component of PED remains dark during the study, as opposed to hyperfluorescence on FA, and the vascular component appears as hyperfluorescence [25].

> **Pearl**
> Consider a diagnosis of RAP in cases with focal intraretinal hemorrhages, cystic macular edema, and a poor response to anti-VEGF therapy.

Polypoidal Vasculopathy

Polypoidal choroidal vasculopathy has been described a peculiar hemorrhagic disorder of the macula, posterior uveal bleeding syndrome, and multiple recurrent retinal pigment epithelium detachments in African-American women [26–29]. Yannuzzi et al. gave the disorder the name idiopathic polypoidal choroidal vasculopathy (IPCV). IPCV presents with multiple, recurrent, detachments of the RPE (serous and hemorrhagic), secondary to leakage and bleeding from choroidal vascular abnormalities. Classically thought of a distinct entity separate from neovascular AMD, some consider IPCV a subtype of AMD. Besides, similar macular appearance of the two entities may share common risk factors and even genetic abnormalities [30].

> **Pearl**
> Although more common in darkly pigmented individuals, IPCV is not only a disease of pigmented females. Consider the diagnosis in cases which lack drusen, have orange-red lesions with peripapillary location, and have multiple hemorrhagic PEDs with a prominent exudative component. Also consider the diagnosis in cases poorly responsive to anti-VEGF therapy.

Originally, IPCV was reported exclusively in females of darkly pigmented races, though recent reports include Caucasian males [31–33]. Female cases still outnumber male ones by a ratio of approximately 5:1. African Americans and Asians are at higher risk of developing IPCV [34]. It remains unclear if IPCV represents a variant of AMD within a different population, or if the conditions are unrelated. IPCV is usually diagnosed in patients who are between the ages of 50 and 65. The two entities can be difficult to distinguish and indocyanine green angiography (ICGA) is essential in making the diagnosis in difficult cases. An IPCV study group attempted to define the condition with a scheme based on fundus examination, ICG

findings, or both. 'Definite' cases were determined if at least one of the following criteria were met:
Protruding elevated orange-red lesions observed by fundus examination
Characteristic polypoidal lesions seen on ICGA
"Probable" cases were determined if at least one of the following criteria were met:
Only an abnormal vascular network is seen in ICG.
Recurrent hemorrhagic and/or serous detachments of the RPE were observed (Fig. 3.9) [35].

Although clinically IPCV may appear similar to AMD in that patients develop multiple RPE detachments, bilateral disease, IPCV is not linked to drusen, it appears reddish (as opposed to grey-green), and does not develop significant fibrous proliferation and disciform scarring as seen in late wet AMD [29, 34]. In contrast to AMD, patients with IPCV have a relapsing-remitting course with long-term preservation of good vision with 50% of eyes having had a favorable visual outcome at two years without treatment [34]. FA can assist in the diagnosis though ICG is the better diagnostic modality to differentiate this entity from AMD. ICGA better highlights the choroidal circulation due to its longer wavelength, which can penetrate the RPE. On ICGA, there is a cluster of leaking polypoidal choroidal vessels usually in the peripapillary area seen in the early phases.

Response to treatment also differs among patients with exudative AMD and IPCV. IPCV seems to have better responses to photodynamic therapy, but a poorer response to the anti-VEGF therapy [36].

Diagnosis

AMD is a clinical diagnosis made by the physician following a comprehensive examination of a patient. Patients with nonexudative (dry) AMD in one or both eyes or unilateral exudative AMD may have no complaints and may be detected on a routine ophthalmic exam. Symptomatic patients with dry AMD usually present with complaints of gradual dulling of vision, which may require brighter lights or magnifying lenses to help with

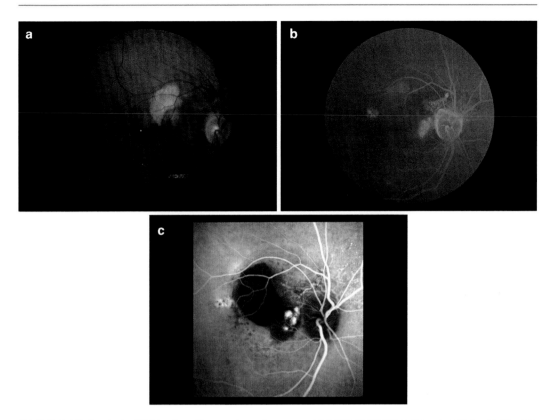

Fig. 3.9 (**a**) Color photo, (**b**) late phase fluorescein angiogram, and (**c**) ICG highlighting the polypoidal vasculature in a patient with idiopathic polypoidal choroidal vasculopathy

activities of daily living. Vision loss may be severe in cases of advanced dry AMD with central geographic or nongeographic atrophy. Despite having good central vision, patients with significant atrophy often have difficulty reading due to central and paracentral scotomas not enabling them to read an entire line of small print or even an entire letter of large print. They also may have difficulty seeing at night or in conditions of low lighting [37, 38]. Patients with wet AMD may complain of distorted vision with wavy lines, central or paracentral scotomas, rapid onset visual loss, or they may not notice any changes [39].

Diagnosis of AMD should include a detailed medical history to evaluate for predisposing conditions such as hypertension, smoking, and family history. This is not only important for the diagnosis of AMD, but also is useful in cases with a diagnostic dilemma to narrow the differential diagnosis. Dilated fundus examination should

be performed and a stereoscopic viewing method such as slit-lamp biomicroscopy with a contact or noncontact lens is essential.

The clinical hallmarks of AMD are drusen. Drusen can be easily recognizable as subretinal yellow material, though drusen may also be very subtle and overlooked. Although the finding of isolated small drusen with distinct borders (hard drusen) in an elderly patient is not worrisome to the clinician, the findings should be documented and followed. Isolated drusen do not account for significant vision loss [10]. Drusen are dynamic and can spontaneously disappear resulting in overlying atrophy of the RPE [40]. Clinically when drusen are either larger than 63 μ(mu)m, associated with other changes such as RPE hyper- and hypopigmentation, with vision loss below 20/30, or when soft drusen begin to coalesce, the dialogue should be started with the patients concerning the diagnosis of dry AMD. Macular changes in AMD are almost always present in both eyes although frequently are asymmetric. Late manifestations of non-neovascular AMD are geographic and non-geographic atrophy of the RPE. Geographic atrophy is a well-demarcated area of retinal thinning that allows for increased visualization of the underlying choroidal vessels. They may be located centrally in the macula, peripapillary, or both.

Ancillary testing of patients with dry AMD may include color fundus photography to aid in the description of drusen and for documenting progression or change. Optical coherence tomography (OCT) and FA may be helpful in ruling out neovascular component or highlighting areas of atrophy. Fundus autofluorescence can delineate areas of atrophy and help in cases when the diagnosis is in question. Patients should be advised to perform monocular amsler grid testing to detect early neovascular changes. Each box represents one degree of visual field, and the grid is testing the central 10° of fixation. Leakage of blood or serum such as in subretinal hemorrhage, subretinal fluid, hard exudates, and macular edema all herald the onset of neovascular AMD. Although hemorrhage has been described in geographic atrophy without CNV, hemorrhage almost always represents neovascular AMD [41].

Clinically, exudative AMD has a multitude of clinical appearances. The hallmark feature of wet AMD is the choroidal neovascularization (CNV). This classically appears as a grayish-green membrane beneath the retina in a macula that has accompanying drusen. Using stereo-ophthalmoscopy, one can appreciate findings such as separation of the retina from underlying RPE (subretinal fluid), sub-RPE fluid (PED), and intraretinal changes (cystoid macular edema). The ophthalmoscopic appearance of CNV, however, is often more subtle. RPE detachments can represent an underlying neovascular complex and appear as a near translucent and well-demarcated subretinal lesion. At times, the only clinical finding of CNV may be subretinal lipid. Other clinical findings found in neovascular AMD include subretinal hemorrhage, vitreous hemorrhage, hemorrhagic RPE detachments, and in the late stages subretinal fibrosis with disciform scars of the macula. Ancillary testing that can assist in the diagnosis of neovascular AMD include OCT to detect subtle sub-RPE and subretinal and retinal

material (fluid, hemorrhage, exudates, fibrosis). FA is particularly useful in diagnosing leakage from a CNV or pooling of an RPE detachment. It is also useful in delineating lesion location, size, and for determining disease activity, progression, and response to treatment. For diagnostic purposes, ICG is useful in atypical cases of neovascular AMD, in cases of idiopathic polypoidal choroidal vasculopathy, retinal angiomatous proliferation, or when the diagnosis is in question.

> **Pearl**
> Consider indocyanine green angiography (ICGA) in cases when the diagnosis of typical exudative AMD is in question or in cases that are poorly responsive to anti-VEGF therapy.

Differential Diagnosis

Because both dry and wet AMD can present in various ways, the differential diagnosis for each entity is fairly large. Subtle features in the history, presentation, personal attributes, family history, fundus appearance, and findings on ancillary testing are essential to differentiate each of the entities. Differentiating these conditions is vitally important as the treatment options and prognosis may vary considerably.

Nonexudative AMD

Central Serous Chorioretinopathy (CSCR)
The classic presentation includes serous retinal detachments, though many patients have focal RPE irregularities thought to be evidence of old episodes. The RPE hypopigmentation can be mistaken for dry AMD. Key differentiating features include younger age in CSCR, 25–50, and the presence of serous retinal detachment in the absence of drusen. OCT is particularly useful in these cases. CSCR in individuals above 50 years of age do have a higher prevalence in females (Fig. 3.10) [42–46].

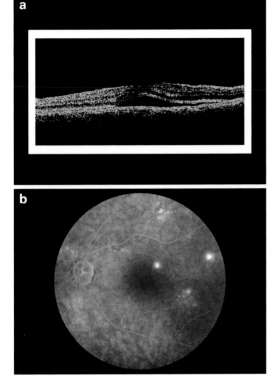

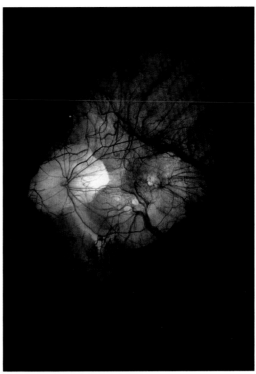

Fig. 3.10 (a) OCT and (b) fluorescein angiogram of a patient with central serous chorioretinopathy with a serous detachment of the fovea on OCT and multiple pinpoint areas of hyperflourescence on fluorescein angiogram

Fig. 3.11 Myopic degeneration in a middle aged woman with spectacle correction of −11.50 diopters

High Myopia

Patients with high myopia can develop retinal and RPE atrophy. The key differentiating features of this condition is the history of significant myopia (at least 6 diopters). Other features include lack of drusen, presence of lacquer cracks (yellow subretinal streaks), macular hyperpigmented spots (Fuchs spot), and optic nerve anomalies including an oblique insertion (tilted) of the optic nerve and an area of white sclera and/or choroidal vessels (myopic crescent) surrounding the optic nerve (Fig. 3.11) [47, 48].

Stargardt's Disease/Fundus Flavimaculatus

Many patients with Stargardt's disease have normal appearing fundi, though patients may have yellow fleck-like deposits at the level of the RPE and atrophic macular changes as in dry AMD. Key differentiating features include: age of vision loss in Stargardt's disease usually occurs in the first several decades and the typical FA findings. Patients with Stargardt's disease often have a "dark choroid" pattern on FA, in which the retinal circulation is highlighted against a hypoflourescent choroid. Bull's eye maculopathy can occur in both Stargardt's disease and dry AMD with GA (Fig. 3.12) [49, 50].

Cuticular Drusen

These drusen are small and numerous and usually initially seen in patients aged 30 to 40, though the patients may not present until they are older. On FA, there is a classic "starry night" pattern, which highlights even more drusen than can be seen on ophthalmoscopy [3].

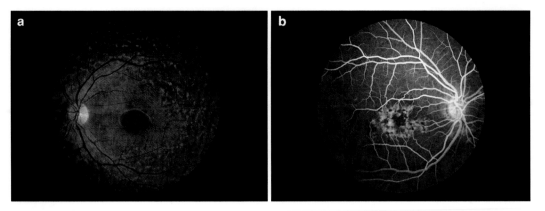

Fig. 3.12 (**a**) Color photo and (**b**) fluorescein angiogram of two patients with Stargardt's disease/Fundus flavimaculatus highlighting retinal flecks and a silent choroid with macular hyperfluorescing lesions

Pattern Dystrophy

Patients with this condition present with yellow, vitelliform lesions in the macula with reticular hyperpigmentation. Key differentiating features include younger patients with pattern dystrophy and the FA findings. FA shows early hypopigmentation and surrounding hyperpigmentation with late staining of vitelliform areas [51–54].

Old Exudative AMD

CNV that has either been treated or involutes can leave atrophic changes. Old subretinal or sub-RPE tissue as seen on clinical exam or on OCT may help to differentiate old CNV from geographic atrophy.

Old Laser Scars

The history of prior laser treatment should be obtainable in these cases. In addition, FA should reveal areas of hypofluorescence that correspond to the laser scars, as opposed to areas of atrophy in AMD that usually are hyperfluorescent.

Other Conditions

Some other conditions that may mimic drusen or dry AMD include:

Hard exudates

Cotton wool spots

Type II membranoproliferative glomerulonephritis [55]

Exudative AMD

Central Serous Chorioretinopathy

Patients with CSCR may have serous retinal detachments or sub-RPE fluid (RPE detachment) and can be mistaken for RPE detachments in wet AMD. Differentiating factors include age (usually ages 25–50), lack of drusen, absence of hemorrhage, and multiple areas of hyper and hypoflourescence on ICGA. The natural history is significantly different with visual recovery being common in CSR [42–46].

Idiopathic Polypoidal Choroidal Vasculopathy

Patients with IPCV are typically elderly and suffer from hypertension just as in wet AMD. Differentiating factors include darkly pigmented individuals, lack of drusen, multiple serosanguinous RPE detachments with a significant lipid component (rare variant of neovascular AMD, as well), minimal fibrous component (rare disciform scar formation), red-orange color of complex (as opposed to grey-green), and choroidal vascular channels terminating in polyp-like structures on ICGA [28–31].

Retinal Angiomatous Proliferation (RAP)

Retinal angiomatous proliferation is often difficult to be fully differentiated from exudative AMD especially in stage 3 and is largely considered a

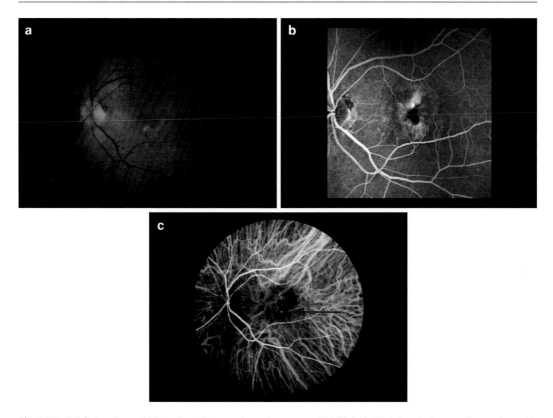

Fig. 3.13 (**a**) Color photo, (**b**) late phase fluorescein angiogram, and (**c**) ICG highlighting the hot spot in a patient with retinal angiomatous proliferation

subset of AMD. Typical features include retinal hemorrhages, prominent cystoid macula edema, elderly (85 years), and Caucasian. ICGA can detect hot spots (Fig. 3.13) [25–27].

Presumed Ocular Histoplasmosis Syndrome (POHS)

Patients with POHS have punched out yellow-white chorioretinal scars in the midperiphery, chorioretinal scarring adjacent to optic nerve/peripapillary atrophy, and CNV. It is more common in the Ohio-Missippi River Valley and in younger individuals (20–50) (Fig. 3.14) [10].

Angioid Streaks

Angioid streaks are bilateral reddish-brown sub-retinal bands radiating from the optic disc representing calcified Bruch's membrane. About 50% of the time, an associated condition such as Ehlers–Danlos, pseudoxanthoma elasticum, Padget's

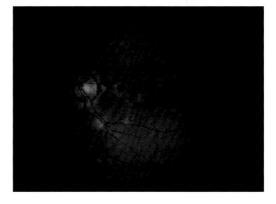

Fig. 3.14 A patient with presumed ocular histoplasmosis syndrome with punched out chorioretinal lesions, peripapillary atrophy, and CNV

disease, and sickle cell disease can be found. Key differentiating features are the peripapillary streaks, which show as window defects on FA due to overlying atrophy (Fig. 3.15) [56, 57].

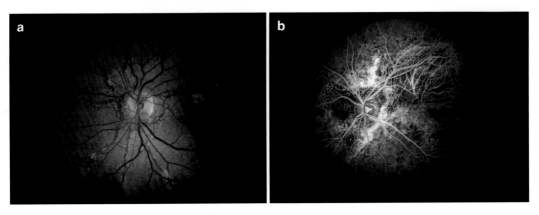

Fig. 3.15 (**a**) Fundus photo and (**b**) fluorescein angiogram CNV due to angioid streaks in a patient with Ehlers–Danlos syndrome

High Myopia

Patients with myopic degeneration may develop macular CNV. The key differentiating feature of this condition is the history of significant myopia (at least 6 diopters). Other features include lack of drusen, lacquer cracks (yellow subretinal streaks), macular hyperpigmented spots representing nonprogressing CNV (Fuchs spot), and optic nerve anomalies including an oblique insertion (tilted) of the optic nerve and an area of white sclera and/or choroidal vessels (myopic crescent) surrounding the nerve (Fig. 3.16) [47, 48].

Cystoid Macular Edema

Patients with neovascular AMD may develop CME. However, some patients diagnosed with cystoid macular edema have undiagnosed occult CNV lesions. This is specifically relevant in patients with the diagnosis of idiopathic CME or post-cataract surgery CME. FA is particularly useful in these patients.

> **Pearl**
> Rule out occult CNV in cases of CME of unknown etiology or CME in the post-operative setting.

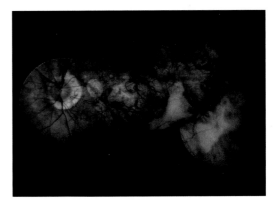

Fig. 3.16 Fundus photo of old CNV due to myopic degeneration

Traumatic Choroidal Rupture

Acutely there is often subretinal hemorrhage in or adjacent to the rupture and CNV can later form on the edge of the rupture site. These patients typically have unilateral findings and a history of significant trauma.

Macular Hemorrhage

Hemorrhage secondary to retinal arterial macroaneurysm, valsalva retinopathy, and trauma can be confused with hemorrhage from AMD. Differentiating features include lack of associated AMD findings, history, and unilateral findings.

CNV Secondary to Laser
A history of prior macular laser would be essential.

Idiopathic
A diagnosis of exclusion in which CNV is present in the absence of any other fundus abnormalities [58].

Summary

AMD is a complex disorder with an extensive differential diagnosis. Using a good clinical exam, history taking, and ancillary testing, the physician can navigate properly to obtain the proper diagnosis. Conditions with similar appearances must be excluded as the treatment and/or prognosis may vary considerably. As our understanding of the disease process improves, we hope an international system of classification will be adopted so clinical trials can be properly compared.

References

1. Kahn HA, Leibowitz HM, Ganley JP, Kini MM, Colton T, Nickerson RS, et al. The Framingham Eye Study II. Association of ophthalmic pathology with single variables previously measured in the Framingham Heart Study. Am J Epidemiol. 1977;106(1):33–41.
2. Gass JDM. Pathogenesis of disciform detachment of the neuroepithelium. II. Idiopathic central serous choroidopathy. Am J Ophthalmol. 1960;63:587–615.
3. Russell SR, Mullins RF, et al. Location, substructure, and composition of basal laminar drusen compared with drusen associated with age-related macular degeneration. Am J Ophthalmol. 2000;129:205–14.
4. Abdelsalam A, Del Priore L, Zarbin MA. Drusen in age-related macular degeneration: pathogenesis, natural course, and laser photocoagulation-induced regression. Surv Ophthalmol. 1999;44(1):1–29. Review.
5. Gass JD. Drusen and disciform macular detachment and degeneration. Arch Ophthalmol. 1973;90(3):206–17.
6. Green WR, McDonnell PJ, Yeo JH. Pathologic features of senile macular degeneration. Ophthalmology. 1985;92(5):615–27.
7. Sarks SH. Council lecture. Drusen and their relationship to senile macular degeneration. Aust J Ophthalmol. 1980;8(2):117–30.
8. Holz FG, Wolfensberger TJ, Piguet B, Gross-Jendroska M, Wells JA, Minassian DC, et al. Bilateral macular drusen in age-related macular degeneration.

9. Prognosis and risk factors. Ophthalmology. 1994;101(9):1522–8.
9. Spraul CW, Grossniklaus HE. Characteristics of Drusen and Bruch's membrane in postmortem eyes with age-related macular degeneration. Arch Ophthalmol. 1997;115(2):267–73.
10. Gass JD. Stereoscopic atlas of macular disease: diagnosis and treatment. 4th ed. St. Louis: Mosby; 1997.
11. Lim JI. Age-related macular degeneration. New York: Marcel Dekkar, Inc.; 2002.
12. Klein R, Klein BE, Jensen SC, Meuer SM. The five-year incidence and progression of age-related maculopathy: the Beaver Dam Eye Study. Ophthalmology. 1997;104(1):7–21.
13. Klein ML, Mauldin WM, Stoumbos VD. Heredity and age-related macular degeneration. Observations in monozygotic twins. Arch Ophthalmol. 1994;112(7):932–7.
14. Macular Photocoagulation Study Group. Risk factors for choroidal neovascularization in the second eye of patients with juxtafoveal or subfoveal choroidal neovascularization secondary to age-related macular degeneration. Arch Ophthalmol. 1997;115(6):741–7.
15. Ferris 3rd FL, Fine SL, Hyman L. Age-related macular degeneration and blindness due to neovascular maculopathy. Arch Ophthalmol. 1984;102(11):1640–2.
16. Sunness JS, Gonzalez-Baron J, Applegate CA, Bressler NM, Tian Y, Hawkins B, et al. Enlargement of atrophy and visual acuity loss in the geographic atrophy form of age-related macular degeneration. Ophthalmology. 1999;106(9):1768–79.
17. Macular Photocoagulation Study Group. Five-year follow-up of fellow eyes of patients with age-related macular degeneration and unilateral extrafoveal choroidal neovascularization. Arch Ophthalmol. 1993;111(9):1189–99.
18. Bressler NM, Frost LA, Bressler SB, Murphy RP, Fine SL. Natural course of poorly defined choroidal neovascularization associated with macular degeneration. Arch Ophthalmol. 1988;106(11):1537–42.
19. Bird AC, Bressler NM, Bressler SB, et al. An international classification and grading system for age-related maculopathy and age-related macular degeneration. Surv Ophthalmol. 1995;39:367–74.
20. Klein R, Klein BE, Linton KL. Prevalence of age-related maculopathy. The Beaver Dam Eye Study. Ophthalmology. 1992;99(6):933–43.
21. The Age-Related Eye Disease Study Research Group. The Age-Related Eye Disease Study system for classifying age-related macular degeneration from stereoscopic color fundus photographs: the Age-Related Eye Disease Study Report Number 6. Am J Ophthalmol. 2001;132:668–81.
22. Jager RD, Mieler WF, Mille JW. Age-related macular degeneration. N Engl J Med. 2008;358:2606–17.
23. Green WR, Gass JDM. Senile disciform degeneration of the macula. Arch Ophthalmol. 1971;100:487–94.
24. Green WR, Enger C. Age-related macular degeneration histopathologic studies: the 1992 Lorenz E. Zimmerman lecture. Ophthalmology. 1993;100:1519–35.

25. Yannuzzi LA, Negrao S, Iida T, et al. Retinal angiomatous proliferation in age-related macular degeneration. Retina. 2001;21:416–34.

26. Borrillo JL, Sivalingam A, Martidis A, et al. Surgical ablation of retinal angiomatous proliferation. Arch Ophthalmol. 2003;121:558–61.

27. Fernandes LH, Freund KB, Yannuzzi LA, et al. The nature of focal areas of hyperfluorescence or hot spots imaged with indocyanine green angiography. Retina. 2002;22:557–68.

28. Stern RM, Zakov N, Zegarra H, et al. Multiple recurrent serous sanguineous retinal pigment epithelial detachments in black women. Am J Ophthalmol. 1985;100:560–9.

29. Yannuzzi LA, Sorenson J, Spaide RF, et al. Idiopathic polypoidal choroidal vasculopathy. Retina. 1990; 10:1–8.

30. Laude A, Cackett PD, Vithana EN, Yeo IY, Wong D, Koh AH, et al. Polypoidal choroidal vasculopathy and neovascular age-related macular degeneration: same or different disease? Prog Retin Eye Res. 2010;29(1):19–29. 2009 Oct 23.

31. Yannuzzi LA, Ciardella AP, Spaide RF, et al. The expanding clinical spectrum of idiopathic polypoidal vasculopathy. Arch Ophthalmol. 1997;115:478–85.

32. Perkovich PT, Zakov N, Berlin LA, et al. An update on multiple recurrent serosanguineous retinal pigment epithelium detachments in black women. Retina. 1990;10:18–26.

33. Lafaut BA, Leyes AM, Snyders B, et al. Polypoidal choroidal vasculopathy in Caucasians. Graefes Arch Clin Exp Ophthalmol. 2000;238:752–9.

34. Uyama M, Wada M, Nagai Y, et al. Polypoidal choroidal vasculopathy: natural history. Am J Ophthalmol. 2002;133:639–48.

35. Japanese Study Group of Polypoidal Choroidal Vasculopathy. Criteria for diagnosis of polypoidal choroidal vasculopathy. Nippon Ganka Gakkai Zasshi. 2005;109:417–27.

36. Chan WM, Lam DS, Lai TY, Liu DT, Li KK, Yao Y, et al. Photodynamic therapy with verteporfin for symptomatic polypoidal choroidal vasculopathy: one-year results of a prospective case series. Ophthalmology. 2004;111:1576–84.

37. Sunness JS, Rubin GS, Applegate CA, Bressler NM, Marsh MJ, Hawkins BS, et al. Visual function abnormalities and prognosis in eyes with age-related geographic atrophy of the macula and good visual acuity. Ophthalmology. 1997;104(10):1677–91.

38. Steinmetz RL, Haimovici R, Jubb C, Fitzke FW, Bird AC. Symptomatic abnormalities of dark adaptation in patients with age-related Bruch's membrane change. Br J Ophthalmol. 1993;77(9):549–54.

39. Fine AM, Elman MJ, Ebert JE, Prestia PA, Starr JS, Fine SL. Earliest symptoms caused by neovascular membranes in the macula. Arch Ophthalmol. 1986;104(4):513–4.

40. Bressler NM, Munoz B, Maguire MG, Vitale SE, Schein OD, Taylor HR, et al. Five-year incidence and disappearance of drusen and retinal pigment epithelial abnormalities. Waterman study. Arch Ophthalmol. 1995;113(3):301–8.

41. Sunness JS, Gonzalez-Baron J, Bressler NM, Hawkins B, Applegate CA. The development of choroidal neovascularization in eyes with the geographic atrophy form of age-related macular degeneration. Ophthalmology. 1999;106(5):910–9.

42. Yannuzzi LA, Shakin JL, Fisher YL, et al. Peripheral retinal detachments and retinal pigment epithelial atrophic tracts secondary to central serous pigment epitheliopathy. Ophthalmology. 1984;91:1554–72.

43. Spaide RF, Campeas L, Haas A, et al. Central serous chorioretinopathy in younger and older adults. Ophthalmology. 1996;103:2070–9; discussion 2079–80.

44. Spaide RF, Hall LS, Haas A, et al. Indocyanine green videoangiography of older patients with central serous chorioretinopathy. Retina. 1996;16:203–13.

45. Marmor MF. New hypotheses on the pathogenesis and treatment of serous retinal detachment. Graefes Arch Clin Exp Ophthalmol. 1988;226:548–52.

46. Tittl MK, Spaide RF, Wong D, et al. Systemic findings associated with central serous chorioretinopathy. Am J Ophthalmol. 1999;128:63–8.

47. Yoshida T, Ohno-Matsui K, Ohtake Y, et al. Myopic choroidal neovascularization: a 10-year follow-up. Ophthalmology. 2003;110(7):1297–305.

48. Johnson DA, Yannuzzi LA, Shakin JL, et al. Lacquer cracks following laser treatment of choroidal neovascularization in pathologic myopia. Retina. 1998;18: 118–24.

49. Armstrong JD, Meyer D, Xu S, et al. Long-term follow up of Stargardt's disease and fundus flavimaculatus. Ophthalmology. 1998;105:448–58.

50. Weleber RG. Stargardt's macular dystrophy. Arch Ophthalmol. 1994;112:752–4.

51. Marmor MF, Byers B. Pattern dystrophy of the pigment epithelium. Am J Ophthalmol. 1977;84:32–44.

52. Hsieh RC, Fine BS, Lyons JS. Patterned dystrophies of the retinal pigment epithelium. Arch Ophthalmol. 1977;95:429–35.

53. Patrinely JR, Lewis RA, Font RL. Foveomacular vitelliform dystrophy, adult type. A clinicopathologic study including electron microscopic observations. Ophthalmology. 1985;92:1712–8.

54. Jaffe GJ, Schatz H. Histopathologic features of adult-onset foveomacular pigment epithelial dystrophy. Arch Ophthalmol. 1988;106:958–60.

55. Kim DD, Mieler WF, Wolf MD. Posterior segment changes in membranoproliferative glomerulonephritis. Am J Ophthalmol. 1992;114(5):593–9.

56. Clarkson JG, Altman RD. Angioid streaks. Surv Ophthalmol. 1982;26:235–46.

57. Lim JI, Bressler NM, Marsh MJ, et al. Laser treatment of choroidal neovascularization in patients with angioid streaks. Am J Ophthalmol. 1993;116: 414–23.

58. Ho AC, Yannuzzi LA, Pisicano K, et al. The natural history of idiopathic subfoveal choroidal neovascularization. Ophthalmology. 1995;102:782–9.

Fundus Imaging of Age-Related Macular Degeneration

Allen Chiang, Andre J. Witkin, Carl D. Regillo, and Allen C. Ho

Key Points

- Digital fundus cameras and confocal scanning laser ophthalmoscopes have increased the efficiency and resolution of fundus photography.
- Autofluorescent images yield information about the functional status of the outer retina and retinal pigment epithelium (RPE).
- Fluorescein angiography remains invaluable for studying retinal vascular anatomy and physiology in eyes with neovascular age-related macular degeneration (AMD).
- Optical coherence tomography (OCT) permits visualization of the vitreoretinal interface, retina, RPE, and choroid, though the implementation of enhanced-depth imaging, in exquisite detail.
- Indocyanine green (ICG) angiography is useful for differentiating neovascular AMD from masquerading conditions.

Introduction

Advancements in fundus imaging technology have contributed immensely to our study and understanding of vitreoretinal disease. Monochromatic and color photography afford an increasingly efficient and reliable way to document fundus findings, having evolved from 35 mm film-based camera systems to high-resolution cameras based on either digital imaging sensors or scanning laser systems. Fluorescein angiography (FA) introduces an added dimension to fundus imaging, providing a means to assess the retinal vascular anatomy and physiology in a manner previously unattainable [1]. Similarly, indocyanine green (ICG) angiography enhances our ability to visualize and analyze the choroidal circulation [2]. In the presence of these dyes, information on other layers of the fundus, particularly the retinal pigment epithelium (RPE), can be obtained indirectly by assessing the degree of increased or decreased transmission of underlying choroidal fluorescence, amount of staining and leakage, and RPE contour via stereoscopic cues. Autofluorescence imaging [3], using several interconnected physiologic principles, provides a means to evaluate the RPE and outer retina on both an anatomic and a functional basis. Optical coherence tomography (OCT) allows ophthalmologists to visualize the vitreoretinal interface as well as the underlying architecture of the retina and the RPE in exquisite cross-sectional detail. Moreover, recent implementations of OCT have permitted improved visualization of the choroid in a number of conditions, including age-related macular degeneration (AMD). Although each of these imaging methods will be discussed individually, in clinical practice they are complementary and often employed simultaneously.

A. Chiang (✉)
Retina Service, Wills Eye Institute/Mid-Atlantic Retina, 840 Walnut St., Suite 1020, Philadelphia, PA, USA
e-mail: chiang.allen@gmail.com

A.C. Ho and C.D. Regillo (eds.), *Age-related Macular Degeneration Diagnosis and Treatment*,
DOI 10.1007/978-1-4614-0125-4_4, © Springer Science+Business Media, LLC 2011

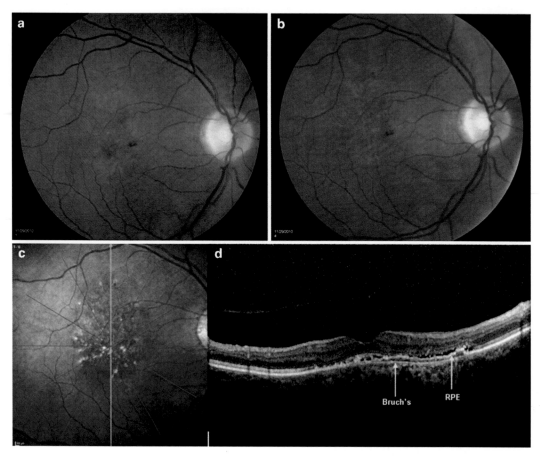

Fig. 4.1 Occult choroidal neovascularization. (**a**) Digital color fundus photograph from an eye with exudative age-related macular degeneration. (**b**) Digital red-free fundus photograph. Note that intraretinal hemorrhage is more clearly highlighted. (**c**) SLO infrared image demonstrates the direction of subsequent OCT image. (**d**) Optical coherence tomography image. The retinal pigment epithelium (RPE) is elevated from Bruch's membrane by a fibrovascular membrane. Shallow subretinal fluid is also evident

Color Photography

Originally, fundus cameras utilized 35 mm photographic film that required a chemical development process in order to reproduce the captured images. More recently, digital photography has supplanted film-based technology as charged coupled devices (CCDs), silicone microprocessors, and digital memory chips have become increasingly more affordable. While the spatial resolution of a film is similar to that of high quality scientific CCDs, other determinants of color image quality including color accuracy, noise, dynamic range, and sensitivity are generally superior with high-resolution color CCDs. Digital images also have other significant advantages; they can instantly be retaken if the initial image capture is of poor quality and they are easy to store, retrieve, and reproduce. Collectively, these attributes make high-resolution digital color photography an efficient and a practical way to record baseline and follow-up images of patients with AMD (Fig. 4.1a).

Monochromatic Photography

When film-based photography was prevalent, a green filter was commonly placed within the imaging light path of the fundus camera in order to produce "red-free" photographs. Green light is advantageous for highlighting small hemorrhages, which appear dark, and for improving the contrast of certain anatomic structures such as blood vessels and the retinal nerve fiber layer (Fig. 4.1b). Even with the arrival of digital imaging, monochromatic photography continued to be used frequently since monochromatic CCDs were initially less expensive and achieved higher resolution than color CCD cameras. However, with the advent of high-resolution color CCDs there is less reason to specifically take a "red-free" image since the green channel of a color photograph can be digitally selected and inspected. Similar analysis of other wavelengths may be useful as well. For example, a particular type of drusen, originally called reticular pseudodrusen, is much easier to see with either infrared or blue light as opposed to red or green light. In the past, a common technique to evaluate patients for the presence of pseudodrusen involved leaving the excitation filter used for fluorescein angiography in place while removing the barrier filter. Now, with digital color photography, it is easy to separate an image into the principle red, green, and blue channels, and the latter has been suggested for improved diagnosis of pseudodrusen [4].

Further advancements have involved a shift beyond the visible light spectrum. Commercially available scanning laser ophthalmoscopes (SLOs), such as one manufactured by Heidelberg Engineering, utilize near-infrared light to create a monochromatic image of the fundus. With near infrared light, the reflectance characteristics of fundus structures differ from that of visible light, and this information has diagnostic value (Fig. 4.1c). For instance, the optic nerve exhibits low reflectivity in near-infrared light and thus appears dark. Conversely, melanin reflects near infrared light, often accounting for the bright appearance of pigmented scars. In line with these physical principles, reticular pseudodrusen are readily visible with this type of SLO imaging.

Autofluorescence Imaging

Autofluorescent images are derived from stimulated emission of light from photoreactive molecular structures, particularly lipofuscin granules, within the RPE (Fig. 4.2a, b) [5–7]. Lipofuscin consists of a diverse group of molecules [7] that accumulate in all post-mitotic

cells as byproducts of the oxidative breakdown and metabolic rearrangement of various biochemical compounds, including polyunsaturated fatty acids and proteins. The retinoids present in lipofuscin are adept at light absorption in the visible light spectrum due to a moderate number of conjugated double bonds intrinsic to their molecular structure. This also forms the molecular basis for the autofluorescence of retinoid molecules, which can be captured either by an SLO or a fundus camera-based system.

Commercial SLO systems employ horizontal and vertical scanning mirrors to scan a specific region of the retina and create raster images viewable on a computer monitor. They utilize 488 nm light to excite lipofuscin and a long-pass filter starting at 500 nm as a barrier. Advantages of current SLO systems include integrated software that automatically adjusts the brightness and contrast of each image, which improves the overall quality of image acquisition, and confocal imaging methodology, which diminishes extra light by focusing detected light through a small pinhole [8]. In this way, greater image resolution is achieved since light only from the conjugate plane is used. Disadvantages of confocal SLO imaging include image noise, some variability from one image to the next, and a potentially variable but unknown alteration by the software in the production of the final image. In contrast, fundus camera-based systems use filters that are placed on the light path in a manner similar to that for fluorescein angiography, but with an excitation filter of 535–585 nm (green) which targets the lower end of the absorption curve for lipofuscin, and a barrier filter of 605–715 nm. Fundus camera-based systems have lower incremental cost, low image noise, higher repeatability, and the ability to capture raw information from the patient. Their major drawback is the absence of automated image optimization. Raw images from fundus camera-based systems are often of lower contrast than the processed images that are automatically produced by confocal SLOs; thus enhancements must be performed manually by the user.

The source of lipofuscin in the RPE is the outer segments of the retinal photoreceptors. The main component of lipofuscin in RPE cells is A2E, which comprises two molecules of

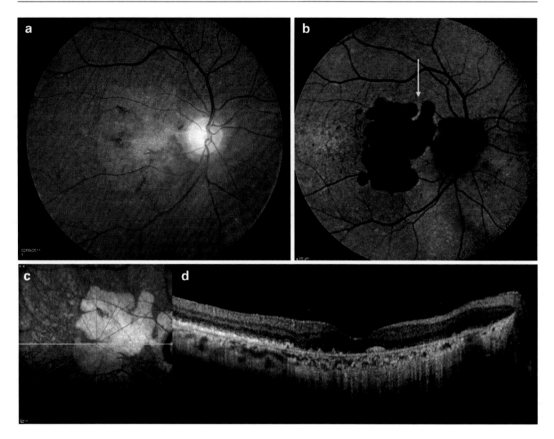

Fig. 4.2 Geographic atrophy. (**a**) Digital color fundus photograph from an eye with geographic atrophy. (**b**) SLO fundus autofluorescence image showing absence of auto-fluorescence in the area of RPE atrophy. Areas of hyper-autofluorescence at the border of the RPE atrophy are seen (*arrow*). (**c**) SLO infrared image demonstrates the direction of subsequent OCT image. (**d**) OCT image shows disappearance of the RPE, with appearance of Bruch's membrane. Increased OCT signal into the chorio-capillaris is apparent underneath areas of RPE atrophy

trans-retinal and one molecule of phosphatidly-ethanolamine. Precursors of A2E, including A2PE-H$_2$, A2PE, and A2-rhodopsin, are each autofluorescent and aggregate in the outer segments of photoreceptors prior to phagocytosis by the RPE [9, 10]. Collectively, the components of lipofuscin inhibit lysosomal protein degradation [11], are photoreactive [12], and are capable of inducing RPE cellular apoptosis [13], specifically blue light-induced apoptosis [14]. In addition, A2E and its precursors are susceptible to oxidative stress and damage [15, 16], resulting from photo-oxidative reactions within the neighboring milieu that proliferate reactive oxygen species and free radicals [17]. Conditions that produce separation of the retina from the RPE impede the physiologic phagocytosis of shed outer segments. Excessive buildup of lipofuscin precedes the degeneration of photoreceptors and associated geographic atrophy and represents a common pathway in the pathogenesis of various monogenetic and complex retinal diseases (Fig. 4.2) [18–20].

> **Pearl**
> Autofluoresence imaging may be useful for following and measuring geographic atrophy.

Optical Coherence Tomography

Optical coherence tomography (OCT) is an imaging technique capable of evaluating the macula in cross-section and with very high detail.

OCT imaging calculates distances within a target tissue by measuring the "echo time delay" of light, or the time it takes for light to be backscattered from the target tissue. This is analogous to an a-scan ultrasound. Multiple OCT "a-scans" may then be taken in a line, to form an image analogous to a b-scan ultrasound image, but using light instead of sound. Because light travels too fast to be detected directly, the echo-time delay must be measured indirectly, using a technique called low coherence interferometry. First, the light signal emanating from the OCT instrument is split in two using a beam splitter. One beam is sent to the eye and the other beam is sent to a reference mirror. The light then reflects back from both the target and the reference to a Michelson interferometer, where the signals combine to form an interference pattern [21, 22].

Low coherence refers to the light source used in OCT. In OCT, the axial and transverse resolutions are uncoupled. The axial resolution is determined by the bandwidth, one of the determinants of temporal coherence, of the light source. Coherence refers to correlation of different physical characteristics of light. Highly coherent light produces minimal interference, while less coherent light produces more complex interference patterns. Previous generations of OCT instruments used superluminescent diode light sources with bandwidths of ~25 um centered near a wavelength of 810 nm, and capable of 10 um axial resolution in the human eye. With wider bandwidth light sources (or less temporally coherent), the interference pattern becomes more complex, and allows for improved ability to localize echoes within a target, thereby increasing axial resolution [23]. Transverse resolution is independent of the bandwidth of the light, and is dependent on the optical focusing of light on the retina. Transverse resolution in commercially available OCT instruments is limited to $10-15$ μm by natural aberrations in the human eye [23, 24].

Interference between the reference and sample arms of the interferometer will only occur if the arms are nearly the exact length, therefore the distance that light travels to and from the reference mirror must equal the distance that light travels when it is reflected from a given intraocular structure. In the original OCT systems (referred to as "time domain" OCT), the position of the reference mirror was continuously moved so that the time delay of the reference light beam matched the time delay of light echoes from various intraocular structures. As the reference mirror was moved, variations in optical reflectivity could be detected within the target tissue. In "Fourier-" or "spectral-domain" OCT systems, the interference signal is detected using a stationary reference arm. Instead of moving the reference arm to detect distances within tissue, multiple depths within tissue may be localized by analyzing the pattern of the interference signal, by taking the Fourier transform of this interference spectrum [25]. Because all light echoes from different axial depths in the sample are measured simultaneously rather than sequentially, imaging can be performed at much greater speeds than in previous "time domain" systems, and a greater wealth of OCT data becomes available.

Another integral component of OCT is the utilization of analysis software. Computer algorithms are used to calculate retinal thickness by automatically delineating the inner and outer retinal borders. When a series of OCT images are obtained through the macula, a topographic map of retinal thickness may be created. Previous time domain OCT (TD-OCT) systems used scanning modes that acquired six linear images centered at the point of fixation, spaced 30° apart and typically 6 mm in length. Newer spectral-domain OCT (SD-OCT) systems create macular maps using a much larger amount of OCT data; typically, a "raster" series of horizontal OCT images are used in macular mapping protocols. These various retinal thickness calculations may be compared to normative databases, or be followed over time or before and after treatment with extreme precision due to registration of a particular point of interest within the macula.

OCT measures changes in optical reflectivity within the retina, and can be useful in analyzing retinal microstructure. Although these optical reflections do not equate to in-vivo retinal structures, a high correlation between OCT and retinal histology has been shown [26, 27]. Nerve fiber layers (retinal nerve fiber layer, inner and outer plexiform layers) are more highly reflective on

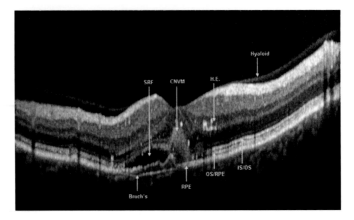

Fig. 4.3 Classic choroidal neovascularization. OCT image demonstrates a partially-detached posterior hyaloid, sub-retinal fluid (SRF), CNV, and hard exudates (HE). The RPE is partially detached from Bruch's membrane in the area of the foveola. Besides the RPE, two other hyper-reflective outer retinal lines are noted. The photoreceptor inner-outer segment junction (IS/OS) is the innermost of these lines, and the outer segment/RPE interdigitation (OS/RPE) is the middle of these lines

OCT, while the cellular layers (ganglion cell layer, inner and outer nuclear layers) are less highly reflective. The external limiting membrane is visible as a moderately-reflective line toward the outer part of the outer nuclear layer. The outer aspect of the neurosensory retina is bounded by three closely-spaced reflective layers [28]. The inner of these two layers represents part of the photoreceptors, likely the junction between the inner and outer segments, and the outermost reflective layer represents the RPE. There is also an apparent layer between the RPE and inner segment/outer segment (IS/OS) junction, which may represent the tips of the photoreceptors or the interdigitation between the RPE and photoreceptor outer segments (Fig. 4.3). Retinal blood vessels are evident in OCT images by their shadowing of deeper retinal structures, as blood is highly-reflective, and scattering of OCT signal. In some cases, the posterior hyaloid is visible as a thin, moderately reflective line anterior to the retina. In areas of RPE loss or detachment, Bruch's membrane may become visible, and in areas of RPE loss, OCT signal is able to penetrate into the choroid and sclera more readily (Fig. 4.4). OCT is also able to clearly delineate choroidal neovascularization (CNV). CNV that appears "classic" on FA typically appear anterior to the RPE, and "occult" CNV appears underneath the RPE.

> **Pearl**
> OCT imaging is an essential diagnostic tool for managing neovascular AMD.

Enhanced Depth Imaging

A limitation of SD-OCT is that the quality of the interference signal is not the same at all tissue depths. At the top of the SD-OCT image (the "zero-delay line"), signal as well as resolution are highest, but further down in the image, signal and resolution are worse due to increasing mismatches in path length. The degradation of image signal is perhaps more significant since it correlates with increasing image darkness. In a standard OCT image, the vitreoretinal interface is placed near the top of the image by the OCT technician, therefore the best OCT imaging capability is in the vitreous, while the poorest OCT signal and resolution are in the outer retina and choroid.

Spaide and colleagues described a technique called enhanced depth imaging OCT (EDI-OCT) that permits imaging of the choroid, and in very high myopes, of the sclera as well [29]. This technique involves pushing the SD-OCT instrument closer to the eye to obtain an inverted image. In contrast to a typical SD-OCT image, deeper

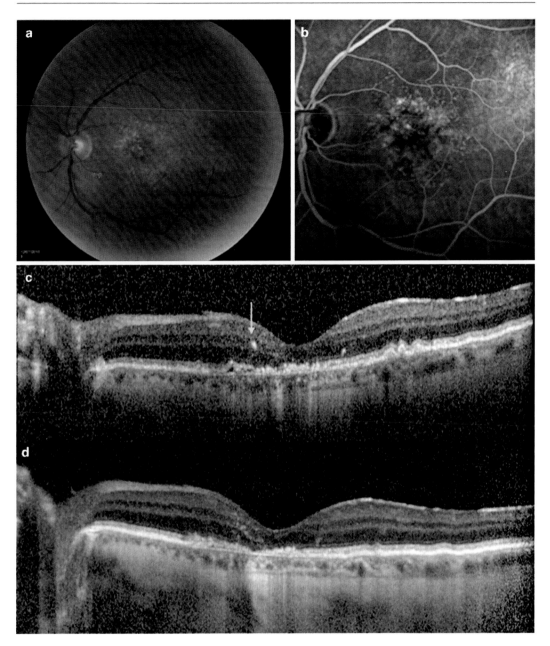

Fig. 4.4 Drusen with pigment epithelial atrophy. (**a**) Digital color fundus photograph from an eye with drusen and central RPE atrophy. (**b**) A mid-phase SLO fluorescein angiogram shows hyperfluorescence of the drusen. (**c**) OCT image demonstrates a focal area of RPE atrophy and corresponding increased signal penetration into the choriocapillaris. Focal elevations of the RPE represent drusen. Intraretinal hyper-reflective lesions likely represent intraretinal migration of RPE pigment (*arrow*). (**d**) Enhanced depth imaging OCT allows clearer visualization of the outer retinal layers and choriocapillaris

structures in the eye are no longer dark in this inverted image owing to a differential in the sensitivity. Clinical applications of EDI-OCT continue to expand and it may add additional information to the diagnosis and analysis of AMD.

Fundus Angiography

Fundus angiography encompasses the diagnostic application of two different dyes that are administered intravenously: fluorescein sodium, which

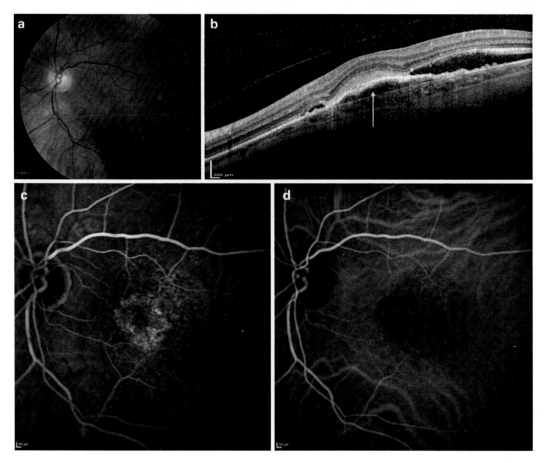

Fig. 4.5 Occult choroidal neovascularization. (a) Digital color fundus photograph from an eye with exudative age-related macular degeneration. (b) OCT image shows an elevation of the sub-foveal RPE (*arrow*) by a fibrovascular membrane. There is a pocket of associated subretinal fluid. (c) SLO mid-phase fluorescein angiogram shows mottled hyperfluorescence without the appearance of well-defined "classic" CNV. (d) SLO ICG angiogram shows a more-clearly demarcated area of hyperfluorescence representing CNV

enables a detailed assessment of the retinal vasculature, and indocyanine green (ICG), which due to its more highly protein-bound nature is more useful for studying the choroidal circulation [1, 2]. Fluorescein angiography preceded ICG angiography and accordingly, its correlation to histopathologic findings is better understood in comparison with ICGA angiography. In addition, the number of clinical indications for its use exceeds that of ICG angiography. Indeed, the clinical significance of many ICG angiographic findings remains either unclear or undefined. Nevertheless, ICG angiography may prove to be helpful when attempting to differentiate neovascular AMD from its various masqueraders, including polypoidal choroidal vasculopathy and central serous chorioretinopathy. Furthermore, it has contributed greatly to our understanding about the pathophysiology of different types of CNV, particularly poorly defined or occult CNV, which may be imaged inadequately by fluorescein angiography (Fig. 4.5) [30].

Fluorescein Dye Characteristics

Fluorescein sodium is a highly water soluble dye with a molecular weight of 376 that is rapidly metabolized to fluorescein monoglucuronide and eliminated via renal excretion. The fluorescein molecule achieves a higher energy state following exposure to blue-green light that is in the range of

465–490 nm, which is the absorption peak of fluorescein excitation. Upon returning to the lower energy state, emission of a longer wavelength (520–530 nm) occurs for every quantum of stimulating light and corresponds to a yellow-green color. Traditional fundus cameras possess two interference bandpass filters, which block out all light except for a specific wavelength. An excitation filter permits imaging blue-green light to pass through and a barrier filter that blocks most of the reflected blue light while allowing yellow-green wavelengths to return unimpeded to the fundus camera's detection system, either 35 mm film or a digital CCD. Little extraneous light is able to reach the detection system because the excitation and barrier filters have minimal overlap with regard to wavelength transmission.

However, it is this small mismatch in the filters that is responsible for the phenomenon of pseudofluorescence, in which nonfluorescent light is imaged. Certain material in the fundus such as hard exudates reflect a large proportion of the excitation light. Transmission of some of this reflected light through the barrier filter is what generates this false fluorescence, which is now largely avoided due to the utilization of modern filters. Nevertheless, after several years of use, these filters will allow increasing degrees of pseudofluorescence as they wear thin. Other substances in the fundus such as lipofuscin and optic nerve head drusen actually fluoresce upon exposure to the excitation light. This distinct phenomenon, referred to as autofluorescence, is captured prior to the injection of any fluorescein dye.

Indocyanine Green Dye Characteristics

ICG, or tricarbocyanine, is a dye that binds tightly to serum proteins, confining it to the intravascular compartment until it is cleared by the liver. Only 60–80% of fluorescein is protein bound as compared with 98% of ICG. ICG is characterized by a peak spectral absorption in the near infrared range of the light spectrum of approximately 800 nm. Emission of fluorescent light in the range of 825–835 nm occurs during its decay following excitation. ICG angiography camera systems incorporate a barrier filter which

blocks reflected light shorter than 825 nm. Light absorption and fluorescence occur within the near infrared spectrum, which allows ICG to provide better visualization through the RPE, shallow hemorrhages, lipid, and serosanguinous fluid. The longer wavelengths involved in ICG angiography as compared with fluorescein angiography convey less extensive scattering and greater penetrance through overlying pigment. Collectively, these attributes permit ICG angiography to deliver enhanced visualization of the choroidal vasculature.

Cameras and Angiography

Cameras that are used in fluorescein angiography are based on either one of two fundamentally different design principles: the scanning laser ophthalmoscope or the fundus camera. As mentioned earlier, SLOs image the fundus by sweeping focused 488 nm laser light across the fundus in a raster pattern and are capable of reconstructing a three-dimensional structure from the acquired raster images. A key feature of the SLO pertains to its application of confocal imaging, which means that only light from a conjugate plane of interest is detected by the image sensor. More specifically, use of point illumination and a spatial pinhole act to eliminate out-of-focus light from tissue planes that are outside the singular plane of interest [31]. Implementation of this optical imaging technique enables SLOs to deliver enhanced optical resolution and the contrast of vascular structures in particular. Another significant advantage of scanning laser systems is the ability to capture images at a high frame rate and in real time. In patients with neovascular AMD, this capability provides a detailed assessment of the microvasculature that feeds and drains a focus of neovascularization during the filling phase, with potential therapeutic implications. Indeed, the selective ablation of feeder vessels of choroidal neovascular membranes with ICG angiography-guided laser photocoagulation appears to be a viable treatment strategy in those patients with extrafoveal feeder vessels [32].

The alternative to the SLO is a fundus camera-based system. Modern fundus cameras utilize a xenon flash to discharge a bank of capacitors and a digital imaging sensor to record the resultant photographs. Images acquired by digital fundus camera systems typically have a higher pixel density and less noise than those obtained with the SLO. However, a digital fundus camera system has some limitations. In particular, the frame rate is limited by the speed at which the system reads and resets the CCD sensor, recharges its capacitors, and writes data to the internal memory cache. As a result, most digital fundus cameras are unable to capture images at more than one or two frames per second. In addition, unlike SLOs, fundus cameras do not have confocal imaging, which means that every source of fluorescence within the optical pathway is imaged. This phenomenon may adversely impact image contrast in comparison with SLO-based systems.

Patient Consent and Instruction

Fluorescein angiography is one of the few invasive diagnostic tests that is commonly performed in the ophthalmologist's office. Accordingly, physicians are obliged to inform patients of the potential risks of fluorescein angiography. In addition, it behooves the physician to review the medical history prior to ordering the test, to identify certain medical conditions such as asthma or uncontrolled hypertension that can increase the likelihood of an adverse reaction. Since fluorescein is excreted via the renal system, it is critical for ophthalmologists to elicit any history of renal disease that would limit a patient's ability to adequately eliminate fluorescein. In such cases, it is prudent to communicate with their nephrologist or primary-care physician prior to proceeding with the test. Regarding women of child-bearing age, it is important to recognize that fluorescein sodium falls into pregnancy category C; adequate animal studies have not been conducted and it is unknown whether it has teratogenic effects. Therefore, it is sensible to avoid fluorescein angiography in a pregnant woman if at all possible.

The most common side effect of fluorescein angiography is that of a generalized yellowish hue to the skin. In addition, patients should be warned that their urine will appear a bright yellow-green color for roughly 24 h. Other common side effects include nausea (about 5%), emesis, and the development of hives (also about 5%) [33, 34]. Fortunately, in a majority of patients the sensation of nausea is transient and resolves over a matter of 10–20 s without treatment. While hives are often mild and typically responsive to treatment with oral diphenhydramine or a similar antihistamine, these patients should be monitored to rule out the development of additional anaphylactoid symptoms. It is important to recognize that patients who experience such side effects are prone to a similar response with repeat fluorescein angiography [33]. On occasion there may be some infiltration of dye into subcutaneous tissue during the injection, which leads to pain and localized skin discoloration; ice is often therapeutic in this situation. In contrast, the constellation of life-threatening adverse effects associated with anaphylactic shock is fortunately very uncommon. The incidence of death after fluorescein injection is estimated to be 1 in 222,000 [34].

Indocyanine green dye was first approved for human use in 1956, for the purpose of studying the hepatic and cardiac systems [35].Therefore, nearly 55 years of data regarding its side effect profile is available. In general, the more common side effects associated with fluorescein angiography occur less frequently with ICG angiography, perhaps because ICG is more highly protein bound and thus less likely to stimulate the chemoreceptor trigger zone. Mild gastrointestinal disturbance, itching, or hives are uncommon with ICG [36–38].Extravasation of injected ICG is painful and can cause a dark green spot that may last for several days. The incidence of death after ICG angiography has been estimated at 1 per 333,000 [34].

ICG contains approximately 5% iodine by weight. More specifically, it contains inorganic iodine, and the risks of administration in patients with allergies to organic iodine is unknown. While patients who are allergic to shellfish are often cautioned against receiving iodine-containing radiocontrast agents, there is little factual evidence to support such a recommendation. Since these patients typically have no difficulty consuming iodized salt, the rationale behind linking radiocontrast agents and ICG or shellfish and the inorganic iodine in ICG preparations would appear to be tenuous at best. On the other hand, patients with renal disease or liver dysfunction may truly have an increased risk for adverse reactions [39]. ICG has not been shown to cross the placental barrier, however formal studies on fetal toxicity have not been performed [38].

While fluorescein and ICG angiography are generally very safe in-office diagnostic procedures, adverse reactions can occur and may occasionally be severe. It is worthwhile to emphasize that patients should be screened carefully for potential risk factors and as with all intravenously administered agents, it is essential that adequate resuscitation facilities and properly trained personnel be available to manage these problems. Particularly for more remote office locations, it is prudent to establish a working protocol that addresses stabilization of a patient until paramedics can arrive. Although there is no official mandate to have written consent for fundus angiography, many ophthalmologists prudently elect to maintain documentation of the informed consent process. At a minimum, each patient should be made aware of the risks and benefits of fundus angiography.

Fluorescein Injection

Solutions containing fluorescein sodium are available in single-use ampules in one of two different volumes and concentrations that are functionally similar: 5 ml of a 10% solution and 2 ml of a 25% solution. The former is commonly used while the latter may be appropriate in cases when a highly sensitive imaging system such as an SLO is used. The fluorescein dye is drawn up into a syringe and connected to a 23-gauge butterfly needle via flexible clear tubing, which allows the individual injecting the dye to be certain that the needle is in the vein due to a small reflux or "flashback" of blood into the tubing.

Selecting an optimal site for injection requires experience and may need to be tailored to the patient's anatomy. A favorable target for injection is the antecubital vein, which is commonly used due to its relatively large size and readily accessible location. In some patients, particularly those who are obese, the veins on the dorsal surface of the hands are often easier to visualize and inject. However, injecting dye into these vessels may be slightly more painful, and rolling of the veins is more likely to occur. Localized ecchymosis following injection is also more readily noticeable. It is important to recognize that although arm-to-choroid and arm-to-retina circulation times are sometimes used to assess ocular perfusion, these measurements may be difficult to interpret since they are influenced by numerous factors including the injection location and the rate of injection.

Fluorescein Technique

Following fluorescein injection, the photographer waits expectantly while focusing on the fundus through the camera's viewfinder. Appearance of the dye in younger individuals typically takes place within 12 s, though it may be mildly delayed in older patients. As soon as fluorescein dye is detected, the photographer begins recording images in rapid sequence. A digital fundus camera system permits the photographer to take as many photographs early after injection as needed, since it is easy and convenient to delete unwanted frames at a later time. Experienced photographers are adept at performing the necessary fine focus and illumination adjustments early on in the angiographic series. After the early phase, stereo pairs of the fundus can be taken of both eyes if desired. There are stereoviewers available for digital angiography, although stereophotography is now less frequently pursued in this era of digital imaging. If the patient has macular disease, the photographer should visually scan the retina peripheral to the vascular arcades in effort to document any abnormalities. Midphase photographs are then acquired 1–2 min later. At about 5 or 6 min after the injection, additional stereo pairs are taken of the macula and any pathologic areas. Many clinicians also request a series of late-phase photographs between 10 and 15 min after fluorescein dye injection.

Indocyanine Green Technique

Dye injection for ICG angiography is performed in a similar fashion to fluorescein angiography. However, the photographer should be poised to record images almost immediately after injection since the choroidal vasculature starts to fill even before the retinal vasculature. Mid-phase photographs are routinely taken at 5 and 10 min after injection while late-phase photographs are taken at the 30 min time point. In general, SLOs record the filling phases with greater temporal resolution than fundus camera systems. However, late-phase image quality is better with fundus camera-based systems.

Fluorescein Angiographic Interpretation

Within the intravascular compartment, approximately 80% of the fluorescein sodium is bound to serum proteins while the other 20% remains unbound; binding alters the absorption and emission spectra only slightly. Unbound fluorescein is freely diffusible, yet diffusion is normally restricted by the blood-retinal barrier, which is part of the blood-ocular barrier and an amalgam of two separate anatomical boundaries that restrict the passage of large molecules into the retina. The retinal pigment epithelium maintains the outer portion of the blood-retinal barrier while the inner blood-retinal barrier is comprised of a single layer of nonfenestrated endothelial cells, which have intercellular tight junctions.

The filling sequence in fluorescein angiography reflects the anatomy of the vasculature supplying the globe, choroid, and retina. Details of retinal circulation are readily visible due to the contrast provided by the underlying RPE. In addition, it fills from a central point and its presence is more or less confined to two dimensions. Initially, the large choroidal vessels begin to fluoresce, approximately 1–2 s prior to the first appearance of dye in the retinal arterioles. This initial phase of fluorescein filling the arterioles is referred to as the "arterial phase" or "early phase". Although the dye moves swiftly through the retinal vessels, an experienced photographer may be able to capture the dye front in one of the early frames as it moves through the retinal arterioles and approaches the capillary bed. Filling of the capillary network introduces an abrupt increase in the retinal fluorescence. In the absence of media opacities, individual perifoveal capillaries are readily apparent. In contrast, it is more difficult to distinguish fine vessels within the lobular choriocapillaris layer. Nevertheless, the choriocapillaris is better visualized on fluorescein angiography than on ICG angiography because the plane of focus for the photographer is shallower during fluorescein angiography.

Over the next few seconds in a healthy individual, the dye reaches the posterior capillary venules and rapidly progresses to fill the larger veins. In elderly patients, however, this arteriovenous transit time may be slightly increased and still considered physiologic. Eventually, the initial bolus of fluorescein dye leaves the ocular circulation, which causes the total fundus fluorescence to fade to some degree. Once the bolus of dye has traveled through the systemic circulation, however, it reappears in the ocular circulation and produces a corresponding increase in fundus fluorescence. This stage of the angiogram is referred to as the "recirculation phase" and occurs within about a minute after the fluorescein injection. Recirculation is readily apparent to the photographer or when reviewing videography from a scanning laser ophthalmoscope, but is less evident when reviewing still frames in isolation. Photographs recorded from 1 to 3 min after fluorescein injection are commonly referred to as mid-phase images. As the dye is cleared from the blood stream by the renal system, the total fluorescence gradually diminishes. This stage of the angiogram is referred to as the "late phase" and applies to images taken after the 5 min time point. In these frames, the fundus appears darker than after the initial dye injection.

The Macula

In fundus imaging, the macula has a characteristic appearance and fluorescence pattern that can be attributed its unique histologic features. Due to an abundance of xanthophyll pigment, which absorbs shorter wavelengths within the visible light spectrum, the macula normally exhibits a yellowish hue on fundus photography. On fluorescein angiography, the macula appears darker than the surrounding areas because RPE cells in the macular region are taller and are packed with a higher concentration of melanin granules than anywhere else in the fundus, which leads to reduced transmission of fluorescent light from the underlying choroidal vessels. Furthermore, there is a physiologic absence of central fluorescence within the retinal capillary network corresponding to the foveal avascular zone.

Deviations from Normal Angiographic Appearance

Hyperfluorescence refers to an abnormally bright area on the fluorescein angiogram, where the fluorescence is in excess of what would be expected on a physiologic angiogram (Table 4.1). One reason for hyperfluorescence is simply when fluorescence is more readily visible. Normally, melanin pigment in the choroid and RPE layers and xanthophyll pigment in the macula block underlying choroidal fluorescence. Focal or generalized attenuation or loss of either of these two layers permits increased transmission and visibility of choroidal fluorescence referred to as transmission or window defects, which appear in the early phase of the angiogram. Another reason for hyperfluorescence is the excess accumulation of fluorescein dye either within vascular abnormalities of the optic disc, retina, or choroid, or within the extravascular space, which is typically observed in the mid to late phases. As an example, CNV demonstrates a network of abnormal vessels as well as a leakage of dye into the surrounding extravascular compartment (Fig. 4.6).

Normally about 45–60 s after injection, fluorescence of the retinal and choroidal vessels begins to wane. By the 10–15 min time point, fluorescein is completely emptied from the retinal and choroidal circulation. With exception to fluorescence of the lamina cribosa or a scleral crescent, any other late-phase hyperfluorescence represents extravascular fluorescein and is referred to as leakage. By convention, fluorescein leakage is further categorized based on its appearance. Fluorescein leakage that flows into well-demarcated anatomic or pathologic spaces is referred to as pooling, while leakage of dye that has diffused into surrounding tissue is called

Table 4.1 Fluorescein hyperfluorescence associated with age-related macular degeneration

Transmitted fluorescence	RPE thinning, atrophy or depigmentation, RPE tear
Abnormal vessels	CNV
Leakage	CNV directly into the subretinal space, leakage through the RPE
Pooling	Neurosensory detachment, pigment epithelial detachment, cystoid macular edema
Staining	Scars, "brushfire" staining at borders of RPE atrophy, perivascular staining (vasculitis)

Table 4.2 Fluorescein hypofluorescence associated with age-related macular degeneration

Blocked retinal fluorescence	Vitreous or retinal hemorrhage
Blocked choroidal fluorescence	Hemorrhage RPE hyperplasia RPE hypertrophy RPE reduplication associated with RPE tear
Vascular filling defects	Occlusion of a vascular bed

staining. Finally, although not usually associated with AMD, there are two other forms of abnormal late fluorescence worth mentioning; one occurs when the dye enters the vitreous and the other when it leaks into the optic nerve head.

There are two main causes of hypofluorescence. Either there is less fluorescein present within the vasculature than expected in a particular fundus region or there is something impeding our view of retinal or choroidal fluorescence (Table 4.2).

Indocyanine Green Angiographic Interpretation

The phases of ICG angiography are similar to those of fluorescein angiography, with the obvious addition of choroidal filling phases. Choroidal filling occurs largely in parallel to retinal vascular filling, yet they are slightly out of phase since the choroidal vasculature starts to fill first in the early phase of the angiogram. Since there is sequential filling of the short posterior ciliary arteries, a "watershed" effect may be seen. The transit phase begins with filling of the medium

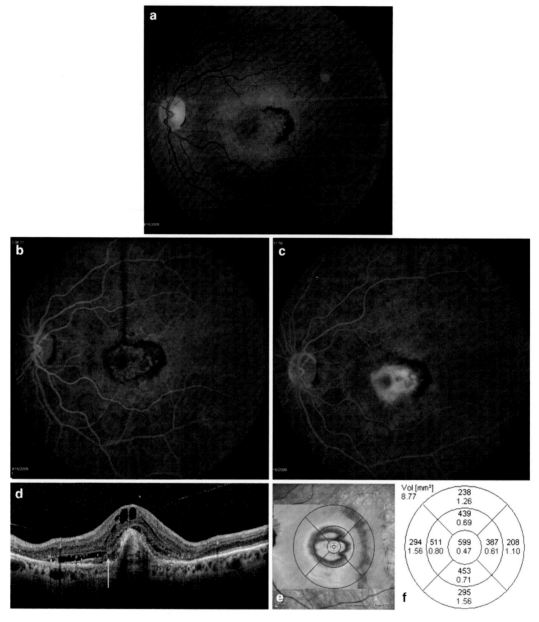

Fig. 4.6 Classic choroidal neovascularization. (**a**) Digital color fundus photograph from an eye with exudative age-related macular degeneration. (**b**) Mid-phase digital fluorescein angiogram shows appearance of a well-demarcated "classic" CNV. Fluorescence is blocked in the area of subretinal hemorrhage. (**c**) Late-phase fluorescein angiogram shows leakage of dye from the CNV. (**d**) OCT image demonstrates a partially-detached posterior hyaloid, intraretinal cystic fluid, subretinal fluid, a subfoveal lesion underlying the RPE, with high reflectivity and shadowing of underlying choroidal structure, and a broader moderately-reflective lesion overlying the RPE (*arrow*), likely representing the "classic" component of the CNV. (**e**) OCT thickness map. (**f**) ETDRS OCT thickness map

choroidal arteries; the choriocapillaris remains dark during this phase. At the peak of the transit phase, the retinal vessels are filled with ICG dye and demonstrate venous laminar flow. The transition to the venous phase is more rapid in the choroid than in the retinal circulation. As the choroidal veins fill during this middle phase, it may become increasingly difficult to distinguish the choroidal arteries as a diffuse, homogenous choroidal fluorescence is observed. It is during this middle phase that hyperfluorescent lesions start to become more evident. In the late phase, which occurs around the 15 min time point, no details of the retinal or choroidal vessels are visible. The large choroidal vessels become hypofluorescent, the optic disc appears dark, and background fluorescence is significantly diminished, all of which allow choroidal vascular abnormalities such as choroidal neovascular membranes to stand out markedly (Fig. 4.7).

Certain terms in fundus angiography relate specifically to ICG imaging. A distinct focus of increasing hyperfluorescence less than one disc diameter in size is referred to as a "hot spot". Hot spots typically represent an area of occult CNV, or polypoidal vasculopathic abnormalities (Fig. 4.8). Another term that is used to describe occult CNV is "placoid hyperfluorescence," which applies to an area of hyperfluorescence that is greater than one disc diameter in size and lacks well-defined borders. These terms reflect the utility of ICG angiography for cases in which occult recurrent or persistent CNV is suspected, but the fluorescein angiography is equivocal.

Non-neovascular Age-Related Macular Degeneration

Drusen

Drusen have been classified into a number of groups on the basis of size and appearance. They may be large (>125 μ(mu)m, about the diameter of an arcade vein near the optic disc) intermediate (63–124 μ(mu)m), or small (<63 μ(mu)m). The RPE overlying a drusen is often thinner, which produces a transmission window defect on FA. Smaller drusen can sometimes appear bright early in a fluorescein angiogram. Basal laminar drusen, or cuticular drusen, appear as a "starry sky" of thousands of bright spots on FA (Fig. 4.9). Occasionally, cuticular drusen may be associated with yellow subfoveal material that mimics vitelliform dystrophy. Soft drusen usually are not readily visible in the early phases of a fluorescein angiogram, but may stain later (Fig. 4.8). Subretinal drusenoid deposits, also known as reticular pseudodrusen, are subretinal drusen that

do not exhibit significant angiographic findings [40]. The biochemical composition of drusen may affect both fluorescein [41] and indocyanine green staining [42].

On OCT, drusen are visualized as moderately-reflective material under the highly reflective RPE layer. Drusen have a relatively homogeneous composition. Typically, drusen lift up the RPE, and in the case of large soft drusen, Bruch's membrane may be visualized (Fig. 4.8). Cuticular drusen are apparent as smaller nodular deposits below the RPE, creating a "saw-tooth" pattern. Reticular pseudodrusen may be visualized anterior to the RPE on OCT. On autofluorescence, soft drusen appear hypoautofluorescent, although they may have a hyperautofluorescent rim. Cuticular drusen and reticular pseudodrusen also may be hypoautofluorescent, although many times they are not apparent on fundus autofluorescence [43].

Pigmentary Abnormalities Including Geographic Atrophy

Focal hyperpigmentation is a risk factor for the development of CNV. Histopathologic correlation of focal hyperpigmentation has demonstrated detached cells containing pigment in the subretinal space. These areas of focal hyperpigmentation also display focal hyperautofluorescence and increased absorption of infrared light, suggesting these cells contain lipofuscin [44]. In addition, the presence of focal hyperpigmentation was found to be highly correlated with retinal angiomatous proliferation in the fellow eye [44]. In cases of focal hyperpigmentation apparent on examination, intraretinal migration of highly-reflective RPE pigment may be visualized on OCT (Fig. 4.4) [45].

Another pigmentary alteration is RPE atrophy, which can occur in sharply-defined areas of severe atrophy, known as geographic atrophy (GA), or in less well-defined, more granular regions of less severe atrophy known as nongeographic atrophy. The outer borders of a region of geographic atrophy are slightly hyperpigmented at the level of the RPE and occasionally hyperautofluorescent [46], suggesting that these cells may contain excess lipofuscin. Of note, areas of

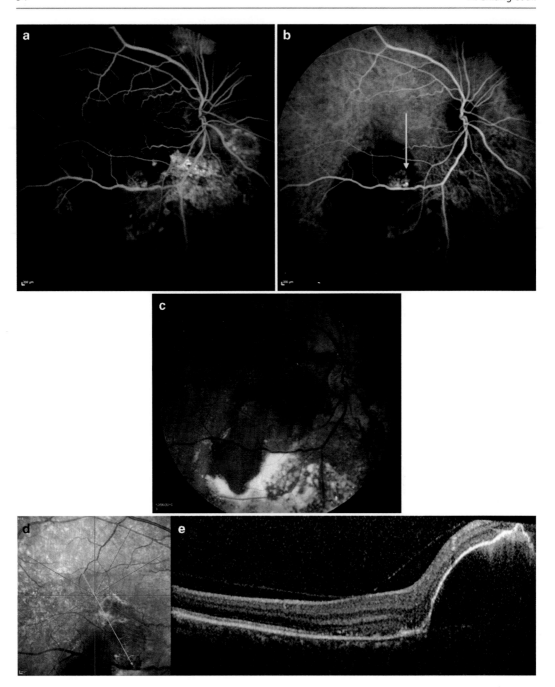

Fig. 4.7 Idiopathic polypoidal choroidal vasculopathy (IPCV). (**a**) SLO mid-phase fluorescein angiogram from an eye with IPCV. Inferior to the disc, there is a large patch of mottled hyperfluorescence representing mostly RPE atrophy, with pinpoint areas of higher fluorescence possibly representing polypoidal lesions. (**b**) SLO ICG angiogram more clearly demonstrates a single polypoidal lesion (*arrow*) with an adjacent large pigment epithelial detachment (PED). (**c**) Digital color fundus photograph demonstrates a large hemorrhagic PED as well as a large amount of hard exudates inferiorly. (**d**) SLO infrared image demonstrates the direction of subsequent OCT image. (**e**) OCT image clearly demonstrates the presence of a large PED, with a partially-detached posterior hyaloid

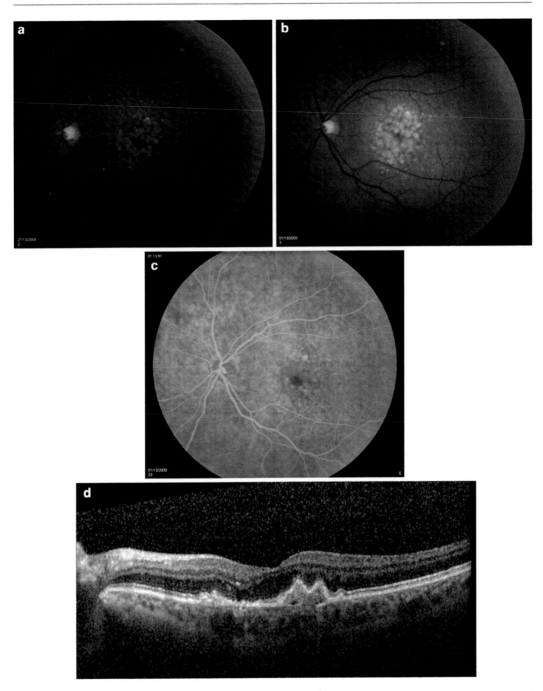

Fig. 4.8 Soft drusen. (**a**) Digital color fundus photograph from an eye soft drusen. (**b**) Digital red-free image demonstrating a bright appearance of the drusen. (**c**) Digital fluorescein angiogram demonstrates difficult visualization of soft drusen. (**d**) OCT image shows focal elevations of the RPE by homogeneous moderately-reflective drusenoid material, and visualization of the underlying Bruch's membrane

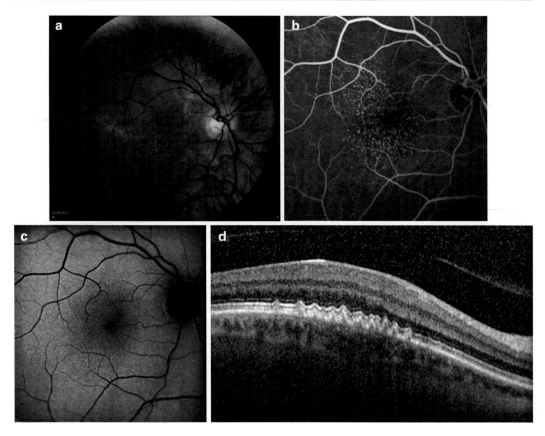

Fig. 4.9 Cuticular drusen. (**a**) Digital red-free fundus photograph from an eye with cuticular drusen. (**b**) SLO fluorescein angiogram demonstrates a "starry-sky appearance, and shows many more drusen than apparent on the red-free photograph. (**c**) SLO fundus autofluorescence demonstrates minimal changes in areas with cuticular drusen. (**d**) OCT shows a "saw-tooth" appearance of the RPE overlying small deposits of drusenoid material

increased hyperautofluorescence at the border of healthy and atrophic RPE represent areas of "sick" RPE at risk for cell death and resultant enlargement of geographic atrophy in the future (Fig. 4.2) [47].

During fluorescein angiography, the appearance early in the fluorescein depends on the amount of retained choriocapillaris. A "window defect" is often apparent in the area of RPE atrophy, with variable appearance of the underlying choroidal vessels. Late in the angiogram, a well-demarcated region of late hyperfluorescence without signs of leakage becomes evident, which is secondary to staining of deeper layers of the eye without normal blockage by overlying pigment. Generally, geographic atrophy shows increasing fluorescence during the early and mid phases of the fluorescein angiogram. More advanced forms of geographic atrophy show early fluorescence of the larger choroidal vessels with a lack of overlying choriocapillaris. Geographic atrophy often appears hypofluorescent during indocyanine green angiography because of the lack of healthy choriocapillaris and overlying RPE, which shows normal physiologic staining late in the angiographic sequence.

On OCT, areas of RPE atrophy appear as focal thinning of the RPE layer with resulting increased penetration of OCT signal into the underlying choriocapillaris and sclera. Overlying areas of RPE atrophy, the inner retinal layers, including the IS/OS junction as well as the outer nuclear layer, may appear thinned or missing [48]. On occasions, retinal pseudocysts may appear overlying areas of geographic atrophy, which likely represent a degenerative process within the retina [49].

Neovascular Age-Related Macular Degeneration

Choroidal Neovascularization

Choroidal neovascularization is a pathophysiologic process that produces specific structural alterations in the macular region that can be readily detected and evaluated with angiography. The new abnormal choroidal vessels proliferate along the inner aspect of Bruch's membrane and penetrate through defects in Bruch's membrane into the sub-RPE space (type 1 neovascularization) or subretinal space (type 2) [50]. The angiographic appearance of CNV varies according to the density, location, and maturity of these new vessels as well as the condition of the surrounding retina and RPE.

CNV and Fluorescein Angiography

Categorization of CNV by classic and occult features on fluorescein angiography was originally introduced by the Macular Photocoagulation Study Group as a grading system for eyes enrolled in the Macular Photocoagulation Study [51]. The term "classic" CNV refers to a well-delineated, discrete focus of hyperfluorescence that manifests during the early phase of the filling sequence [51–53]. Although visualization of dye within the actual abnormal capillary network is possible, it is not mandatory for the diagnosis of classic CNV (Figs. 4.6 and 4.10). In contrast, the term "occult" CNV encompasses two hyperfluorescent patterns on fluorescein angiography: fibrovascular pigment epithelial detachments (PEDs) and late leakage of undetermined source (Figs. 4.1 and 4.5) [51–53]. The first pattern usually shows stippled hyperfluorescent dots in the early phase of the angiogram and a notched border. Pooling of dye within the PED occurs over the course of the angiogram and late-phase leakage may be observed around the margin of the PED. The second pattern is characterized by ill-defined late choroidal-based leakage in the absence of any identifiable classic CNV or fibrovascular PED in earlier phases of the angiogram. Interestingly, OCT examination has introduced valuable data

that has added to our understanding of these angiographic findings. For example, it appears that actually the majority of eyes with occult CNV on the basis of fluorescein and ICG angiography have a fibrovascular PED [54].

It is not uncommon for both classic and occult CNV features to be present in one lesion. In this situation, the lesion is characterized in accordance with the relative area of each type of CNV. For example, if a lesion is 75% classic and 25% occult, it would be defined as being predominantly classic. Conversely, if the lesion is 25% classic and 75% occult, the lesion would be called predominantly occult. Lesions with classic CNV occupying less than 50% of the total area are referred to as minimally classic lesions. Historically, these descriptive terms were particularly useful in the era of photodynamic therapy for neovascular AMD as a reliable and reproducible way to classify lesions.

> **Pearl**
> Fluorescein angiography remains the gold standard angiograph test for the detection of CNV. ICG angiography may be useful in some cases of neovascular AMD or its variants.

CNV and Indocyanine Green Angiography

In general, ICG angiography does not image classic CNV as dramatically as fluorescein angiography; it does not show prominent leakage likely due to the higher protein-binding affinity of ICG. Conversely, areas of occult CNV that appear very poorly defined on fluorescein angiography may be more well defined on ICG angiography (Fig. 4.5). In spite of this, there is still variability; certain areas of occult CNV appear as relatively large plaques of hyperfluorescence while others exhibit minimal hyperfluorescent abnormalities.

Clinically, ICG angiography is utilized with less frequency than fluorescein angiography, yet it remains very helpful for differentiating occult CNV secondary to neovascular AMD from three potential masqueraders in particular: retinal

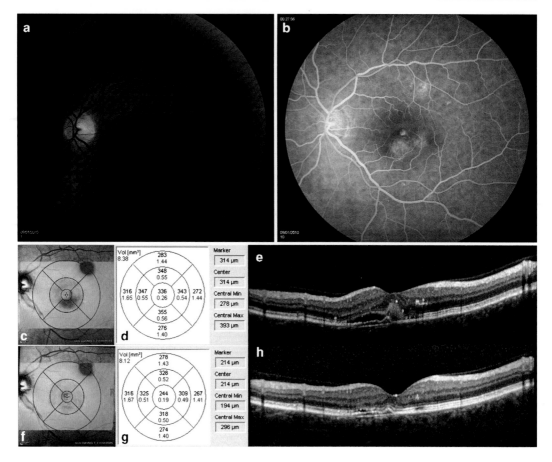

Fig. 4.10 Classic choroidal neovascularization, before and after treatment. (**a**) Digital color fundus photograph from an eye with exudative age-related macular degeneration. (**b**) Digital fluorescein angiography demonstrates several areas of mottled hyperfluorescence as well as a more discreet small classic CNV. (**c**) OCT map at initial visit. (**d**) ETDRS map and thickness measurements from initial visit. (**e**) OCT image from the initial visit (this is the same image as in Fig. 4.3). (**f**) OCT map after 2 injections of intravitreal ranibizumab. (**g**) ETDRS map and thickness measurements from the same visit. (**h**) OCT image from the same follow-up visit demonstrates resolution of much of the subretinal fluid, and disappearance of subretinal hyper-reflective CNV

angiomatous proliferation (RAP), central serous chorioretinopathy (CSCR), and polypoidal choroidal vasculopathy (PCV). RAP lesions are characterized by a retinal-choroidal anastomosis and are considered a distinct subtype of neovascular AMD [55], also referred to as "type 3" neovascularization. RAP lesions are often more easily visualized with ICG angiography than fluorescein angiography [56]. While this may not be relevant with regard to anti-vascular endothelial growth factor (VEGF) therapy, which appears to be effective for RAP lesions [57], it supports the observation that thermal laser photocoagulation alone is unsuccessful as a long-term treatment strategy [58].

The second main use of ICG angiography is to differentiate occult CNV due to AMD from central serous chorioretinopathy (CSCR). In CSCR, the choroidal vessels appear dilated in the early filling phase of the angiogram. Mid-phase images usually show multifocal areas of choroidal vascular hyperpermeability, followed by silhouetting of the larger vessels in the late phase.

Finally, ICG angiography is often essential for making the diagnosis of PCV, which is a distinct abnormality of the choroidal vasculature that is more common in the Asian and African-American populations, though it can occur in Caucasians. PCV is characterized by three-dimensional, branching, dilated inner choroidal vessels with reddish-orange, aneurismal projections at the terminal aspects of the lesion [59]. PCV commonly presents with variably sized serous or serosanguineous detachments of neurosensory retina and RPE detachments. The polypoidal lesions are usually located at the margin of the PED, may range in size, and may be accompanied by overlying RPE atrophy, RPE hyperplasia, and subretinal fibrosis (Fig. 4.7) [60]. In the early phase of the ICG angiogram, the polypoidal vessels may exhibit pulsations [61]. Thereafter, increasing choroidal vascular hyperpermeability is often detectable and in the late phase, ICG stains exudation in the inner choroid and retina due to its high affinity for fibrin [59].

Retinal Pigment Epithelial Detachment

Although PEDs related to confluent drusen may occur in the setting of non-neovascular AMD [62], most PEDs are related to CNV. On fundus photography, these PEDs are kidney bean shaped with a "notch" that typically signifies the presence of an underlying occult CNV. Other findings that would suggest occult CNV include: blood or other exudative material within or adjacent to the PED, an irregular PED contour, and ill-defined late leakage or irregular, heterogeneous filling of the PED on fluorescein angiography. Adequate visualization of CNV on fluorescein angiography is often precluded by the melanin in the RPE and the intense hyperfluorescence within the PED that is due to rapidly accumulating dye. For this reason, the presence of a large PED has typically been an exclusion criterion in most studies of the treatment of neovascular AMD. In this situation, ICG angiography is a useful adjunct since it is not impeded by the presence of pigment or dye within a PED. With ICG, the full extent of the CNV within a notched PED can be readily distinguished. Similarly, in large PEDs without a notch, an underlying focus of CNV is often identified with ICG although not apparent on fluorescein angiography.

Analysis by EDI-OCT of the internal characteristics of fibrovascular PEDs secondary to AMD has demonstrated that the CNV proliferates along the undersurface of the RPE detachment [63]. Contraction of the CNV has been associated with the formation of RPE tears, which may occur as part of the natural history of the disease [64, 65]. In addition, it is possible that anti-VEGF therapy may potentiate RPE tear formation in patients with fibrovascular PEDs [66, 67].

Tears of the RPE have a characteristic appearance on fundus photography and fluorescein angiography, although their size, location with respect to the foveola, and the associated visual acuity may vary [68]. Classically, there is a denuded area of exposed choroid adjacent to the dehisced RPE, which is scrolled back towards the CNV. The bare area is hyperfluorescent in the early phase of the angiogram due to a transmission window defect. Moreover, leakage from the underlying CNV may be visualized as the study progresses into the late phase, though the scrolled RPE may mask this hyperfluorescence to a certain degree. The scrolled RPE has been referred to as "doubly hypofluorescent" and "doubly autofluorescent" in light of what is essentially a vertical summation of pigment and lipofuscin, respectively. Based on OCT and autofluorescence imaging, it appears that the denuded area may eventually be repopulated by RPE cells that are devoid of melanin, with potential for visual recovery [69].

Retinal Vascular Contribution to the Exudative Process

Over the last decade, eyes with neovascular lesions that exhibit a retinal vascular anastomosis to CNV have received increasing attention in effort to better understand the anatomic structure of the anastomotic connection. This condition was first described by Hartnett and coworkers as deep retinal vascular anomalous complexes (RVAC) [70]. It was subsequently renamed retinal angiomatous proliferation (RAP) by Yannuzzi and colleagues [55]. Still later, Gass and colleagues [71] proposed that these eyes have a chorioretinal anastomosis with occult choroidal neovascularization (OCRA).

Of these proposed acronyms, RAP is most commonly used in clinical practice.

Clinically, these lesions are often accompanied by focal hyperpigmentation. Other findings that may be present include microaneurysms, retinal vascular telangiectasias, dot intraretinal hemorrhages, right-angle venules and arterioles, and PEDs. Although a direct communication between the abnormal retinal vascular complex and the choroid is usually present, in a minority of patients the neovascular lesion may originate within the retina as a primary angiomatous complex without evidence of choroidal involvement [50]. In spite of the potential variation that may exist in the underlying pathophysiology, lesions that involve retinal vascular proliferation are considered to be a distinct subgroup of neovascular AMD for which anti-VEGF-based therapies appear to be effective [57].

Fundus Imaging Characteristics of Therapies for Neovascular AMD

Thermal Laser

Thermal laser photocoagulation, generally reserved for the treatment of extrafoveal or juxtafoveal CNV lesions [72], is a relic of the pre-anti-VEGF era when treated eyes often experienced a decline in visual acuity [73]. Patients treated with thermal laser are typically seen two and four weeks later with repeat fluorescein angiography. Previous laser treatment is discernible by hypofluorescence in the center of the lesion during the early and mid phases of the angiogram. Lingering subretinal fluid and focal hyperfluorescent leakage at the margin of the treated lesion on the angiogram are indicative of persistent CNV. In contrast, late staining of the lesion, particularly in the center without involvement of the edge, is commonly observed and does not usually necessitate additional laser treatment.

Recurrence of neovascularization following thermal laser treatment, which is defined by the appearance of new vessels six or more weeks later, is rather common [73]. Fundus and angiographic findings are variable and may include visible signs of exudation such as blood and lipid,

new focal area of hyperfluorescence at the margin of a previously treated area, or stippled hyperfluorescence with or without pronounced thickening at the level of the RPE, which would suggest new growth of occult CNV. Recurrences after thermal laser often occur in fovea-centric fashion, thus other forms of treatment are indicated.

Photodynamic Therapy

The area of neovascularization one week following PDT generally appears dark on ICG angiography due to a profound reduction of perfusion in the entire photosensitized area and surrounding choroid as well [74]. Interestingly, this is usually not observed in patients who have a retinal vascular contribution to the CNV. After treatment, choroidal reperfusion occurs gradually over several weeks, beginning with the larger vascular stumps first, followed by smaller vessels [74]. Identification of these larger stumps on ICG angiography provided a rationale for feeder vessel treatment using thermal laser, with the aim of preventing reperfusion of the abnormal vascular structure.

In the main clinical trials of PDT for neovascular AMD, patients received regular 3-month follow-up visits with fluorescein angiography. Leakage on angiography three months after treatment served as an indication for retreatment, however this was not referred to as a recurrence since this was observed in almost all cases in the phase one and two studies [75, 76]. Indeed, at three-month follow-up in the Treatment of Age-Related Macular Degeneration With Photodynamic Therapy Trial (TAP), 90% of patients still demonstrated leakage from CNV and were retreated accordingly [77]. Since PDT with verteporfin selectively occludes vessels within CNV but does not actually generate thermal damage, this short-lived cessation of leakage is not unexpected. In general, a variable number of periodic retreatments are necessary to maintain cessation of leakage and achieve reduction of lesion size. Although PDT is no longer employed as monotherapy in clinical practice, its use in combination with anti-VEGF therapy remains under investigation in clinical trials. Combination therapy for neovascular AMD will be presented in a later chapter.

Anti-VEGF Therapy

CNV lesions do not recede or disappear with anti-VEGF therapy, however they do demonstrate less leakage on fluorescein angiography [78]. In general, the size of these lesions is stabilized with continued treatment. Treated eyes also demonstrate less fibrosis and decreased retinal thickness on OCT. Such improvements in anatomical outcomes have been demonstrated in CNV lesions of various clinical phenotypes and reflect the functional outcomes achieved in the pivotal MARINA and ANCHOR trials [78]. Currently, monthly intravitreal anti-VEGF injections remain the gold standard for neovascular AMD. Yet, due to the relatively invasive nature of fluorescein angiography and its potential adverse effects, it is generally not performed on a frequent basis by most treating physicians. Instead, OCT is commonly used to monitor the status of a patient (Fig. 4.10).

Not surprisingly, the treatment burden imposed by monthly injections has prompted a myriad of investigations into the efficacy of various alternative dosing regimens. The current norm in clinical practice with ranibizumab or bevacizumab is to implement an initiation/induction phase followed by an individualized maintenance phase that is modeled after one of two basic approaches: PRN [79–81] or treat and extend [82], which involves treating a patient at every visit, but extending the follow-up duration in the absence of exudation on OCT. However, the ideal evidence-based alternative treatment strategy remains elusive. This topic and other treatment approaches will be discussed in more detail in subsequent chapters.

References

1. Spaide R. Fluorescein angiography. Philadelphia: W.B. Saunders Co.; 1999.
2. Tittl M, Slakter J, Spaide R, Sorenson J, Guyer DR. Indocyanine green videoangiography. Philadelphia: W.B. Saunders Co.; 1999.
3. Holz FG, Schmitz-Valckenberg S, Spaide R, Bird AC. Atlas of fundus autofluorescence imaging. Dordrecht: Springer; 2007.
4. Cohen SY, Dubois L, Tadayoni R, Delahaye-Mazza C, Debibie C, Quentel G. Prevalence of reticular pseudodrusen in age-related macular degeneration with newly diagnosed choroidal neovascularisation. Br J Ophthalmol. 2007;91(3):354–9.
5. Delori FC, Dorey CK, Staurenghi G, Arend O, Goger DG, Weiter JJ. In vivo fluorescence of the ocular fundus exhibits retinal pigment epithelium lipofuscin characteristics. Invest Ophthalmol Vis Sci. 1995;36(3):718–29.
6. von Ruckmann A, Fitzke FW, Bird AC. Distribution of fundus autofluorescence with a scanning laser ophthalmoscope. Br J Ophthalmol. 1995;79(5):407–12.
7. Eldred GE, Katz ML. Fluorophores of the human retinal pigment epithelium: separation and spectral characterization. Exp Eye Res. 1988;47(1):71–86.
8. Webb RH, Hughes GW, Delori FC. Confocal scanning laser ophthalmoscope. Appl Opt. 1987;26(8): 1492–9.
9. Liu J, Itagaki Y, Ben-Shabat S, Nakanishi K, Sparrow JR. The biosynthesis of A2E, a fluorophore of aging retina, involves the formation of the precursor, A2-PE, in the photoreceptor outer segment membrane. J Biol Chem. 2000;275(38):29354–60.
10. Fishkin N, Jang YP, Itagaki Y, Sparrow JR, Nakanishi K. A2-rhodopsin: a new fluorophore isolated from photoreceptor outer segments. Org Biomol Chem. 2003; 1(7):1101–5.
11. Eldred GE. Lipofuscin fluorophore inhibits lysosomal protein degradation and may cause early stages of macular degeneration. Gerontology. 1995;41 Suppl 2:15–28.
12. Gaillard ER, Atherton SJ, Eldred G, Dillon J. Photophysical studies on human retinal lipofuscin. Photochem Photobiol. 1995;61(5):448–53.
13. Suter M, Reme C, Grimm C, Wenzel A, Jaattela M, Esser P, et al. Age-related macular degeneration. The lipofusion component N-retinyl-N-retinylidene ethanolamine detaches proapoptotic proteins from mitochondria and induces apoptosis in mammalian retinal pigment epithelial cells. J Biol Chem. 2000;275(50): 39625–30.
14. Sparrow JR, Nakanishi K, Parish CA. The lipofuscin fluorophore A2E mediates blue light-induced damage to retinal pigmented epithelial cells. Invest Ophthalmol Vis Sci. 2000;41(7):1981–9.
15. Dillon J, Wang Z, Avalle LB, Gaillard ER. The photochemical oxidation of A2E results in the formation of a 5,8,5',8'-bis-furanoid oxide. Exp Eye Res. 2004; 79(4):537–42.
16. Avalle LB, Wang Z, Dillon JP, Gaillard ER. Observation of A2E oxidation products in human retinal lipofuscin. Exp Eye Res. 2004;78(4):895–8.
17. Sparrow JR, Zhou J, Ben-Shabat S, Vollmer H, Itagaki Y, Nakanishi K. Involvement of oxidative mechanisms in blue-light-induced damage to A2E-laden RPE. Invest Ophthalmol Vis Sci. 2002;43(4):1222–7.
18. Dorey CK, Wu G, Ebenstein D, Garsd A, Weiter JJ. Cell loss in the aging retina. Relationship to lipofuscin

accumulation and macular degeneration. Invest Ophthalmol Vis Sci. 1989;30(8):1691–9.

19. Holz FG, Bellman C, Staudt S, Schutt F, Volcker HE. Fundus autofluorescence and development of geographic atrophy in age-related macular degeneration. Invest Ophthalmol Vis Sci. 2001;42(5):1051–6.

20. Wing GL, Blanchard GC, Weiter JJ. The topography and age relationship of lipofuscin concentration in the retinal pigment epithelium. Invest Ophthalmol Vis Sci. 1978;17(7):601–7.

21. Hee MR, Izatt JA, Swanson EA, Huang D, Schuman JS, Lin CP, et al. Optical coherence tomography of the human retina. Arch Ophthalmol. 1995; 113(3):325–32.

22. Huang D, Swanson EA, Lin CP, Schuman JS, Stinson WG, Chang W, et al. Optical coherence tomography. Science. 1991;254(5035):1178–81.

23. Drexler W, Sattmann H, Hermann B, Ko TH, Stur M, Unterhuber A, et al. Enhanced visualization of macular pathology with the use of ultrahigh-resolution optical coherence tomography. Arch Ophthalmol. 2003;121(5):695–706.

24. Drexler W, Morgner U, Ghanta RK, Kartner FX, Schuman JS, Fujimoto JG. Ultrahigh-resolution ophthalmic optical coherence tomography. Nat Med. 2001; 7(4):502–7.

25. Wojtkowski M, Bajraszewski T, Gorczynska I, Targowski P, Kowalczyk A, Wasilewski W, et al. Ophthalmic imaging by spectral optical coherence tomography. Am J Ophthalmol. 2004;138(3):412–9.

26. Anger EM, Unterhuber A, Hermann B, Sattmann H, Schubert C, Morgan JE, et al. Ultrahigh resolution optical coherence tomography of the monkey fovea. Identification of retinal sublayers by correlation with semi-thin histology sections. Exp Eye Res. 2004;78(6):1117–25.

27. Gloesmann M, Hermann B, Schubert C, Sattmann H, Ahnelt PK, Drexler W. Histologic correlation of pig retina radial stratification with ultrahigh-resolution optical coherence tomography. Invest Ophthalmol Vis Sci. 2003;44(4):1696–703.

28. Srinivasan VJ, Monson BK, Wojtkowski M, Bilonick RA, Gorczynska I, Chen R, et al. Characterization of outer retinal morphology with high-speed, ultrahigh-resolution optical coherence tomography. Invest Ophthalmol Vis Sci. 2008;49(4):1571–9.

29. Spaide RF, Koizumi H, Pozzoni MC. Enhanced depth imaging spectral-domain optical coherence tomography. Am J Ophthalmol. 2008;146(4):496–500.

30. Guyer DR, Yannuzzi LA, Slakter JS, Sorenson JA, Hanutsaha P, Spaide RF, et al. Classification of choroidal neovascularization by digital indocyanine green videoangiography. Ophthalmology. 1996;103(12): 2054–60.

31. Pawley JB, editor. Handbook of biological confocal microscopy. Berlin: Springer; 2006.

32. Desatnik H, Treister G, Alhalel A, Krupsky S, Moisseiev J. ICGA-guided laser photocoagulation of feeder vessels of choroidal neovascular membranes in

age-related macular degeneration. Indocyanine green angiography. Retina. 2000;20(2):143–50.

33. Fox IJ, Wood EH. Applications of dilution curves recorded from the right side of the heart or venous circulation with the aid of a new indicator dye. Proc Staff Meet Mayo Clin. 1957;32(19):541–50.

34. Kwiterovich KA, Maguire MG, Murphy RP, Schachat AP, Bressler NM, Bressler SB, et al. Frequency of adverse systemic reactions after fluorescein angiography. Results of a prospective study. Ophthalmology. 1991;98(7):1139–42.

35. Yannuzzi LA, Rohrer KT, Tindel LJ, Sobel RS, Costanza MA, Shields W, et al. Fluorescein angiography complication survey. Ophthalmology. 1986;93(5): 611–7.

36. Hope-Ross M, Yannuzzi LA, Gragoudas ES, Guyer DR, Slakter JS, Sorenson JA, et al. Adverse reactions due to indocyanine green. Ophthalmology. 1994;101(3): 529–33.

37. Obana A, Miki T, Hayashi K, Takeda M, Kawamura A, Mutoh T, et al. Survey of complications of indocyanine green angiography in Japan. Am J Ophthalmol. 1994;118(6):749–53.

38. Fineman MS, Maguire JI, Fineman SW, Benson WE. Safety of indocyanine green angiography during pregnancy: a survey of the retina, macula, and vitreous societies. Arch Ophthalmol. 2001;119(3):353–5.

39. Costa DL, Huang SJ, Orlock DA, Freund KB, Yannuzzi LA, Spaide RF, et al. Retinal-choroidal indocyanine green dye clearance and liver dysfunction. Retina. 2003;23(4):557–61.

40. Zweifel SA, Spaide RF, Curcio CA, Malek G, Imamura Y. Reticular pseudodrusen are subretinal drusenoid deposits. Ophthalmology. 2010;117(2):303–12.e1.

41. Pauleikhoff D, Zuels S, Sheraidah GS, Marshall J, Wessing A, Bird AC. Correlation between biochemical composition and fluorescein binding of deposits in Bruch's membrane. Ophthalmology. 1992;99(10): 1548–53.

42. Arnold JJ, Quaranta M, Soubrane G, Sarks SH, Coscas G. Indocyanine green angiography of drusen. Am J Ophthalmol. 1997;124(3):344–56.

43. Spaide RF, Curcio CA. Drusen characterization with multimodal imaging. Retina. 2010;30(9):1441–54.

44. Spaide RF. Fundus autofluorescence and age-related macular degeneration. Ophthalmology. 2003;110(2): 392–9.

45. Ho J, Witkin AJ, Liu J, Chen Y, Fujimoto JG, Schuman JS, et al. Documentation of intraretinal retinal pigment epithelium migration via high-speed ultrahigh-resolution optical coherence tomography. Ophthalmology. 2011;118(4):687–93. Epub 2010 Nov 20.

46. Holz FG, Bellmann C, Margaritidis M, Schutt F, Otto TP, Volcker HE. Patterns of increased in vivo fundus autofluorescence in the junctional zone of geographic atrophy of the retinal pigment epithelium associated with age-related macular degeneration. Graefes Arch Clin Exp Ophthalmol. 1999;237(2):145–52.

47. Holz FG, Bellman C, Staudt S, et al. Fundus autofluorescence and development of geographic atrophy in
age-related macular degeneration. Invest Ophthalmol
Vis Sci. 2001;42:1051–6.
48. Bearelly S, Chau FY, Koreishi A, Stinnett SS, Izatt JA,
Toth CA. Spectral domain optical coherence tomography imaging of geographic atrophy margins.
Ophthalmology. 2009;116(9):1762–9.
49. Cohen SY, Dubois L, Nghiem-Buffet S, et al. Retinal
pseudocysts in age-related geographic atrophy. Am J
Ophthalmol. 2010;150(2):211–7. e1.
50. Klein ML, Wilson DJ. Clinicopathologic correlation
of choroidal and retinal neovascular lesions in age-
related macular degeneration. Am J Ophthalmol.
2011;151(1):161–9.
51. Subfoveal neovascular lesions in age-related macular
degeneration. Guidelines for evaluation and treatment
in the macular photocoagulation study. Macular
Photocoagulation Study Group. Arch Ophthalmol.
1991 Sep;109(9):1242–57.
52. Solomon SD, Bressler SB, Hawkins BS, Marsh MJ,
Bressler NM. Guidelines for interpreting retinal photographs and coding findings in the Submacular
Surgery Trials (SST): SST report no. 8. Retina.
2005;25(3):253–68.
53. Barbazetto I, Burdan A, Bressler NM, Bressler SB,
Haynes L, Kapetanios AD, et al. Photodynamic therapy of subfoveal choroidal neovascularization with
verteporfin: fluorescein angiographic guidelines for
evaluation and treatment – TAP and VIP report No. 2.
Arch Ophthalmol. 2003;121(9):1253–68.
54. Coscas F, Coscas G, Souied E, Tick S, Soubrane G.
Optical coherence tomography identification of occult
choroidal neovascularization in age-related macular
degeneration. Am J Ophthalmol. 2007;144(4):592–9.
55. Yannuzzi LA, Negrao S, Iida T, Carvalho C,
Rodriguez-Coleman H, Slakter J, et al. Retinal
angiomatous proliferation in age-related macular
degeneration. Retina. 2001;21(5):416–34.
56. Massacesi AL, Sacchi L, Bergamini F, Bottoni F. The
prevalence of retinal angiomatous proliferation in
age-related macular degeneration with occult choroidal neovascularization. Graefes Arch Clin Exp
Ophthalmol. 2008;246(1):89–92.
57. Hemeida TS, Keane PA, Dustin L, Sadda SR,
Fawzi AA. Long-term visual and anatomical outcomes
following anti-VEGF monotherapy for retinal angiomatous proliferation. Br J Ophthalmol. 2010;94(6):701–5.
58. Bearelly S, Espinosa-Heidmann DG, Cousins SW.
The role of dynamic indocyanine green angiography
in the diagnosis and treatment of retinal angiomatous
proliferation. Br J Ophthalmol. 2008;92(2):191–6.
59. Imamura Y, Engelbert M, Iida T, Freund KB,
Yannuzzi LA. Polypoidal choroidal vasculopathy:
a review. Surv Ophthalmol. 2010;55(6):501–15.
60. Sho K, Takahashi K, Yamada H, Wada M, Nagai Y,
Otsuji T, et al. Polypoidal choroidal vasculopathy:
incidence, demographic features, and clinical characteristics. Arch Ophthalmol. 2003;121(10):1392–6.

61. Okubo A, Ito M, Sameshima M, Uemura A,
Sakamoto T. Pulsatile blood flow in the polypoidal
choroidal vasculopathy. Ophthalmology. 2005;112(8):
1436–41.
62. Casswell AG, Kohen D, Bird AC. Retinal pigment
epithelial detachments in the elderly: classification
and outcome. Br J Ophthalmol. 1985;69(6):397–403.
63. Spaide RF. Enhanced depth imaging optical coherence tomography of retinal pigment epithelial detachment in age-related macular degeneration. Am J
Ophthalmol. 2009;147(4):644–52.
64. Hoskin A, Bird AC, Sehmi K. Tears of detached retinal pigment epithelium. Br J Ophthalmol. 1981;65(6):
417–22.
65. Gass JD. Pathogenesis of tears of the retinal pigment
epithelium. Br J Ophthalmol. 1984;68(8):513–9.
66. Chiang A, Chang LK, Yu F, Sarraf D. Predictors of
anti-VEGF-associated retinal pigment epithelial tear
using FA and OCT analysis. Retina. 2008;28(9):
1265–9.
67. Chan CK, Meyer CH, Gross JG, Abraham P, Nuthi
AS, Kokame GT, et al. Retinal pigment epithelial
tears after intravitreal bevacizumab injection for neovascular age-related macular degeneration. Retina.
2007;27(5):541–51.
68. Sarraf D, Reddy S, Chiang A, Yu F, Jain A. A new
grading system for retinal pigment epithelial tears.
Retina. 2010;30(7):1039–45.
69. Peiretti E, Iranmanesh R, Lee JJ, Klancnik Jr JM,
Sorenson JA, Yannuzzi LA. Repopulation of the retinal pigment epithelium after pigment epithelial rip.
Retina. 2006;26(9):1097–9.
70. Hartnett ME, Weiter JJ, Staurenghi G, Elsner AE. Deep
retinal vascular anomalous complexes in advanced age-
related macular degeneration. Ophthalmology. 1996;
103(12):2042–53.
71. Gass JD, Agarwal A, Lavina AM, Tawansy KA. Focal
inner retinal hemorrhages in patients with drusen: an
early sign of occult choroidal neovascularization and
chorioretinal anastomosis. Retina. 2003;23(6):741–51.
72. Krypton laser photocoagulation for neovascular lesions
of age-related macular degeneration. Results of a randomized clinical trial. Macular Photocoagulation Study
Group. Arch Ophthalmol. 1990 Jun;108(6):816–24.
73. Laser photocoagulation of subfoveal neovascular
lesions in age-related macular degeneration. Results of
a randomized clinical trial. Macular Photocoagulation
Study Group. Arch Ophthalmol. 1991 Sep;109(9):
1220–31.
74. Schmidt-Erfurth U, Michels S, Barbazetto I, Laqua H.
Photodynamic effects on choroidal neovascularization and physiological choroid. Invest Ophthalmol Vis
Sci. 2002;43(3):830–41.
75. Schmidt-Erfurth U, Miller JW, Sickenberg M,
Laqua H, Barbazetto I, Gragoudas ES, et al.
Photodynamic therapy with verteporfin for choroidal
neovascularization caused by age-related macular
degeneration: results of retreatments in a phase 1 and
2 study. Arch Ophthalmol. 1999;117(9):1177–87.

76. Miller JW, Schmidt-Erfurth U, Sickenberg M, Pournaras CJ, Laqua H, Barbazetto I, et al. Photodynamic therapy with verteporfin for choroidal neovascularization caused by age-related macular degeneration: results of a single treatment in a phase 1 and 2 study. Arch Ophthalmol. 1999;117(9):1161–73.

77. Photodynamic therapy of subfoveal choroidal neovascularization in age-related macular degeneration with verteporfin: one-year results of 2 randomized clinical trials—TAP report. Treatment of age-related macular degeneration with photodynamic therapy (TAP) Study Group. Arch Ophthalmol. 1999 Oct;117(10): 1329–45.

78. Sadda SR, Stoller G, Boyer DS, Blodi BA, Shapiro H, Ianchulev T. Anatomical benefit from ranibizumab treatment of predominantly classic neovascular age-related macular degeneration in the 2-year anchor study. Retina. 2010;30(9):1390–9.

79. Spaide R. Ranibizumab according to need: a treatment for age-related macular degeneration. Am J Ophthalmol. 2007;143(4):679–80.

80. Fung AE, Lalwani GA, Rosenfeld PJ, Dubovy SR, Michels S, Feuer WJ, et al. An optical coherence tomography-guided, variable dosing regimen with intravitreal ranibizumab (Lucentis) for neovascular age-related macular degeneration. Am J Ophthalmol. 2007;143(4):566–83.

81. Boyer DS, Heier JS, Brown DM, Francom SF, Ianchulev T, Rubio RG. A Phase IIIb study to evaluate the safety of ranibizumab in subjects with neovascular age-related macular degeneration. Ophthalmology. 2009;116(9):1731–9.

82. Brown DM, Regillo CD. Anti-VEGF agents in the treatment of neovascular age-related macular degeneration: applying clinical trial results to the treatment of everyday patients. Am J Ophthalmol. 2007;144(4):627–37.

Therapy of Nonexudative Age-Related Macular Degeneration

Annal D. Meleth, Veena R. Raiji, Nupura Krishnadev, and Emily Y. Chew

Key Points

- Age-related macular degeneration (AMD) has multifactorial etiology. Nutrition, cigarette smoking, and plasma homocysteine may be modifiable risk factors that provide therapeutic targets in the management of AMD.
- Data regarding therapeutic interventions for primary prevention of AMD are limited and thus far inconclusive.
- A limited number of randomized controlled trials are available to validate observational data regarding risk factors and potential therapeutic interventions for AMD.
  - The Age-Related Eye Disease Study (AREDS) demonstrated that daily oral supplementation of a combination of antioxidant vitamins and zinc has been shown to reduce progression to advanced AMD among patients who are at intermediate to high risk of progression of disease [1].
  - The Women's Antioxidant and Folic Acid Cardiovascular Study (WAFACS) demonstrated that daily long-term supplementation with folic acid, pyridoxine, B12, and cyanocobalamin reduced risk of advanced AMD in a population of female healthcare professionals with, or at risk for, cardiovascular disease.
- The more efficacious combination of nutrients and antioxidants has not yet been determined.
- Preliminary observational data suggests that omega-3 fatty acids and carotenoids, specifically lutein and zeaxanthin, may play a role in prevention and treatment of AMD. At present, there is insufficient data from randomized controlled clinical trials to make therapeutic recommendations.

Introduction

Age related macular degeneration (AMD) is the leading cause of blindness among adults over the age of 65 in the Western world. The prevalence of AMD is expected to increase dramatically, from 1.75 million in 2000 to 2.95 million in 2020, due to the rapidly aging population [2]. Given the large and now increasing burden of disease, the identification of modifiable risk factors and new avenues for preventive treatment has become increasingly important. The pathogenesis of macular degeneration is multi-factorial with genetic, environmental, and physiologic components. The retina is uniquely susceptible to oxidative damage, given its high metabolic activity and daily exposure to light. In addition, the presence of large numbers of lipids with double bonds makes it an ideal target for reactive oxygen species. The increasing incidence of macular degeneration with advancing age may be related to gradual

A.D. Meleth (✉)
Department of Epidemiology and Clinical Applications, National Eye Institute/National Institutes of Health, 10 Center Drive, Bethesda, MD 20892, USA
e-mail: echew@nei.nih.gov

A.C. Ho and C.D. Regillo (eds.), *Age-related Macular Degeneration Diagnosis and Treatment*,
DOI 10.1007/978-1-4614-0125-4_5, © Springer Science+Business Media, LLC 2011

dysfunction and degeneration of retinal tissues as oxidative damage accumulates. This cumulative damage may result in physiologic dysfunction, in addition to impaired auto-regulation with restricted exchange and processing of nutrients and metabolic byproducts with progressive disease. Nutrients which may modulate this oxidative damage include lutein, zeaxanthin, beta-carotene, C, E, and B vitamins, and zinc [3–7]. A growing body of scientific evidence also implicates inflammatory processes in the pathogenesis and progression of macular degeneration [8]. Clinical evidence suggests a role for a combination of antioxidants in reducing progression of AMD and a potential role for omega-3 fatty acids and macular xanthophylls in the prevention and treatment of macular degeneration. The Age Related Eye Disease Study 2 (AREDS2) will further examine the role of these micronutrients in the treatment of AMD.

The data regarding the impact of modifiable risk factors and micronutrients on macular degeneration comes from both large observational studies and a small number of randomized controlled trials. Major studies that have studied the impact of micronutrients in macular degeneration include the Age Related Eye Disease Study, the Rotterdam Study, and the Blue Mountain Eye Disease study.

AREDS

The Age-Related Eye Disease Study (AREDS) was a multicenter randomized placebo-controlled trial designed to assess the impact of an antioxidant and micronutrient combination on the incidence and progression of AMD and age-related cataract. The AREDS supplement contained 15 mg beta-carotene, 500 mg Vitamin C, 400 IU Vitamin E, 80 mg zinc oxide, and 2 mg of copper as cupric oxide. Participants were stratified into four categories of AMD of varying severities of disease as well as rates of progression to advanced AMD:

- *Category 1*: none to few drusen; 0.44% developed advanced AMD by year 5.
- *Category 2*: Extensive small drusen, pigment abnormalities, or at least 1 intermediate size druse; 1.3% probability of progression to advanced AMD by year 5.

- *Category 3*: Extensive intermediate drusen, large drusen, or noncentral geographic atrophy (GA); 18% probability of progression. Patients within category 3 who had bilateral large drusen or noncentral GA in at least 1 eye at enrollment were 4 times more likely to progress to AMD than the remaining participants in category 3; 27% vs. 6% in 5 years.
- *Category 4*: Advanced AMD in one eye or patients with vision loss due to nonadvanced AMD in 1 eye; 43% probability of progression to advanced AMD in 5 years.

The AREDS found that there was a 27% reduction in risk of progression of disease in participants taking AREDS supplements in Categories 3 and 4. Patients with category 1 or 2 AMD had a very low risk of progression to advanced AMD; 0.4% and 1.3%, respectively. Due to the low event rate, it was not possible to establish a treatment effect for the AREDS formulation for these participants. The widespread use of the AREDS supplements in appropriate patients can have significant impacts on cost and overall morbidity in the population [9]. Mortality rates are higher in patients with AMD in a number of studies. This is likely secondary to the shared risk factors that also affect mortality. Patients with advanced AMD also had higher rates of cardiovascular deaths in the AREDS trial [10, 11]. Interestingly, participants taking zinc supplements, either alone or in combination with other antioxidants, had improved survival in the AREDS than those not taking zinc (RR 0.78; 95% CI, 0.41–1.47) [11]. Overall mortality among AREDS participants taking supplementation was reduced by 14% (RR 0.86, CI 0.65–1.12) [11, 12].

Pearl
AREDS [13]
- Randomized placebo controlled trial
- Designed to assess impact of antioxidant and micronutrient combination on:
  ○ Incidence of progression of AMD
  ○ Incidence of progression of cataract

(continued)

Pearl (continued)
- AREDS supplement: 15 mg beta-carotene, 500 mg Vitamin C, 400 IU Vitamin E, 80 mg zinc oxide, 2 mg copper (as cupric oxide)
- Results:
  - 27% reduction in progression to advanced AMD in patients taking AREDS supplement with *intermediate to high risk* of progression:
    - Extensive intermediate size drusen
    - At least 1 large druse
    - Noncentral geographic atrophy in one or both eyes
    - Advanced AMD or vision loss due to AMD in 1 eye
  - The widespread use of the AREDS supplements in appropriate patients can have significant impacts on cost and overall morbidity in the population [9]
  - Patients with advanced AMD also had higher rates of cardiovascular deaths in the AREDS trial [10, 11]
    - Overall, patients in AREDS on supplementation had a 14% reduction in mortality risk (RR 0.86, CI 0.65–1.12) [11, 12]

Carotenoids

Beta-Carotene

Beta-carotene is a carotenoid, which is not found in high concentrations in the macula. Major sources of beta-carotene in the diet include cantaloupe, citrus fruits, carrots, and broccoli [14–16]. Beta-carotene was the major carotenoid used in the AREDS trial due to availability of a supplement and presence of several trials underway investigating the impact of beta-carotene supplementation on cancer and cardiovascular disease [13]. The AREDS, as reviewed above, showed that supplementation with combination high-dose

zinc, 15 mg beta-carotene, vitamins C and E, and copper was associated with a reduction in risk of advanced AMD among patients with Stage 3 or greater AMD. [13]. Other data regarding a potential therapeutic role for beta-carotene in AMD has been mixed. A trial examining supplementation of 20 mg of beta-carotene and 50 mg of alpha-tocopherol in a Finnish population failed to demonstrate a significant effect on the incidence of AMD [17]. Subsequent observational data has been mixed regarding the role of beta-carotene. In the Blue Mountain Eye Study, beta-carotene was a risk factor for the development of incident neovascular AMD [18] (RR 2.4 when comparing top tertile of intake with bottom tertile). In the Rotterdam study, beta-carotene when combined with Vitamin E and zinc showed a protective effect on incident AMD (adjusted RR 0.65, 95% CI 0.46–0.92). In univariate analysis, beta-carotene alone was not shown to have a significant effect on the development of AMD [19]. A similar multivariate analysis performed studied dietary intake in the AREDS population, and found that patients taking combination antioxidants with zinc, omega-3 fatty acids, and macular carotenoids had a reduced risk of both early and advanced AMD. Dietary beta-carotene was not found to be a significant contributor in this analysis or in the Physicians Health Study Cohort [20, 21].

Important data from large randomized controlled clinical trials demonstrated an increased lung cancer risk with beta-carotene supplementation [22, 23] using higher doses (20–30 mg) of beta-carotene than the AREDS formulation (15 mg). The Physicians Health Study, a randomized controlled trial of beta-carotene (50 mg every other day) vs. placebo did not show a significant difference in mortality in the treated and untreated groups [24].

Given the above data, it is evident that much remains to be learned regarding a role for beta-carotene in the treatment of AMD. It is unclear whether beta-carotene has a beneficial effect when not used in combination with antioxidants and zinc in the treatment of macular degeneration. It is also unclear what dose of beta-carotene would be ideal, if used for therapy of AMD. The AREDS2 will attempt to address this issue by including two formulations without beta-carotene in the secondary randomization of the study [3, 25].

Macular Xanthophylls

The retinal carotenoids, lutein and zeaxanthin, are selectively concentrated in the macula. They represent the major source of macular pigment and are responsible for the yellow appearance of the macula lutea. They are derived entirely from the diet, as humans cannot synthesize them de novo [26]. The average western diet contains 1.3–3 mg/day of lutein and zeaxanthin combined, with lutein representing the majority of intake [14, 15]. Lutein is primarily derived from green leafy vegetables, such as spinach, kale, and collard greens, while zeaxanthin is primarily found in corn, orange peppers, and citrus fruit. Both are found in high concentrations in egg yolk [16]. Due to their high number of double bonds, the macular carotenoids are capable of quenching reactive oxygen species, limiting oxidative stress and increasing membrane stability. The macular pigments may also act as filters for blue light and limit retinal photo-stress [26–28].

Macular pigment can be measured using a variety of noninvasive techniques. Data correlating age with macular pigment levels or presence of AMD have been equivocal [29]. These data are likely noisy due to the multitude of factors that affect uptake and distribution of these carotenoids in vivo. A recent large cross-sectional study in a homogenous Caucasian population showed a reduction in macular pigment with age and in patients with risk factors for macular degeneration (family history, tobacco use) [29]. A prospective study demonstrated that dietary supplementation of lutein and zeaxanthin increased macular pigment optical density (MPOD) most in patients with a low baseline MPOD. These changes, however, did not correlate with a change in serum concentration of the macular pigments [30]. In another recent interventional trial, lutein and zeaxanthin supplementation increased serum levels of

lutein, zeaxanthin and macular pigment levels by approximately 15% [31].

A small prospective study examining dose ranges and adverse effects of supplementation with lutein and zeaxanthin showed an increase in serum levels of the carotenoids, which was unaffected by other serum antioxidant vitamin concentrations or co-supplementation of long-chained polyunsaturated fatty acids. In the same study, serum concentrations rose in response to supplementation over three months and then stabilized. No adverse effects of supplementation were demonstrated with lutein supplementation up to 10 mg per day; however, these studies tended to be small in sample size with limited follow-up. [32]. These data suggest that changes in serum levels of lutein and zeaxanthin do not necessarily correlate with a change in MPOD [30, 32].

A number of studies have examined the association between risk of macular degeneration and supplementation with the macular xanthophylls. The majority of data suggests a protective role of the macular carotenoids in macular degeneration. An analysis of dietary intake in the AREDS using a compound score taking into consideration consumption of Vitamins C and E, zinc, lutein, zeaxanthin, docosahexaenoic acid, eicosapentaenoic acid, and low-dietary glycemic index (dGI) showed a higher intake of these nutrients was associated with a lower risk of both early and advanced AMD (OR = 0.727 for drusen, and 0.616 for advanced AMD) [20]. When comparing the highest with the lowest quintiles of intake in the AREDS population, lutein and zeaxanthin intake was independently inversely associated with neovascular AMD (OR 0.65), geographic atrophy (OR, 0.45), and large or extensive intermediate drusen (OR, 0.73) [33].

Among participants in the Blue Mountain Eye Disease Study, those in the top tertile of intake for lutein and zeaxanthin intake had a reduced risk of incident neovascular AMD (RR, 0.35), and those with above median intakes had a reduced risk of indistinct soft or reticular drusen (RR, 0.66) [34]. A large retrospective cross-sectional cohort study within the Nurses Health Study showed a statistically nonsignificant

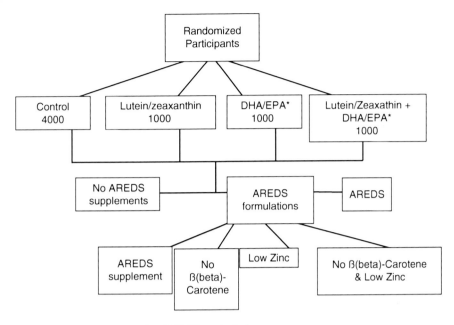

Fig. 5.1 Age-related eye disease study 2 (AREDS2) study design

reduction in incident neovascular AMD with increased consumption of lutein and zeaxanthin. These participants were also less likely to smoke and consumed more omega-3 fatty acids [35]. In 2006, the Carotenoids in Age-Related Macular Degeneration Study (CAREDS) concluded that lutein- and zeaxanthin-rich diets may protect against intermediate AMD in female patients less than 75 years of age [36]. A large population-based study, the Pathologies Oculaires Liees – a l'Age (POLA) study – was also strongly suggestive of a protective role of the xanthophylls, particularly zeaxanthin, among patients with the highest dietary intake for protection against AMD and cataract [37]. The Eye Disease Case Control Study also showed a 43% lower risk for AMD among patients with the highest quintile of carotenoid intake compared with those in the lowest quintile [38].

The Food and Drug Administration conducted a review of the literature in 2006 regarding lutein/zeaxanthin supplementation, which concluded that the current data is not yet strong enough to support treatment recommendations with lutein and zeaxanthin [39]. This view was also espoused by the most recent Cochrane Review on supplementation for slowing the progression of macular degeneration [4].

Given the large body of data suggesting a possible protective effect of lutein and zeaxanthin on macular degeneration and the need for further clarification regarding a potential therapeutic role for these xanthophylls in the treatment of AMD, the Age Related Eye Disease Study 2 (AREDS2) includes two randomization arms with lutein and zeaxanthin supplementation. One arm of the randomization includes lutein 10 mg and zeaxanthin 2 mg only, while the second arm also includes the omega-3 fatty acids (docosohexanoeic acid [350 mg] and eicosapentanoic acid [650 mg]) (Fig. 5.1, Table 5.1) [25].

Fatty Acids

The long-chain polyunsaturated fatty acids (LCPUFAs) and docosahexaenoic acid (DHA) are present in high concentrations in the outer

Table 5.1 The four AREDS formulations to be tested in the second randomization of AREDS2

	1	2	3	4
Vitamin C	500 mg	500 mg	500 mg	500 mg
Vitamin E	400 IU	400 IU	400 IU	400 IU
Beta-carotene	15 mg	0 mg	0 mg	15 mg
Zinc oxide	80 mg	80 mg	25 mg	25 mg
Cupric oxide	2 mg	2 mg	2 mg	2 mg

segments of photoreceptors. DHA, synthesized from the dietary precursors, alpha-linoleic acid (ALA), and eicosapentaenoic acid (EPA), is an important structural component of retinal membranes and is constantly shed throughout the visual cycle [40]. Dietary LCPUFAs are primarily derived from oily fish (tuna, sardines, salmon, mackerel, herring, and trout) [40] and ALA is primarily derived from plant-based foods (flaxseed, flaxseed oil, walnuts, walnut oil, soybeans, soybean oil, pumpkin seeds, rapeseed (canola) oil, and olive oil).

Evidence is growing regarding the potential mechanisms by which LCPUFAs may be involved in the pathogenesis of AMD, as several LCPUFA–derived mediators are implicated in immunomodulation and inflammatory responses [41–46]. Ocular inflammation results in the cleavage of membrane-bound LCPUFAs and the production of multiple paracrine and autocrine mediators of retinal inflammation, neovascularization, and cell survival [42, 43, 47, 48], all of which play a role in the pathogenesis of AMD.

A number of studies have shown an inverse relationship between rates of AMD and intake of omega-3 LCPUFAs. The dietary ancillary study of the Eye Disease Case Control Study (EDCCS) showed a reduced risk of neovascular AMD with increased dietary intake of omega-3 LCPUFAs and fish (OR 0.6 for both when comparing highest with lowest quintiles) [38]. A cross-sectional population-based study in a European population showed a 53% reduced risk of neovascular macular degeneration in participants who ate fish more than once per week [49]. The results of a meta-analysis showed that fish intake of twice or more per week compared with intake less that once per month was associated with a 37% reduction in

risk of early AMD. A protective effect was also demonstrated against late AMD [50]. A secondary analysis of the United States twin study also showed that fish consumption and omega-3 fatty acid intake reduce the risk of AMD [51]. Supplementation has been demonstrated to increase serum concentration of EPA, though the clinical significance of this is not yet known [52].

Higher intakes of DHA and EPA were associated with a lower risk of progression to advanced AMD in the AREDS population, independent of AREDS supplementation [53]. Participants with the highest intake of omega-3 long-chain polyunsaturated fatty acids were approximately half as likely to have neovascular AMD at baseline (for DHA+EPA, OR: 0.65, 95% CI 0.50–0.85) [54]. They were also less likely to progress over a six-year period from bilateral drusen to central geographic atrophy than participants with the lowest intake of these LCPUFAs (OR: 0.65, 95% CI 0.45–0.92) [54, 55]. In a nested cohort study of AREDS, patients with moderate to high risk of advanced AMD and the highest consumption of omega-3 fatty acids demonstrated a 30% reduction in incident advanced AMD [48].

In the Blue Mountain Eye Study, a reduction in 10-year incident early AMD was shown with dietary intake of one serving of fish per week or greater [34]. Another large Australian cohort study also showed that higher omega-3 fatty acid intake was inversely associated with early AMD when the highest and lowest quartiles were compared [56]. Conversely, the third National Health and Nutrition Examination Survey did not show a statistically significant association between fish intake and prevalence of AMD [57]. In their meta- analysis of omega-3 fatty acid consumption and risk of AMD, Chong et al. concluded that consumption of omega-3 fatty acids may be associated with a lower risk of AMD but overall, evidence was insufficient to recommend supplementation for primary prevention in the general population [50].

There is a growing body of clinical and scientific evidence that supports a role for omega-3 fatty acids in the pathogenesis and progression of AMD. As this evidence accumulates, the need for a large multi-center randomized controlled trial is apparent. The AREDS2 will address the effect of DHA + EPA supplementation (1 g/day) on the secondary prevention of AMD [25].

Vitamin E

Vitamin E is present in the retina in the form of alpha-tocopherol [58]. It is a potent antioxidant and free-radical scavenger that has been investigated as a potential disease modifying agent in AMD. Dietary sources of Vitamin E include whole grains, fortified cereals, and nuts [59].

Vitamin E intervention in the Vitamin E Cataract and Age-Related Maculopathy (VECAT) Study showed no effect of Vitamin E supplementation on the incidence of early or late AMD, although a slight reduction in hypopigmentation was shown in patients with early AMD [60]. Other data regarding intake of Vitamin E and risk of AMD have been mixed. High dietary intake of Vitamin E was shown to reduce risk of incident AMD in Physician's Health Study, though this finding was not statistically significant. (RR 0.87) [61]. In contrast, participants in the highest tertiles of Vitamin E intake in the Blue Mountain Eye Study had a higher risk of late AMD than those in the lowest tertile of consumption, though this trend was also not significant [18]. Vitamin E was not shown to have any effect on the incidence of AMD in the Eye Disease Case Control Study [38]. The AREDS formulation contained 400 IU of Vitamin E and when used in combination with Vitamins C, zinc, and beta-carotene, was shown to reduce the risk of advanced AMD in participants at intermediate risk of progression [13]. In the Rotterdam Study, a reduced risk of incident

AMD was shown with increased dietary intake of Vitamin E [19].

A large meta-analysis of trials examining the impact of Vitamin E on mortality showed a minimally increased risk of mortality with Vitamin E supplementation both when used alone or in combination with beta-carotene and Vitamin A (RR 1.04) [62]. AREDS mortality analyses did not show any increased risk of death with AREDS supplementation [11].

Vitamin C

Vitamin C is a water-soluble glucose-derived molecule, which plays an important role in collagen, catecholamine, and neurohormone synthesis. Additionally, it serves as an antioxidant by scavenging free radicals and detoxifying them in the retina and other neural tissue [63]. Vitamin C plays an important role in immune function, iron absorption, and vitamin E regeneration [64]. Dietary consumption is required since it is not produced endogenously. It is found primarily in citrus fruits, tomatoes, potatoes, red and green peppers, broccoli, kiwi, and strawberries [19, 64].

Vitamin C is found in rod outer segments and Muller cells and protects Vitamin E (alpha-tocopherol), which is an important retinal membrane component, from UV irradiation-induced oxidation [65]. Vitamin C also allows Vitamin E regeneration, thus improving its anti-oxidant effects on the retina [66].

One prominent study did not demonstrate a significant association between above and below-median intake of Vitamin C and incident AMD [18]. However, another study has shown that an above-median intake of vitamin C, when combined with vitamin E, beta-carotene, and zinc, was associated with a 35% reduced risk of incident AMD when compared with below-median intake of at least one of these nutrients [19]. Overall, data regarding a potential therapeutic role for Vitamin C in AMD is limited. A protective effect may be related to an improvement in overall systemic oxidative status.

Pearl

Rotterdam [34]

- Population-based prospective cohort study
- Designed to assess frequency and determinants of common diseases
- A validated food frequency questionnaire (FFQ) was used to assess the intake of a number of common nutrients
- Results:
  - A lower risk of incident AMD was shown among patients with energy-adjusted above-median dietary consumption of vitamin A, C, E, zinc, and beta-carotene when compared with patients with below-median consumption [34].

Zinc

Zinc is primarily stored in muscle, bone, skin, hair, and liver of adults [67], and is primarily found in oysters, red meat, poultry, beans, nuts, whole grains, crab, lobster, and dairy products. Grain and plant bioavailability is less than that from animal sources [68]. Zinc and other metals (such as copper) play an important role in the visual cycle and photoreceptor survival [69] and is found primarily in pigment-rich ocular structures (retina, choroid, retinal pigment epithelium (RPE)). As a cofactor and major constituent of several important enzymes (carbonic anhydrase, alcohol dehydrogenase, Cu, Zn-superoxide dismutase), zinc plays an active role in rhodopsin synthesis (through interactions with Vitamin A), protein stabilization, modification of photoreceptor plasma membranes, modulation of synaptic transmission, and protection against cellular stress-signaling pathways [67, 69, 70]. In the RPE, zinc helps to induce metallothionein synthesis, which may help in the removal of hydroxyl radicals [67]. Animal studies have demonstrated a connection between zinc deficiency and anencephaly, anophthalmia, microphthalmia, and impaired immune function [70–72]. In humans, zinc deficiency has been linked to night-blindness, AMD, impaired dark adaption, and other pigmentary retinopathies [67, 70, 73–75]. Furthermore, zinc levels in the neural retina and choroid have been shown to vary with age [69]. In male patients, zinc has been shown to decline with age in the neural retina and increases with age in the choroid. No age-related change has been demonstrated in the RPE [69, 75]. Primates with early onset macular degeneration were found to have decreased levels of zinc [76]; however, studies regarding the role of zinc in AMD in humans have been conflicting.

A positive treatment effect from oral zinc supplementation has been speculated for some time [77]. A study by Newsome et al. in 2008 showed that oral supplementation with zinc-monocysteine (25 mg twice daily) improved macular function (visual acuity, contrast sensitivity) in patients with dry AMD over placebo [78]. The AREDS study showed an odds reduction for the development of advanced AMD as well as for the progression of intermediate AMD to advanced AMD [13]. Confirmed by the Blue Mountains Eye Study, patients with >15.8 mg/day of zinc supplementation (the highest tertile of intake) were 46% less likely to develop early AMD and 44% less likely to develop any AMD [18]. The Beaver Dam Eye Study showed an inverse association between zinc intake and the incidence of pigmentary abnormalities, but demonstrated no significant inverse associations between zinc intake and incidence of early AMD [79]. In patients with the exudative form of AMD in one eye, oral zinc substitution was found to have no short-term (24 months) effect on the course of AMD [80]. Serum zinc levels were assessed in the AREDS where an increase of 17% was found in patients taking zinc-containing formulations. This effect was seen at both 1 and 5 years [81]. Patients taking zinc were more likely to have been hospitalized for genitourinary complaints than those who were not on zinc formulations (7.5 vs. 4.9% for both men and women and 8.6% vs. 4.4% for men alone) [13]. Recent data has suggested that patients homozygous for the risk-conferring phenotype of complement factor H (Y402H/Y402H) have a reduced treatment response to zinc [82].

Pearl
Blue Mountain Eye Study
- Population-based prospective cohort study
- Designed to assess frequency and risk factors for common eye diseases
- Validated FFQ used to determine intake of nutrients
- Results:
  ○ Participants in the top tertile of intake for lutein/zeaxanthin had a reduced risk of incident neovascular AMD and a reduced risk of indistinct soft or reticular drusen [34]
  ○ Beta-carotene was a risk factor for the development of incident neovascular AMD [18]
  ○ Reduction in 10-year incident early AMD was shown with dietary intake of one serving of fish per week or greater [34]
  ○ Homocysteine levels >15micromol/L in patients less than 75 years of age was associated with an increased likelihood of AMD [83]

Folate/B-Vitamins

Folate, Vitamin B12, and Vitamin B6 are all water-soluble, naturally occurring vitamins. Folic acid is found primarily in green, leafy vegetables, citrus fruits, beans, and peas. It is important in cell division, especially in the production of erythrocytes and the metabolism of homocysteine. Breads, cereals, and other grain products are often fortified with folate [84]. Vitamin B12 (cyanocobalamin) is found naturally in fish, meat, poultry, eggs, and milk products. It plays an important role in erythrocyte formation, DNA synthesis, neurologic function, and homocysteine metabolism. Vitamin B6 is found in fortified cereals, beans, meat, poultry, fish, fruits, and vegetables [84]. It plays an important role in erythrocyte metabolism, neurologic function, immune

function, and hemoglobin oxygen capacity. Homocysteine is a highly reactive intermediary amino acid in methionine metabolism and requires adequate levels of folate, Vitamin B12, and Vitamin B6 for adequate trans-sulfuration and remethylation [85–87].

When homocysteine levels are increased (>15 micromol/l), damage of vascular endothelium through the release of free radicals is possible, as is the promotion of smooth muscle proliferation, and a hypercoaguable state [83, 85, 88]. Homocysteine levels have been shown to increase with age and are higher in men [85]. Hyperhomocysteinemia has been shown to be an independent risk factor for cardiovascular disease, cerebrovascular disease, peripheral vascular disease, atherosclerosis, and thrombosis [85, 87, 88]. In addition to the known effects of homocysteine on vessels, toxicity to ganglion cells neurons and aberrations in redox thiol status causing increased pro-oxidant levels has been demonstrated [86, 89]. Nowak et al. showed that patients with AMD had elevated levels of homocysteine when compared with control groups, and no significant difference in B12 and folate levels [86]. However, Heuberger showed no relation between levels of homocysteine and AMD and an inverse relationship between folate and soft drusen in non-Hispanic blacks [86]. The toxic effects of homocysteine as well as atherosclerosis have become suspected risk factors in the pathogenesis of AMD [86, 87, 90]. In a model proposed by Friedman et al., AMD and atherosclerosis share risk factors and pathogenic mechanisms, which result in the deposition of lipid in the sclera and Bruch's membrane, which may lead to decreased choroidal blood flow, elevation of choriocapillary pressure, drusen, and fragmentation of Bruch's membrane. Patients with advanced AMD have been shown to have decreased choriocapillary density and diameter, compared with normal maculae [91]. The Rotterdam Eye Study showed that patients younger than 85 years with plaques in the carotid bifurcation had a 4.7 increased prevalence odds of neovascular macular degeneration [92].

Results of the Women's Antioxidant and Folic Acid Cardiovascular Study (WAFACS) showed that, based on 7.3 years of follow-up, those who received supplementation with folic acid, pyridoxine, and cyanocobalamin had a 35–40% decreased risk of AMD, first evident after two years of supplementation. AMD was self-reported with a confirmatory questionnaire sent to the treating physician in the WAFACS; due to this study design, true AMD rates may be difficult to ascertain [93]. The Blue Mountains Eye Study showed that homocysteine levels >15micromol/l in patients less than 75 years of age was associated with an increased likelihood of AMD and that hyperhomocysteinemia was a more significant risk factor when vitamin B12 levels are low [83]. Axer-Siegel et al. showed that homocysteine levels were 27.9% higher in patients with neovascular AMD compared with those with dry AMD and 21.9% higher compared with those in the control group. The mean homocysteine level in neovascular AMD was 16.5 nmol/l compared with 11.9 nmol/l in dry AMD and 12.5 nmol/l in controls. This suggests that elevated homocysteine is associated with exudative neovascular AMD, but not dry AMD [85]. Treatment with folate, pyridoxine, and cyanocobalamin have been shown to reduce plasma homocysteine levels [93, 94]. Specifically, supplementation of folate alone can reduce plasma homocysteine by 13–25% [95, 96]. In addition to their role in homocysteine metabolism, folate and the B vitamins may also exert an independent protection against AMD, possibly through their antioxidant effects and ability to help restore endothelial nitrous oxide levels to vasculature, thereby improving vascular reactivity and reducing atherogenticity of endothelium [94, 97, 98]. The WAFACS provides promising initial data that requires further validation prior to becoming a universal treatment recommendation.

AREDS2

A significant amount of data has emerged since the first AREDS suggesting a potential disease-modifying role for omega-3 fatty acids and the macular xanthophylls lutein and zeaxanthin in AMD. The AREDS2 will help to further delineate the role of these micronutrients in preventing progression to advanced AMD in patients at intermediate to high risk of progression [99].

The AREDS2 is a multi-center placebo-controlled randomized controlled trial with the primary aim of evaluating whether high-dose supplementation with omega-3 LCPUFAs and/or lutein with zeaxanthin will prove useful as a treatment for AMD. Lutein and Zeaxanthin were considered for the original AREDS formulation due to their histological and biophysical properties and the epidemiologic data; however, at the time neither carotenoid was available for commercial manufacture. In addition, in a second randomization, the AREDS2 will help to determine whether eliminating beta-carotene and reducing the dose of zinc in the AREDS formulation have any effect on the efficacy of treatment (Fig. 5.1). In contrast to AREDS, AREDS2 will include only participants at intermediate risk of progression or higher. Approximately 4,000 patients have been enrolled who have either (1) bilateral large drusen or (2) large drusen in one eye and advanced AMD (neovascular AMD or central geographic atrophy) in the fellow eye. The primary outcome measure in AREDS2 is progression to advanced AMD. The study will follow the participants through year 5.

Summary

Management of nonexudative AMD remains a dilemma with limited therapeutic options. Data regarding primary prevention of AMD shows promise, but at present, there is insufficient evidence to recommend nutritional supplements to prevent onset of AMD in a general population or even those with family history but no evidence of AMD. The AREDS trial provided compelling evidence, which demonstrated that a combination of Vitamin C, E, beta-carotene, zinc, and copper reduces the risk of advanced AMD in patients with intermediate risk of progression. Individual composition and dosing of this supplement regimen requires refinement. Data suggests that hyperhomocysteinemia may be a risk factor for AMD and initial trial data suggests supplementation with B6, B12, and folate may reduce risk of advanced AMD. Further replications are required. Significant observational data exists regarding disease-modifying characteristics of macular pigments and long-chain fatty acids in AMD; however, no randomized controlled trials have specifically addressed this issue. The AREDS2 trial will add to the evidence base and provide further clarification regarding these issues.

References

1. Age-Related Eye Disease Study Research Group. A randomized, placebo-controlled, clinical trial of high-dose supplementation with vitamins C and E and beta carotene for age-related cataract and vision loss: AREDS report no. 9. Arch Ophthalmol. 2001;119(10): 1439–52.
2. Friedman DS, O'Colmain BJ, Munoz B, et al. Prevalence of age-related macular degeneration in the United States. Arch Ophthalmol. 2004;122(4): 564–72.
3. Coleman H, Chew E. Nutritional supplementation in age-related macular degeneration. Curr Opin Ophthalmol. 2007;18(3):220–3.
4. Evans JR. Antioxidant vitamin and mineral supplements for slowing the progression of age-related macular degeneration. Cochrane Database Syst Rev. 2006(2):CD000254.
5. Evans JR, Henshaw K. Antioxidant vitamin and mineral supplementation for preventing age-related macular degeneration. Cochrane Database Syst Rev. 2000(2):CD000253.
6. Evans JR, Henshaw K. Antioxidant vitamin and mineral supplements for preventing age-related macular degeneration. Cochrane Database Syst Rev. 2008(1): CD000253.
7. Johnson EJ. Age-related macular degeneration and antioxidant vitamins: recent findings. Curr Opin Clin Nutr Metab Care. 2010;13(1):28–33.
8. Ding X, Patel M, Chan CC. Molecular pathology of age-related macular degeneration. Prog Retin Eye Res. 2009;28(1):1–18.
9. Bressler NM, Bressler SB, Congdon NG, et al. Potential public health impact of Age-Related Eye Disease Study results: AREDS report no. 11. Arch Ophthalmol. 2003;121(11):1621–4.
10. Borger PH, van Leeuwen R, Hulsman CA, et al. Is there a direct association between age-related eye diseases and mortality? The Rotterdam Study. Ophthalmology. 2003;110(7):1292–6.
11. Clemons TE, Kurinij N, Sperduto RD. Associations of mortality with ocular disorders and an intervention of high-dose antioxidants and zinc in the Age-Related

Eye Disease Study: AREDS Report No. 13. Arch Ophthalmol. 2004;122(5):716–26.
12. Chew EY, Clemons T. Vitamin E and the age-related eye disease study supplementation for age-related macular degeneration. Arch Ophthalmol. 2005; 123(3):395–6.
13. Age-Related Eye Disease Study Research Group. A randomized, placebo-controlled, clinical trial of high-dose supplementation with vitamins C and E, beta carotene, and zinc for age-related macular degeneration and vision loss: AREDS report no. 8. Arch Ophthalmol. 2001;119(10):1417–36.
14. Nebeling LC, Forman MR, Graubard BI, Snyder RA. Changes in carotenoid intake in the United States: the 1987 and 1992 National Health Interview Surveys. J Am Diet Assoc. 1997;97(9):991–6.
15. Nebeling LC, Forman MR, Graubard BI, Snyder RA. The impact of lifestyle characteristics on carotenoid intake in the United States: the 1987 National Health Interview Survey. Am J Public Health. 1997;87(2): 268–71.
16. Sommerburg O, Keunen JE, Bird AC, van Kuijk FJ. Fruits and vegetables that are sources for lutein and zeaxanthin: the macular pigment in human eyes. Br J Ophthalmol. 1998;82(8):907–10.
17. Teikari JM, Laatikainen L, Virtamo J, et al. Six-year supplementation with alpha-tocopherol and beta-carotene and age-related maculopathy. Acta Ophthalmol Scand. 1998;76(2):224–9.
18. Tan JS, Wang JJ, Flood V, Rochtchina E, Smith W, Mitchell P. Dietary antioxidants and the long-term incidence of age-related macular degeneration: the Blue Mountains Eye Study. Ophthalmology. 2008; 115(2):334–41.
19. van Leeuwen R, Boekhoorn S, Vingerling JR, et al. Dietary intake of antioxidants and risk of age-related macular degeneration. JAMA. 2005;294(24): 3101–7.
20. Chiu CJ, Milton RC, Klein R, Gensler G, Taylor A. Dietary compound score and risk of age-related macular degeneration in the age-related eye disease study. Ophthalmology. 2009;116(5):939–46.
21. Christen WG, Manson JE, Glynn RJ, et al. Beta carotene supplementation and age-related maculopathy in a randomized trial of US physicians. Arch Ophthalmol. 2007;125(3):333–9.
22. The effect of vitamin E and beta carotene on the incidence of lung cancer and other cancers in male smokers. The Alpha-Tocopherol, Beta Carotene Cancer Prevention Study Group. N Engl J Med. Apr 14 1994;330(15):1029–35.
23. Omenn GS, Goodman GE, Thornquist MD, et al. Effects of a combination of beta carotene and vitamin A on lung cancer and cardiovascular disease. N Engl J Med. 1996;334(18):1150–5.
24. Hennekens CH, Buring JE, Manson JE, et al. Lack of effect of long-term supplementation with beta carotene on the incidence of malignant neoplasms and cardiovascular disease. N Engl J Med. 1996;334(18): 1145–9.

25. AREDS2 Manual of Procedures www.areds2.org. Accessed on 01/05/2010.
26. Loane E, Kelliher C, Beatty S, Nolan JM. The rationale and evidence base for a protective role of macular pigment in age-related maculopathy. Br J Ophthalmol. 2008;92(9):1163–8.
27. Snodderly DM, Auran JD, Delori FC. The macular pigment. II. Spatial distribution in primate retinas. Invest Ophthalmol Vis Sci. 1984;25(6):674–85.
28. Snodderly DM, Brown PK, Delori FC, Auran JD. The macular pigment. I. Absorbance spectra, localization, and discrimination from other yellow pigments in primate retinas. Invest Ophthalmol Vis Sci. 1984;25(6): 660–73.
29. Nolan JM, Stack J, OD O, Loane E, Beatty S. Risk factors for age-related maculopathy are associated with a relative lack of macular pigment. Exp Eye Res. 2007;84(1):61–74.
30. Trieschmann M, Beatty S, Nolan JM, et al. Changes in macular pigment optical density and serum concentrations of its constituent carotenoids following supplemental lutein and zeaxanthin: the LUNA study. Exp Eye Res. 2007;84(4):718–28.
31. Schalch W, Cohn W, Barker FM, et al. Xanthophyll accumulation in the human retina during supplementation with lutein or zeaxanthin – the LUXEA (LUtein Xanthophyll Eye Accumulation) study. Arch Biochem Biophys. 2007;458(2):128–35.
32. Rosenthal JM, Kim J, de Monasterio F, et al. Dose-ranging study of lutein supplementation in persons aged 60 years or older. Invest Ophthalmol Vis Sci. 2006;47(12):5227–33.
33. SanGiovanni JP, Chew EY, Clemons TE, et al. The relationship of dietary carotenoid and vitamin A, E, and C intake with age-related macular degeneration in a case-control study: AREDS Report No. 22. Arch Ophthalmol. 2007;125(9):1225–32.
34. Tan JS, Wang JJ, Flood V, Mitchell P. Dietary fatty acids and the 10-year incidence of age-related macular degeneration: the Blue Mountains Eye Study. Arch Ophthalmol. 2009;127(5):656–65.
35. Cho E, Hankinson SE, Rosner B, Willett WC, Colditz GA. Prospective study of lutein/zeaxanthin intake and risk of age-related macular degeneration. Am J Clin Nutr. 2008;87(6):1837–43.
36. Moeller SM, Parekh N, Tinker L, et al. Associations between intermediate age-related macular degeneration and lutein and zeaxanthin in the Carotenoids in Age-related Eye Disease Study (CAREDS): ancillary study of the Women's Health Initiative. Arch Ophthalmol. 2006;124(8):1151–62.
37. Delcourt C, Carriere I, Delage M, Barberger-Gateau P, Schalch W. Plasma lutein and zeaxanthin and other carotenoids as modifiable risk factors for age-related maculopathy and cataract: the POLA Study. Invest Ophthalmol Vis Sci. 2006;47(6):2329–35.
38. Seddon JM, Ajani UA, Sperduto RD, et al. Dietary carotenoids, vitamins A, C, and E, and advanced age-related macular degeneration. Eye Disease Case-Control Study Group. JAMA. 1994;272(18):1413–20.
39. Trumbo PR, Ellwood KC. Lutein and zeaxanthin intakes and risk of age-related macular degeneration and cataracts: an evaluation using the Food and Drug Administration's evidence-based review system for health claims. Am J Clin Nutr. 2006;84(5):971–4.
40. SanGiovanni JP, Chew EY. The role of omega-3 long-chain polyunsaturated fatty acids in health and disease of the retina. Prog Retin Eye Res. 2005;24(1):87–138.
41. Bannenberg G, Arita M, Serhan CN. Endogenous receptor agonists: resolving inflammation. Sci World J. 2007;7:1440–62.
42. Bazan NG. Cell survival matters: docosahexaenoic acid signaling, neuroprotection and photoreceptors. Trends Neurosci. 2006;29(5):263–71.
43. Bazan NG. Neurotrophins induce neuroprotective signaling in the retinal pigment epithelial cell by activating the synthesis of the anti-inflammatory and anti-apoptotic neuroprotectin D1. Adv Exp Med Biol. 2008;613:39–44.
44. Serhan CN. Systems approach to inflammation resolution: identification of novel anti-inflammatory and pro-resolving mediators. J Thromb Haemost. 2009;7 Suppl 1:44–8.
45. Serhan CN, Chiang N, Van Dyke TE. Resolving inflammation: dual anti-inflammatory and pro-resolution lipid mediators. Nat Rev Immunol. 2008;8(5): 349–61.
46. Weylandt KH, Kang JX. Rethinking lipid mediators. Lancet. 2005;366(9486):618–20.
47. Mukherjee PK, Marcheselli VL, Serhan CN, Bazan NG. Neuroprotectin D1: a docosahexaenoic acid-derived docosatriene protects human retinal pigment epithelial cells from oxidative stress. Proc Natl Acad Sci USA. 2004;101(22):8491–6.
48. Sangiovanni JP, Agron E, Meleth AD, et al. {omega}-3 Long-chain polyunsaturated fatty acid intake and 12-y incidence of neovascular age-related macular degeneration and central geographic atrophy: AREDS report 30, a prospective cohort study from the Age-Related Eye Disease Study. Am J Clin Nutr. 2009; 90(6):1601–7.
49. Augood C, Chakravarthy U, Young I, et al. Oily fish consumption, dietary docosahexaenoic acid and eicosapentaenoic acid intakes, and associations with neovascular age-related macular degeneration. Am J Clin Nutr. 2008;88(2):398–406.
50. Chong EW, Kreis AJ, Wong TY, Simpson JA, Guymer RH. Dietary omega-3 fatty acid and fish intake in the primary prevention of age-related macular degeneration: a systematic review and meta-analysis. Arch Ophthalmol. 2008;126(6):826–33.
51. Seddon JM, George S, Rosner B. Cigarette smoking, fish consumption, omega-3 fatty acid intake, and associations with age-related macular degeneration: the US Twin Study of Age-Related Macular Degeneration. Arch Ophthalmol. 2006;124(7): 995–1001.
52. Huang LL, Coleman HR, Kim J, et al. Oral supplementation of lutein/zeaxanthin and omega-3 long chain polyunsaturated fatty acids in persons aged

60 years or older, with or without AMD. Invest Ophthalmol Vis Sci. 2008;49(9):3864–9.

53. Chiu CJ, Klein R, Milton RC, Gensler G, Taylor A. Does eating particular diets alter the risk of age-related macular degeneration in users of the Age-Related Eye Disease Study supplements? Br J Ophthalmol. 2009; 93(9):1241–6.

54. SanGiovanni JP, Agron E, Clemons TE, Chew EY. Omega-3 long-chain polyunsaturated fatty acid intake inversely associated with 12-year progression to advanced age-related macular degeneration. Arch Ophthalmol. 2009;127(1):110–2.

55. SanGiovanni JP, Chew EY, Clemons TE, et al. The relationship of dietary lipid intake and age-related macular degeneration in a case-control study: AREDS Report No. 20. Arch Ophthalmol. 2007;125(5): 671–9.

56. Chong EW, Robman LD, Simpson JA, et al. Fat consumption and its association with age-related macular degeneration. Arch Ophthalmol. 2009;127(5): 674–80.

57. Heuberger RA, Mares-Perlman JA, Klein R, Klein BE, Millen AE, Palta M. Relationship of dietary fat to age-related maculopathy in the Third National Health and Nutrition Examination Survey. Arch Ophthalmol. 2001;119(12):1833–8.

58. Katz ML, Robison Jr WG. Light and aging effects on vitamin E in the retina and retinal pigment epithelium. Vis Res. 1987;27(11):1875–9.

59. Supplements OoD. Vitamin E. http://dietary-supplements.info.nih.gov/factsheets/. Accessed on 01/05/2010.

60. Taylor HR, Tikellis G, Robman LD, McCarty CA, McNeil JJ. Vitamin E supplementation and macular degeneration: randomised controlled trial. BMJ. 2002; 325(7354):11.

61. Christen WG, Ajani UA, Glynn RJ, et al. Prospective cohort study of antioxidant vitamin supplement use and the risk of age-related maculopathy. Am J Epidemiol. 1999;149(5):476–84.

62. Bjelakovic G, Nikolova D, Gluud LL, Simonetti RG, Gluud C. Mortality in randomized trials of antioxidant supplements for primary and secondary prevention: systematic review and meta-analysis. JAMA. 2007;297(8):842–57.

63. Hosoya K, Nakamura G, Akanuma S, Tomi M, Tachikawa M. Dehydroascorbic acid uptake and intracellular ascorbic acid accumulation in cultured Muller glial cells (TR-MUL). Neurochem Int. 2008;52(7): 1351–7.

64. Supplements OoD. Vitamin C. http://dietary-supplements.info.nih.gov/factsheets/. Accessed on 01/05/2010.

65. Friedman PA, Zeidel ML. Victory at C. Nat Med. 1999;5(6):620–1.

66. Stoyanovsky DA, Goldman R, Darrow RM, Organisciak DT, Kagan VE. Endogenous ascorbate regenerates vitamin E in the retina directly and in combination with exogenous dihydrolipoic acid. Curr Eye Res. 1995;14(3):181–9.

67. Grahn BH, Paterson PG, Gottschall-Pass KT, Zhang Z. Zinc and the eye. J Am Coll Nutr. 2001;20 (2 Suppl):106–18.

68. Supplements OoD. Zinc. http://dietary-supplements.info.nih.gov/factsheets/. Accessed on 01/05/2010.

69. Wills NK, Ramanujam VM, Kalariya N, Lewis JR, van Kuijk FJ. Copper and zinc distribution in the human retina: relationship to cadmium accumulation, age, and gender. Exp Eye Res. 2008;87(2):80–8.

70. Karcioglu ZA. Zinc in the eye. Surv Ophthalmol. 1982;27(2):114–22.

71. Cunningham-Rundles S, Cunningham-Rundles C, Dupont B, Good RA. Zinc-induced activation of human B lymphocytes. Clin Immunol Immunopathol. 1980;16(1):115–22.

72. Hurley LS, Swenerton H. Congenital malformations resulting from zinc deficiency in rats. Proc Soc Exp Biol Med. 1966;123(3):692–6.

73. Morrison SA, Russell RM, Carney EA, Oaks EV. Zinc deficiency: a cause of abnormal dark adaptation in cirrhotics. Am J Clin Nutr. 1978;31(2):276–81.

74. Prasad AS. Discovery of human zinc deficiency and studies in an experimental human model. Am J Clin Nutr. 1991;53(2):403–12.

75. Tate DJ, Miceli MV, Newsome DA, Alcock NW, Oliver PD. Influence of zinc on selected cellular functions of cultured human retinal pigment epithelium. Curr Eye Res. 1995;14(10):897–903.

76. Olin KL, Golub MS, Gershwin ME, Hendrickx AG, Lonnerdal B, Keen CL. Extracellular superoxide dismutase activity is affected by dietary zinc intake in nonhuman primate and rodent models. Am J Clin Nutr. 1995;61(6):1263–7.

77. Newsome DA, Swartz M, Leone NC, Elston RC, Miller E. Oral zinc in macular degeneration. Arch Ophthalmol. 1988;106(2):192–8.

78. Newsome DA. A randomized, prospective, placebo-controlled clinical trial of a novel zinc-monocysteine compound in age-related macular degeneration. Curr Eye Res. 2008;33(7):591–8.

79. VandenLangenberg GM, Mares-Perlman JA, Klein R, Klein BE, Brady WE, Palta M. Associations between antioxidant and zinc intake and the 5-year incidence of early age-related maculopathy in the Beaver Dam Eye Study. Am J Epidemiol. 1998;148(2):204–14.

80. Stur M, Tittl M, Reitner A, Meisinger V. Oral zinc and the second eye in age-related macular degeneration. Invest Ophthalmol Vis Sci. 1996;37(7):1225–35.

81. Age-Related Eye Disease Study Research Group. The effect of five-year zinc supplementation on serum zinc, serum cholesterol and hematocrit in persons randomly assigned to treatment group in the age-related eye disease study: AREDS Report No. 7. J Nutr. 2002;132(4):697–702.

82. Klein ML, Francis PJ, Rosner B, et al. CFH and LOC387715/ARMS2 genotypes and treatment with antioxidants and zinc for age-related macular degeneration. Ophthalmology. 2008;115(6):1019–25.

83. Rochtchina E, Wang JJ, Flood VM, Mitchell P. Elevated serum homocysteine, low serum vitamin

B12, folate, and age-related macular degeneration: the Blue Mountains Eye Study. Am J Ophthalmol. 2007;143(2):344–6.

84. Supplements OoD. Folate/B12. http://dietary-supplements.info.nih.gov/factsheets/. Accessed on 01/05/2010.

85. Axer-Siegel R, Bourla D, Ehrlich R, et al. Association of neovascular age-related macular degeneration and hyperhomocysteinemia. Am J Ophthalmol. 2004; 137(1):84–9.

86. Heuberger RA, Fisher AI, Jacques PF, et al. Relation of blood homocysteine and its nutritional determinants to age-related maculopathy in the third National Health and Nutrition Examination Survey. Am J Clin Nutr. 2002;76(4):897–902.

87. Nowak M, Swietochowska E, Wielkoszynski T, et al. Homocysteine, vitamin B12, and folic acid in age-related macular degeneration. Eur J Ophthalmol. 2005;15(6):764–7.

88. Woo KS, Chook P, Lolin YI, Sanderson JE, Metreweli C, Celermajer DS. Folic acid improves arterial endothelial function in adults with hyperhomocystinemia. J Am Coll Cardiol. 1999;34(7):2002–6.

89. Moore P, El-sherbeny A, Roon P, Schoenlein PV, Ganapathy V, Smith SB. Apoptotic cell death in the mouse retinal ganglion cell layer is induced in vivo by the excitatory amino acid homocysteine. Exp Eye Res. 2001;73(1):45–57.

90. van Leeuwen R, Ikram MK, Vingerling JR, Witteman JC, Hofman A, de Jong PT. Blood pressure, atherosclerosis, and the incidence of age-related maculopathy: the Rotterdam Study. Invest Ophthalmol Vis Sci. 2003;44(9):3771–7.

91. Ramrattan RS, van der Schaft TL, Mooy CM, de Bruijn WC, Mulder PG, de Jong PT. Morphometric analysis of Bruch's membrane, the choriocapillaris,

and the choroid in aging. Invest Ophthalmol Vis Sci. 1994;35(6):2857–64.

92. Vingerling JR, Dielemans I, Bots ML, Hofman A, Grobbee DE, de Jong PT. Age-related macular degeneration is associated with atherosclerosis. The Rotterdam Study. Am J Epidemiol. 1995;142(4): 404–9.

93. Christen WG, Glynn RJ, Chew EY, Albert CM, Manson JE. Folic acid, pyridoxine, and cyanocobalamin combination treatment and age-related macular degeneration in women: the Women's Antioxidant and Folic Acid Cardiovascular Study. Arch Intern Med. 2009;169(4):335–41.

94. Hayden MR, Tyagi SC. Homocysteine and reactive oxygen species in metabolic syndrome, type 2 diabetes mellitus, and atheroscleropathy: the pleiotropic effects of folate supplementation. Nutr J. 2004;3:4.

95. Age-Related Eye Disease Study Research Group. Dose-dependent effects of folic acid on blood concentrations of homocysteine: a meta-analysis of the randomized trials. Am J Clin Nutr. 2005;82(4):806–12.

96. Doshi SN, McDowell IF, Moat SJ, et al. Folic acid improves endothelial function in coronary artery disease via mechanisms largely independent of homocysteine lowering. Circulation. 2002;105(1):22–6.

97. Moat SJ, Lang D, McDowell IF, et al. Folate, homocysteine, endothelial function and cardiovascular disease. J Nutr Biochem. 2004;15(2):64–79.

98. Verhaar MC, Wever RM, Kastelein JJ, van Dam T, Koomans HA, Rabelink TJ. 5-methyltetrahydrofolate, the active form of folic acid, restores endothelial function in familial hypercholesterolemia. Circulation. 1998;97(3):237–41.

99. Chew E. Age-related Eye Disease Study 2 Protocol. https://web.emmes.com/study/areds2/resources/areds2_protocol.pdf. Accessed on 01/05/2010.

Management of Neovascular AMD

6

Fernando M. Penha and Philip J. Rosenfeld

Key Points

- VEGF is the most important regulator of angiogenesis and a potent promoter of vascular permeability in different ocular diseases, including AMD. For this reason, VEGF is a key target in treating ocular neovascularization.
- Two anti-VEGF agents have achieved regulatory approval, with others in clinical trials.
- Clinical trials have shown that intravitreal ranibizumab is safe drug and effective, being the first agent to promote visual acuity improvement in patients with wet AMD.
- Bevacizumab, a monoclonal antibody against VEGF, was approved for intravenous, systemic therapy for different types of cancer. It has been used off-label as an intravitreal injection in wet AMD since 2005 with clinical results similar to ranibizumab.
- CATT head-to-head trial comparing bevacizumab versus ranibizumab demonstrated that they have similar outcomes when the same treatment regimen is applied.

- New promising anti-VEGF drugs (VEGF-Trap, KH902, and Pazopanib) are in ongoing clinical trials.

Introduction

Exudative eye diseases, including neovascular age-related macular degeneration (AMD), diabetic retinopathy with macular edema (DME), and retinal vein occlusion (RVO), are the primary causes of clinically significant vision loss in the developed world, particularly among the working and elderly populations [1–3]. In the United States, neovascular AMD is the leading cause of irreversible blindness among those over the age of 65, affecting at least 1.75 million individuals [4]. The neovascular form of AMD is responsible for most of the severe vision loss associated with the diseases. Neovascular AMD arises from the nonexudative form of AMD and is characterized by the growth of abnormal blood vessels in the macula, which arise either from the choroidal circulation and penetrate through Bruch's membrane (known as choroidal neovascularization (CNV)) or arise primarily from the retinal circulation (known as retinal angiomatous proliferation (RAP)). Both forms of neovascularization cause disruption of the normal outer retinal and inner choroidal anatomy resulting from fibrovascular proliferation and the accumulation of fluid in the subretinal pigmented epithelium (sub-RPE) space, the subretinal space, and within the retina [5, 6].

F.M. Penha (✉)
Department of Ophthalmology, Bascom Palmer
Eye Institute, University of Miami, 900 NW 17 St.,
Miami, FL 33136, USA
e-mail: fpenha@med.miami.eduf; penha@me.com

A.C. Ho and C.D. Regillo (eds.), *Age-related Macular Degeneration Diagnosis and Treatment*,
DOI 10.1007/978-1-4614-0125-4_6, © Springer Science+Business Media, LLC 2011

Angiogenesis

An Overview of VEGF

Vascular endothelial growth factor (VEGF) plays an important role in normal angiogenesis as well as pathological neovascularization and vascular exudation in oncology and exudative eye diseases. While normal and pathologic angiogenesis involve a complex balance of positive and negative regulators, VEGF-A, also referred to as VEGF, is one of the most important positive regulators of angiogenesis [7] and vascular permeability [8, 9].

VEGF-A Isoforms

VEGF-A is a member of the VEGF family of growth factors that also includes VEGF-B, VEGF-C, VEGF-D, platelet derived growth factor (PDGF), and placental growth factor (PlGF), which have different binding affinities for the three VEGF receptors: VEGFR1, VEGFR2, and VEGFR3 [10, 11]. VEGF-A also binds to neuropilin-1, a membrane protein on developing neurons that plays a role in embryonic neural blood vessel formation as well as neural tip guidance [12, 13]. Alternative RNA splicing of the human VEGF-A gene results in the formation of four major isoforms ($VEGF_{121}$, $VEGF_{165}$, $VEGF_{189}$, and $VEGF_{206}$) and at least five minor isoforms ($VEGF_{145}$, $VEGF_{148}$, $VEGF_{162}$, $VEGF_{165b}$, and $VEGF_{183}$). $VEGF_{121}$ is freely diffusible, while $VEGF_{189}$ is found in the extracellular matrix; $VEGF_{165}$ exists in both diffusible and matrix-bound forms [14]. Physiologic protease degradation of VEGF also results in biologically active breakdown products that contain fewer than 121 amino acids [14, 15].

Vascular Endothelial Growth Factor-A: Physiological and Pathological Response

VEGF-A Physiological Response

VEGF has different functions in the angiogenesis cascade. VEGF regulates both endothelial cell mitosis [7] and survival rate [16], and acts as a chemo-attractant for bone marrow-derived endothelial progenitor cells [17]. Moreover, VEGF induces the upregulation of extracellular matrix-degrading enzymes, such as metalloproteinases (MMPs) [18] and plasminogen activator [19], as well as nitric oxide [20], a downstream mediator of VEGF signaling [21].

In addition to promoting angiogenesis, VEGF-A also affects vascular permeability. VEGF-A is the most potent known inducer of vascular permeability, approximately 50,000 times more potent than histamine [9]. VEGF-mediated vascular permeability results from the formation of pores in the vascular endothelial cells [22] and the disruption of intercellular junctions between these cells [23]. The angiogenic and vascular permeability effects of VEGF-A on the endothelium are mediated by the transmembrane receptor VEGFR2 [flk-1/kinase insert domain receptor (KDR)] and involve diverse downstream signaling partners, such as the Src family kinases and/or protein tyrosine phosphatases, which result in the disruption and uncoupling of junctions between endothelial cells [24]. This, in turn, leads to the extravasation of fluid, proteins, and circulating inflammatory cells [24]. In neovascular ocular diseases, the edema from new, permeable blood vessels as well as established vessels can disrupt the retinal anatomy and separate the retina from underlying structures, which is in part responsible for the vision loss associated with CNV and macular exudation.

VEGF also plays a role in promoting inflammation. Inflammation involves the release of various cytokines at specific sites in the body by inflammatory cells such as T cells, B cells, macrophages, natural killer cells, neutrophils, and granulocytes. These proinflammatory cytokines include tumor necrosis factor (TNF)-a, interleukin (IL)-6, IL-8, and IL-1a, IL-1b, and oncostatin M, which participate in a cascade of events leading to increased levels of VEGF-A, the promotion of local angiogenesis, and worsening inflammation.

VEGF-A Response in Retinal Diseases
Evidence from preclinical and clinical studies implicates VEGF-A in the pathogenesis of neovascular eye diseases. In streptozotocin-induced diabetic rats, VEGF-A gene expression was

significantly increased in the ganglion and inner nuclear retinal cell layers compared with control rats [25]. Laser-induced RVO in rabbits [26] and monkeys [27] also led to increased VEGF-A mRNA expression, and VEGF-A protein expression has been localized to ischemic regions of the retinal layers affected by laser treatment [26]. Furthermore, VEGF-A inhibition prevented retinal neovascularization in an ischemia-induced mouse model [28] and iris neovascularization in a monkey model [29]. VEGF-A inhibition also prevented laser-induced CNV in monkeys and shortened the duration of CNV [30].

In clinical studies, increased levels of VEGF-A expression were found in the RPE [31], subfoveal fibroblasts [32], and surgically excised CNV [33] from eyes of neovascular AMD patients. VEGF-A is also over-expressed in the aqueous and vitreous fluid of patients with subretinal neovascularization, diabetic retinopathy, retinal vein occlusions, iris neovascularization, retinal detachment, and retinopathy of prematurity (ROP) [34–37] and in all retinal nuclear layers of eyes with ischemic central retinal vein occlusions [38]. The consistent association of pathologic ocular neovascularization with increased VEGF-A expression provided a strong rationale for exploring the therapeutic potential of anti-VEGF drugs in neovascular AMD.

Genetic case-controlled studies have shown that the VEGF gene may influence an individual's tendency to develop AMD [39]. Analyses of single nucleotide polymorphisms (SNPs) in the VEGF-A promoter and gene have associated specific VEGF-A haplotypes with neovascular AMD [40]. In particular, the VEGF SNP 936C/T [when present with the complement factor H (CFH) Y402H] has been associated with an increased risk of developing wet AMD [41].

> **Pearl**
> VEGF-A is implicated as the major angiogenic growth factor in different exudative ocular diseases, including neovascular AMD. Moreover, VEGF-A is the most potent known inducer of vascular permeability, approximately 50,000 times more potent than histamine [9].

Antiangiogenic Drugs

Drugs that inhibit VEGF-A include pegaptanib sodium (MACUGEN; Eyetech, Inc.) and ranibizumab (LUCENTIS; Genentech/Roche), which are approved by the Food and Drug Administration (FDA) for the treatment of choroidal neovascularization (CNV) secondary to AMD. Of the two agents, ranibizumab offers substantial clinical benefit in the treatment of neovascular AMD. A third anti-VEGF agent, bevacizumab (AVASTIN; Genentech/Roche), is used off label for neovascular AMD and other exudative ocular diseases. These anti-VEGF agents, as well as others in clinical development, have shown great potential to treat eye diseases characterized by exudation and neovascularization.

Pegaptanib

Drug Overview
The first and only FDA-approved aptamer in ophthalmology is pegaptanib sodium. Approved in December 2004, pegaptanib is indicated for the treatment of neovascular AMD. By definition, aptamers are oligonucleotides or peptide molecules that bind a specific target molecule, acting as chemical antibodies [42]. The commercially available pegaptanib sodium for injection is a sterile, clear, preservative-free aqueous solution supplied in a single-dose, prefilled syringe containing 0.3 mg of active drug.

Pegaptanib is a selective anti-VEGF agent that acts in the extracellular space inhibiting the isoforms of VEGF that are at least 165 amino acids in length while not binding $VEGF_{121}$ and the smaller proteolytic breakdown products that are biologically active [43]. The selectivity of pegaptanib derives from its interaction with cysteine-137, an amino acid that is contained within the 55 amino-acid heparin-binding domain of VEGF [43, 44], which is not present in the smaller isoforms and breakdown products [44–46]. The rationale for this selectivity is that the drug, at least in theory, will block only the $VEGF_{165}$ isoform and larger isoforms, which were postulated to be the main isoforms involved in pathologic conditions while preserving a wide range of VEGF-mediated physiological processes associated with the smaller isoforms [47–51].

Published Trials

The landmark phase III VEGF Inhibition Study In Ocular Neovascularization (VISION) trials were multicenter, dose-ranging studies that enrolled subjects with a wide range of neovascular lesions, including all angiographic subtypes and lesions up to 12 disc areas in size (including blood, scar, or atrophy, and neovascularization). Patients in the study had a best corrected visual acuity (VA) of 20/40–20/320 in their study eye [52, 53]. Subjects received sham injections or injections of intravitreal pegaptanib sodium (0.3, 1, or 3 mg) every 6 weeks for 54 weeks for the first year of the study.

In the combined trials, 1,186 subjects were enrolled and the results showed that intravitreal pegaptanib sodium decreased the loss vision, with 70% of treated patients losing fewer than 15 letters of visual acuity compared with 55% of controls [53, 54]. Moreover, 6% of pegaptanib sodium-treated patients gained at least 15 letters compared with 2% of the patients in the control group [53]. Fluorescein angiography at 30 and 54 weeks showed that the pegaptanib-treated group had a significant reduction ($P<0.01$) in the rate of growth in the total area of their CNV and in the severity of leakage compared with the control group [53]. The 0.3 mg dose appeared more effective than the 1 mg or 3 mg doses, so the 0.3 mg became the FDA-approved dose.

Bevacizumab

Drug Overview

Research from the 1980s and 1990s has shown that VEGF inhibition using a murine and humanized monoclonal antibody against VEGF markedly suppressed tumor growth in vivo, thereby setting the stage for the development of bevacizumab. Bevacizumab is a humanized monoclonal antibody (IgG1) against human VEGF-A that selectively inhibits all isoforms and bioactive proteolytic breakdown products of VEGF-A. Bevacizumab is

an immunoglobulin G molecule that is comprised of amino acid sequences, which are about 93% human and 7% murine. FDA-approved in 2004 as treatment for metastatic colorectal cancer, bevacizumab was given intravenously at a dose of 5 mg/kg and infused every two weeks in combination with 5-fluorouracil. Additional phase III clinical trials with bevacizumab have since resulted in FDA approval for the treatment of breast, lung, kidney, and brain cancers [55]. No evidence of an antibody immunogenic response to bevacizumab has been found in any clinical trials, confirming the success of the humanization technique.

Bevacizumab is commercially available as 100 and 400 mg preservative-free, single-use vials in a volume of 4 or 16 mL (25 mg/mL). The 100 mg product is formulated in 240 mg α(alpha),α(alpha)-trehalose dihydrate, 23.2 mg sodium phosphate (monobasic, monohydrate), 4.8 mg sodium phosphate (dibasic, anhydrous), and 1.6 mg polysorbate 20, and should be diluted in water prior to intravenous infusion. For off-label ophthalmic use, bevacizumab is not diluted, but rather dispensed into individual syringes for intravitreal injection and the volume (dose) of injection ranges from 0.05 mL (1.25 mg) to 0.1 mL (2.5 mg).

The intravitreal pharmacokinetics of monoclonal antibodies was initially studied in monkeys and rabbits and found to be about 5.6 days [56, 57]. Bevacizumab has since been studied experimentally in rabbits and is shown to have a half-life of 4.32 days [58]. When 1.25 mg was injected in rabbits, concentrations of over 10 μ(mu)g/mL bevacizumab were maintained in the vitreous for at least 30 days. Additional animal studies in rabbits and monkeys suggest a half-life of bevacizumab in the range of four–six days [59, 60]. A human study reported that the half-life of intravitreal bevacizumab was approximately three days, and also showed that a single dose of intravitreal bevacizumab was likely to provide complete intravitreal VEGF blockade for a minimum of four weeks [61]. Another human study has suggested a half-life of 6.7 days while yet another study has reported a half-life of as long as 9.8 days [62, 63]. The exact half-life of bevacizumab in the eye is uncertain at this time and may vary depending on the extent of vitreous liquefication and the phakic status of the eye.

Bevacizumab has a molecular weight of approximately 149 kDa and there was a question of whether such a large molecule could penetrate the retina. Han et al. were the first to show that a full-length immunoglobulin was capable of penetrating the rabbit retina after an intravitreal injection [64]. Subsequently, Sharar et al. used qualitative immunofluorescence to show that intravitreal bevacizumab was able to completely penetrate the retina by 24 h and was essentially absent at four weeks after an injection [65] Moreover, Dib et al. demonstrated subretinal detection of bevacizumab after an intravitreal injection in rabbit eyes. They detected bevacizumab molecules in the subretinal space of all six eyes studied 2 h after an intravitreal bevacizumab injection of 0.05 mL (1.25 mg), suggesting that the molecule could rapidly diffuse through the retina [66].

Published Studies

Although systemic bevacizumab (5 mg/kg) was shown to reduce leakage from CNV, decrease central retinal thickness (CRT) using optical coherence tomography (OCT), and significantly improve vision in neovascular AMD [67–70], the intravenous use of bevacizumab for neovascular AMD was never widely adopted because the intravitreal approach uses up to 500-fold less drug, is much less expensive, and is perceived to be safer due to the smaller dose of drug. In the first-reported case [71] of intravitreal bevacizumab, a patient with recurrent CNV secondary to AMD, who had previously been treated with verteporfin photodynamic therapy (PDT) in combination with triamcinolone acetonide and then treated with pegaptanib injections, was shown to experience a reduction in retinal thickness with resolution of subretinal fluid using OCT imaging and the visual distortion resolved within one week following a single injection of 1.0 mg bevacizumab. Subsequently, several retrospective [72–86] and prospective [73, 87–97] studies of intravitreal bevacizumab (dose range 1.0–2.5 mg) in neovascular AMD patients have been published, all demonstrating clinically significant

improvement in mean visual acuity, reduction in fluorescein angiographic leakage, resolution of OCT-visualized edema in up to 90% of bevacizumab-treated patients, and apparent overall clinical safety (see example of treatment effect in Fig. 6.1). Most studies have been small (up to 100 patients), uncontrolled studies with different retreatment criteria and outcome measures.

A randomized, prospective clinical trial compared verteporfin PDT with bevacizumab (2.5 mg) for the treatment of predominantly classic CNV secondary to AMD and found that at month 6, all 32 eyes (100%) receiving bevacizumab lost fewer than15 letters of visual acuity compared with 73.3% of the PDT-receiving eyes ($P=0.002$) [98]. The OCT outcomes were significantly better at 3 and 6 months in patients treated with bevacizumab versus the PDT group ($P=0.04$ and $P=0.002$, respectively). The study showed overall benefit of treatment with bevacizumab compared with PDT. Another study showed the effect of previous PDT treatment on the response to bevacizumab injections. The authors compared treatment-naïve eyes (80) with eyes previously treated with PDT (29) and showed that both groups had equal anatomic and functional improvements. However, the eyes previously treated with PDT required fewer injections (4.22) when compared with treatment-naïve eyes (6.13) [99]. The rationale of using combined therapy is to either reduce the number of anti-VEGF injections in wet AMD [98–100], or to improve the efficacy of anti-VEGF treatment in cases of exudative maculopathy such as polypoidal choroidal vasculopathy [100]. Combined therapy is now being evaluated by several prospective randomized trials and Chapter 7 discusses this topic in greater detail.

Systemic and ocular adverse events (AEs) attributable to intravitreal bevacizumab have been rare with the most common ocular side effects being endophthalmitis, uveitis, submacular hemorrhage, and RPE tears. In a recent retrospective safety assessment of intravitreal bevacizumab involving 1,173 patients, there were 18 (1.5%) reported systemic AEs, including five deaths (0.4%) and the ocular AEs included subconjunctival hemorrhage [838 cases (19% of 4,303

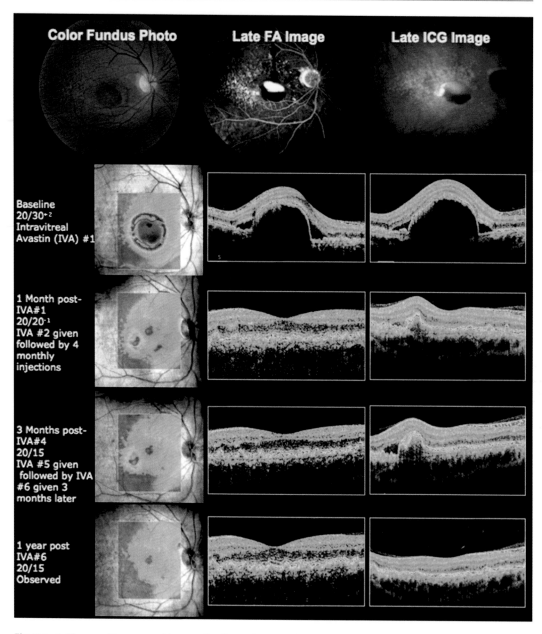

Fig. 6.1 A 72-year-old woman with age-related macular degeneration diagnosed with an occult lesion and a vascularized retinal pigment epithelium detachment (PED) in the right eye. She received four-monthly bevacizumab injections and then was treated every three months. Color fundus images with late-phase images of the fluorescein and indocyanine angiograms at baseline are shown. Optical coherence tomography (OCT) responses from baseline to one year after the last bevacizumab injection are shown. Horizontal (*left*) and vertical (*right*) OCT B-scans through the central macula and visual acuity are shown. Resolution of the PED was observed at the last follow-up visit

injections)], increased intraocular pressure (IOP), endophthalmitis, and tractional retinal detachment [seven cases (0.16%)] each [85]. The low rates of systemic complications in these studies were consistent with the rates of these life-threatening adverse events in the general, untreated population and those reported in an earlier survey of 5,228 patients [101].

Ranibizumab

Drug Overview

Ranibizumab is a humanized antigen-binding fragment (Fab) derived from the same murine monoclonal antibody as bevacizumab. As with bevacizumab, ranibizumab binds VEGF-A at the same location and inhibits all isoforms of VEGF-A as well as the bioactive proteolytic breakdown products of VEGF-A. The binding of ranibizumab to VEGF-A prevents the interaction of VEGF-A with VEGFR1 and VEGFR2 on the surface of endothelial cells, reducing endothelial cell proliferation, vascular leakage, and new blood vessel formation [102]. Compared with the original Fab from the Fab on the humanized monoclonal antibody, ranibizumab contains six amino acid substitutions; five variable domain substitutions, and one constant domain substitution at the C-terminus of the heavy chain. Ranibizumab is a smaller molecule than bevacizumab with a molecular weight of only 48 kD. Like full-length monoclonal antibodies, the Fab molecules have been shown to easily penetrate the retina [57]. When compared with bevacizumab, there were no apparent differences in the retinal penetration and the ocular safety of ranibizumab in rabbit eyes [103]. Ranibizumab (10 mg/mL) is available in 0.3-mL vials and approved by the FDA for monthly intravitreal injections using a volume (dose) of 0.05 mL (0.5 mg) in patients with neovascular AMD.

Published Trials

Level I evidence supporting the use of ranibizumab for the treatment of neovascular AMD includes the published Phase III trials known as the MARINA (Minimally Classic/Occult Trial of the Anti-VEGF Antibody Ranibizumab in the treatment of Neovascular AMD) [104] and ANCHOR (Anti-VEGF Antibody for the Treatment of Predominantly Classic CNV in AMD) [105, 106] trials as well as additional quality-of-life and subgroup analyses [107–111]. In addition, the Phase IIIb trials, including the PIER (A Phase IIIb, Multicenter, Randomized, Double-Masked, Sham Injection-Controlled Study of the Efficacy and Safety of Ranibizumab in Subjects with Subfoveal Choroidal Neovasularization with or without Classic CNV Secondary to Age-Related Macular Degeneration) [112], and SAILOR (Safety and Tolerability of Ranibizumab in Naive and Previously Treated Subjects With CNV Secondary to AMD) [113] trials. Smaller open-label prospective trials such as the PrONTO (Prospective OCT Imaging of Patients with Neovascular AMD Treated with Intraocular Lucentis) study provided additional important dosing information [114, 115].

The pivotal phase III MARINA [104] and ANCHOR [105] trials established ranibizumab as the first FDA-approved drug that prevents vision loss and improves vision in the majority of patients with all subtypes of neovascular AMD. At 12 and 24 months in the MARINA trial, 90–95% of patients treated with 0.3 or 0.5 mg ranibizumab lost fewer than 15 letters of visual acuity compared with 53–64% of control patients; also at 12 and 24 months, 25–34% of ranibizumab-treated patients gained at least 15 letters of visual acuity compared with 4–5% of control patients [104]. The ANCHOR trial, which compared ranibizumab with PDT, had similar findings at 12 and 24 months: 90–96% of the ranibizumab-treated versus 64–66% of the PDT-treated patients lost fewer than 15 letters of visual acuity, whereas 34–41% of the ranibizumab group versus 6% of the PDT group gained more than 15 letters [105].

Analyses of fluorescein angiographic data from both the MARINA and ANCHOR studies also revealed statistically significant decreases in area of CNV, leakage from CNV, area of serous sensory retinal detachment (SSRD), and formation of disciform scar/subretinal fibrosis at both 12 and 24 months after ranibizumab treatment [105, 116]. A retrospective analysis of OCT/fluorescein angiography outcomes prospectively collected in a subset of 46 patients from the MARINA study showed a statistically significant decrease at 12 months in mean foveal center point thickness of the ranibizumab-treated group compared with the sham-treated group [116].

Clinical studies such as the PIER Study, the SAILOR Study, and the PrONTO Study have investigated alternative, less-frequent ranibizumab dosing strategies in an attempt to lower rates of injections while achieving the same visual acuity outcomes. The two-year phase I/II open label PrONTO trial evaluated an OCT-guided, variable dosing regimen of monthly intravitreal ranibizumab (0.5 mg) for three months followed by intravitreal ranibizumab as needed based on OCT-defined retreatment criteria in 40 patients with all subtypes of neovascular AMD [114] (Examples of different OCT-guided treatment approaches can be seen in Figs. 6.2 and 6.3). At the first year, 95% (38/40) of treated patients had lost less than 15 letters of visual acuity; 35% (14/40) of treated patients had gained at least 15 letters of visual acuity, and the mean increase in visual acuity was 9.3 letters. The mean number of injections for the first year was 5.6 (range 3–13); the most common reason for reinjection was a loss of at least five letters of visual acuity in association with presence of macular fluid. The earliest signs of recurrent fluid in the macula following cessation of treatment were detectable using OCT (Fig. 6.3) [117]. At 12 months after treatment, the mean central retinal thickness (CRT) as measured by OCT decreased by 178 microns ($P < 0.001$). At 24 months, the results were virtually identical with a mean visual acuity change of 11.1 letters, a mean CRT/OCT decrease of 215 microns, and a mean number of injections of 10 (range 3–25) over two years [114]. The PrONTO trial showed that for future clinical trials and clinical practice, it might be possible to use qualitative OCT to determine the basis for retreatment.

The two-year PIER trial [112] examined the efficacy and safety of 0.3 or 0.5 mg ranibizumab monthly for three months followed by quarterly dosing. The first-year data showed that a significantly greater proportion of patients receiving ranibizumab lost less than 15 letters of visual acuity (83.3% of patients in the 0.3 mg group and 90.2% of patients in the 0.5 mg group) compared with 49.2% of patients in the sham-treated group ($P < 0.0001$ for each dose level versus sham). However, there was no significant difference in the proportion of patients who gained at least 15 letters: 11.7 and 13.1% of treated patients (0.3 and 0.5 mg, respectively) compared with 9.5% in the sham group. Although the overall safety profile of ranibizumab in the PIER trial was similar to the first year of the MARINA and ANCHOR trials, the efficacy outcomes of the PIER trial were less beneficial than the MARINA and ANCHOR trials most likely because some patients required more frequent dosing than quarterly dosing to achieve maximal benefit. On the basis of the PrONTO and PIER trials, OCT-guided retreatment appears more promising than less-frequent fixed-interval dosing for all patients if the goal is to achieve the same excellent outcomes as monthly dosing while reducing the number of overall injections (Fig. 6.4). Another strategy to decrease the treatment burden is to use the treat-and-extend strategy. In this approach, patients are treated at every monthly visit until there is no longer any fluid in the macula, and then the visit interval is extended by about two weeks and injections are given at every visit. The interval is extended until fluid is detected at a follow-up visit or a fixed interval of every three months is achieved [118, 119].

> **Pearl**
>
> Ranibizumab is the most effective anti-VEGF drug approved by the FDA for the treatment of wet AMD. Several studies are exploring different doses and treatment intervals with ranibizumab as well the combination of ranibizumab with other treatment modalities. To date, anti-VEGF therapy alone, given at a dose of 0.5 mg, either given as a monthly injection or given as needed based on OCT surveillance, results in the best visual acuity outcomes.

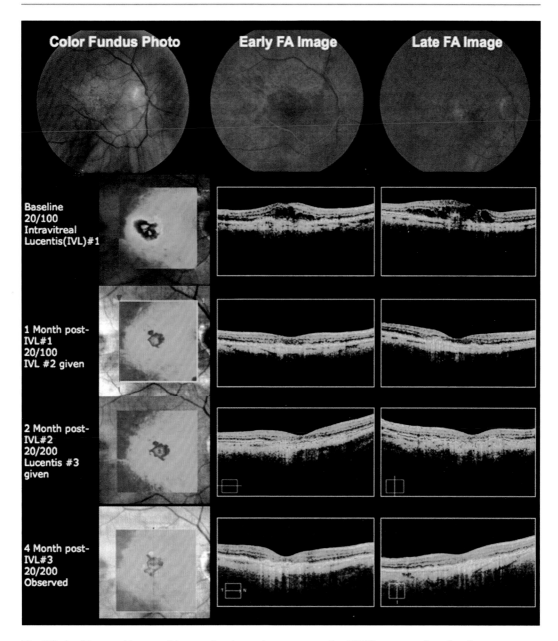

Fig. 6.2 An 83-year-old man with age-related macular degeneration diagnosed with an occult lesion in the right eye. He received the three ranibizumab injections using a treat and extend strategy without recurrence. Color fundus images with early- and late-phase fluorescein angiographic images at baseline are shown. Optical coherence tomography (OCT) response from baseline to one year after the last ranibizumab injections are shown. Horizontal (*left*) and vertical (*right*) OCT B-scans through the central macula and visual acuity are shown. The patient had a good anatomical improvement without gain of visual acuity after the intravitreal injections

Safety Data

After two years of follow-up, MARINA and ANCHOR showed that the most common ocular complications were presumed endophthalmitis (1.3% of eyes in MARINA; 1.4% of eyes in ANCHOR) and uveitis (1.3% of eyes in MARINA; 0.7% of eyes in ANCHOR) [104–106]. A recent review evaluated the safety data from the 3,252

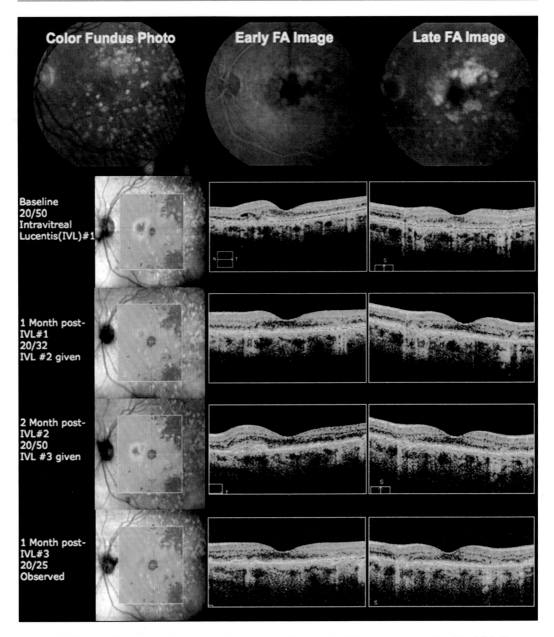

Fig. 6.3 A 78-year-old woman with age-related macular degeneration diagnosed with an occult lesion in the left eye. She received the three ranibizumab injections using a treat and extend strategy with recurrence. Color fundus images with early- and late-phase of fluorescein angiogram at baseline are shown. Optical coherence tomography (OCT) responses from baseline are shown. Horizontal (*left*) and vertical (*right*) OCT B-scans through the central macula and visual acuity are shown. The patient had a good anatomical and functional response after the second injection. However, the intraretinal fluid recurred just before the third injection. This patient should be followed closely to avoid lost of visual acuity

patients in ANCHOR, MARINA, PIER, and SAILOR (level I evidence), who had received over 28,500 intravitreal ranibizumab injections. The rate per injection of presumed endophthalmitis (0.05%) and serious intraocular inflammation (0.03%) were low [120].

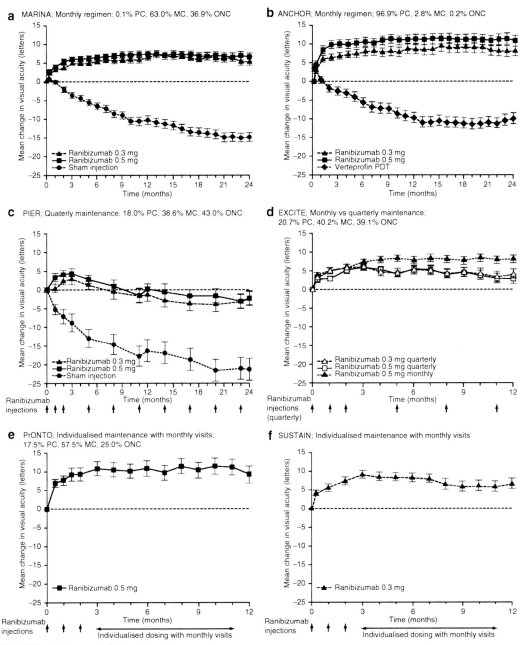

The LOCF method was used to impute missing data.
Vertical bars are ± 1 standard error of the mean.
LOCF = last observation carried forward; PC=predominantly classic; PDF=photodynamic therapy; MC=minimally classic; ONC=occult (with no classic)

Fig. 6.4 Mean change from baseline in best-corrected visual acuity by month for ranibizumab trials: (**a**) MARINA, (**b**) ANCHOR, (**c**) PIER, (**d**) EXCITE, (**e**) PrONTO, (**f**) SUSTAIN (Reprinted from Mitchell et al. [120]. With permission from BMJ Publishing Group Ltd)

The rate of systemic adverse events, including nonfatal myocardial infarction, nonfatal stroke, and death from a vascular or unknown cause, were similar in both trials [104–106]. In MARINA, the rates were 3.8% (sham), 4.6% (0.3 mg of ranibizumab), and 4.6% (0.5 mg of ranibizumab), and in ANCHOR the rates were 4.2% (verteporfin PDT), 4.4% (0.3 mg of ranibizumab), and 5.0% (0.5 mg of ranibizumab). The recently completed Safety Assessment of Intravitreal Lucentis for AMD (SAILOR) trial showed higher stroke rates with increased dosage (0.7% and 1.2% for the 0.3 and 0.5 mg groups, respectively), but the difference was not statistically significant [113]. Incidence of stroke was higher with preexisting risk factors, particularly a previous stroke history (2.7% (0.3 mg) and 9.6% (0.5 mg)) or arrhythmia. Finally, frequencies of cardiovascular events and ocular serious AEs were similar for the two dose groups [112, 113]. According to those trials, the incidence of stroke with ranibizumab is low, but needs to be continuously monitored in ongoing post marketing studies. Moreover, it is important to discuss the benefit–risk profile with individual patients, particularly those with a history of, or risk factors for, heart attack and stroke [120].

Upcoming Clinical Trials

The EXCITE study directly compared the PIER quarterly regimen (0.3 and 0.5 mg) against monthly injections (0.3 mg) [121]. Mean visual acuity (VA) gain over baseline was observed for the whole 12-month trial in all groups. At month 12, compared with month 3, the VA gain was slightly decreased with quarterly dosing (−1.9 and −2.8 letters with 0.3 and 0.5 mg of ranibizumab, respectively). By comparison, in the group receiving monthly ranibizumab at a dose of 0.3 mg, the month 12 VA was slightly increased by + 0.8 letters (NCT00275821).

The SAILOR trial was a single masked, multicenter phase IIIb study to evaluate the safety and tolerability of two doses of intravitreal ranibizumab in patients with neovascular AMD. SAILOR Cohort 1 investigated three loading doses followed by quarterly monitoring visits and injections guided by VA (loss of five-letter loss or more) and OCT criteria such as an increase of 100 μ(mu) in CRT. The mean VA change increased from baseline over the first three injections, but then decreased to a mean gain over baseline of 2.3 letters for both ranibizumab doses, a better result than in PIER, but suboptimal when compared with ANCHOR and MARINA [120].

The Study of Ranibizumab in Patients with Subfoveal Choroidal Neovascularization Secondary to Age-Related Macular Degeneration (SUSTAIN) trial evaluated three 0.3 mg loading doses, followed by as-needed injection according to the same criteria used in the SAILOR trial [120, 122, 123] The interim analysis of 69 patients showed that at 12 months, most of the VA gain obtained during the first three months was maintained. The final results using this flexible regimen are pending.

What happens after two years of treatment? All the studies with intravitreal injections of ranibizumab have the longest follow-up of 24 months. In the HORIZON extension trial of MARINA and ANCHOR, 61% of patients needed some additional treatments in the third year. Moreover, better VA and anatomical outcomes after two years predicted a longer time to retreatment in this period. However, some patients lost VA and this loss might be related to undertreatment during the extension period [124].

There are also two clinical trials that are evaluating the high-dose regimen (2.0 mg) of ranibizumab for wet AMD. The SAVE trial is a phase I/II study, that will evaluate the safety, tolerability, and efficacy of 2.0 mg ranibizumab. Patients with nine or more injections/year with recurrent fluid on OCT are eligible for this study. After three loading doses, the subjects will be randomized between a regimen of every four or six weeks according to the presence of any fluid or hemorrhage on OCT or clinical exam (NCT01025332). The HARBOR trial is currently enrolling patients without previous treatment and will compare monthly with an as-needed regimen of intravitreal ranibizumab injections of 0.5 mg versus 2.0 mg (NCT00891735). Results of those trials are expected at the end of 2011 and 2013, respectively.

In summary, monthly intravitreal injections of ranibizumab over two years remains the gold standard for treatment and is the only long-term level I evidence supporting the use of pan-VEGF inhibition for the treatment of neovascular AMD. Fixed-interval dosing of greater than one-month intervals has failed to yield visual acuity outcomes that are as good as monthly dosing. OCT-guided variable dosing regimens show more promise than fixed interval dosing in that the studies appear to achieve a sustained improvement in visual acuity compared with baseline, and fewer injections are required compared with monthly dosing. A treat-and-extend regimen in which a dry macula is maintained and the treatment intervals are extended may be another alternative to monthly dosing, but prospective trials using this regimen are underway. Trials using higher doses of ranibizumab (2.0 mg) could potentially reduce the number of injections per year with the same visual acuity outcomes as monthly dosing.

Head-to-Head Trials: Ranibizumab Versus Bevacizumab

The current studies show that ranibizumab is the most effective treatment of neovascular AMD based on level I evidence. However, as previously described, small prospective and mainly retrospective studies have shown excellent anatomical and functional outcomes with bevacizumab. Ranibizumab and bevacizumab are derived from the same monoclonal antibody, but bevacizumab has relatively low cost and some studies have even showed that it has greater intravitreal half life compared with ranibizumab.

A retrospective study compared patients treated with bevacizumab (324 eyes) versus ranibizumab (128 eyes) [125]. After 12 months, both treatments improved visual acuity with no statistical difference (27.3% and 20.2%, respectively). Regarding the number of injections, the bevacizumab group required fewer injections than ranibizumab after one year (4.4 versus 6.2, respectively) [125]. Another retrospective study evaluated 84 patients that were being treated with bevacizumab and then switched to ranibizumab after ranibizumab became commercially available [126]. After the same follow-up length for both treatment modalities, the best-obtained VA

(20/63), the mean VA at the final visit (20/80), and the monthly number of injections (0.66) were the same [126]. These preliminary results from retrospective studies suggest that the clinical effect of both drugs is similar. However, all these data need to be confirmed by prospective randomized studies.

The National Eye Institute-sponsored large, randomized controlled trial comparing ranibizumab and bevacizumab (Comparison of AMD Treatment Trials (CATT) was published recently in the New England Journal of Medicine (Martin DF, Maguire MG et al. Ranibizumab and bevacizumab for neovascular age-related macular degeneration. N Engl J Med. 2011 19;364(20): 1897-908). A predefined secondary endpoint of the study was the cost of treatment. Cost and efficacy are the basis for the off-label use of bevacizumab in neovascular AMD. In the United States, relative drug costs for the two agents are estimated at US$50 for bevacizumab compared with US$2,036 for ranibizumab. This trial has enrolled 1,200 patients and successfully compared the two drugs and two different dosing regimens: monthly regimen versus an "as-needed" regimen (i.e., drug injected only when evidence of exudation was present). The study showed that monthly injections of either ranibizumab or bevacizumab were equivalent, resulting in the same visual acuity and fluorescein angiographic outcomes after one year of follow-up. Moreover, ranibizumab administered monthly or "as needed" resulted in equivalent visual acuity outcomes, and "as-needed" dosing of bevacizumab and ranibizumab were shown to be equivalent. However, the "as-neeeded bevacizumab regimen was not as good as monthly injections of either bevacizumab or ranibizumab. The comparison proved inconclusive. This outcome could be explained in part by a subgroup of patients having a less durable treatment effect and thus more frequent injections were required. (Rosenfeld PJ. Bevacizumab versus ranibizumab for AMD. N Engl J Med 2011 19;364(20): 1966-7) It is important to remember that the CATT study addressed the question of efficacy, but the study was insufficiently powered to evaluate the differences in drug-related adverse events. The results from the second year of CATT and from at at least five other large randomized trials worldwide comparing bevacizumab and ranibizumab are expected to address the long term efficacy and safety both drugs.

> **Pearl**
>
> The CATT, a head-to-head trial comparing the efficacy of monthly injections of bevacizumab or ranibizumab in eyes of patients with neovascular AMD, showed that both drugs were equivalent.

Promising VEGF Inhibitors

Aflibercept (VEGF-Trap Eye or Eyelea) is a soluble fusion protein, which combines ligand-binding elements taken from the extracellular components of VEGF receptors 1 and 2 fused to the Fc portion of IgG1 [127]. Experimental data showed that VEGF Trap should penetrate to all retinal layers [128] and it has at least a 200-fold higher affinity than ranibizumab [129]. Unlike the currently available anti-VEGF dugs that inhibit just VEGF-A, VEGF-Trap binds also VEGF-B, and PlGF [129, 130]. VEGF Trap-Eye has undergone Phase 1 and 2 clinical trials in wet AMD, and is presently in Phase 3 clinical testing. The Phase 1 and 2 studies, known as CLEAR-IT (CLinical Evaluation of Antiangiogenesis in the Retina Intravitreal Trial), showed safety and a functional and anatomical improvement specially with a dose of 0.5 and 2 mg [131]. In terms of visual acuity, monthly and quarterly dosing did not result in substantially different results at eight weeks. However, monthly dosing was numerically superior to quarterly dosing at 12 weeks, although not statistically significant [132]. VEGF Trap Eye might be a new anti-VEGF treatment that requires fewer intravitreal injections. In the ongoing phase 3 VIEW 1 and VIEW 2 studies (VEGF Trap-Eye: Investigation of Efficacy and Safety in Wet AMD), VEGF Trap Eye is being compared with the standard monthly 0.5 mg ranibizumab dosing regimen (NCT00509795).

Dosing monthly or every two months, VEGF Trap Eye was non-inferior to monthly 0.5 mg ranibizumab and therefore may be an effective treatment option for neovascular AMD potentially less frequent injections.

KH902 (Chengdu Kanghong Biotechnology) is also a fusion protein that combines ligand-binding elements taken from the extracellular domains of VEGF receptors 1(Flt-1) and 2 (KDR) to the Fc portion of IgG1 [133]. However, different from VEGF Trap, KH902 also includes the extra extracellular domain four of VEGF receptor 2(KDRd4), which may stabilize the three-dimensional structure and increase the efficiency of dimerization [134]. KH902 has a much higher affinity for VEGF due to this extra extracellular domain and may have a longer half life in the vitreous [133, 135]. In-vivo experiments have shown that intravitreal KH902 was able to inhibit leakage and growth of CNV in rhesus monkeys without signs of toxicity at doses of 300 and 500 μ(mu)g [133]. A phase 1 study showed that intravitreal injections up to 1.0 mg of KH902 were well tolerated with VA improvement of >15 letters (3 lines) in 57.2% of patients and a macular thickness reduction of 104 μm after 42 days [136].

Pazopanib (GW786034; GlaxoSmithKline) is a multi-targeted receptor tyrosine kinase inhibitor that has been formulated as an eye drop for the treatment of neovascular AMD. Pazopanib acts by downstream inhibition of receptor activation by VEGF (1, 2 and 3), PDGF (α(alpha) and β(beta)), and stem cell growth factor (c-Kit), resulting in a multi-targeted drug against neovascular diseases [137]. Experimental data showed safety and laser-induced CNV regression after oral [138] and topical [139] administration in mice. A safety and tolerability study in healthy volunteers showed tolerance for the 2 and 4 mg/mL doses used up top three times daily for 14 days [140]. An ongoing phase II study is investigating a 2 and 5 mg/mL dose given three times daily and a 5 mg/mL dose given four times daily for 28 days in neovascular AMD patients (NCT00733304).

Pearl
The next generation of anti-VEGF agents may be more effective by binding VEGF with higher affinity, by blocking the signaling of the VEGF-receptor, or by targeting different VEGF-related and pro-angiogenic proteins. Effectiveness may be improved based on VA improvements or the requirement for fewer injections.

Conclusion

Over the past decade, great advances have occurred in the management of neovascular AMD; from laser photocoagulation to verteporfin PDT and then on to the use of anti-VEGF-A drugs to inhibit neovascularization and prevent vision loss. Three such agents — pegaptanib sodium, ranibizumab, and bevacizumab — have been used successfully for this purpose with bevacizumab and ranibizumab gaining the most acceptance and clinical success. Based on phase III clinical trial data, ranibizumab has been shown to be the most effective and safe anti-VEGF drug for the treatment of all forms of CNV in neovascular AMD. However, bevacizumab is the more frequently used treatment throughout the world based on the perception that bevacizumab has similar efficacy and safety, but at a much lower cost. This perception will be tested by the ongoing comparative clinical trials. Data from ongoing trials comparing different treatment regimens, higher doses of drugs, and higher affinity drugs will be forthcoming over the next few years and should greatly improve the overall treatment burden for both the patient and the clinician. Whether these regimens, doses, and higher affinity drugs increase visual acuity outcomes remains to be determined.

References

1. Bird AC, Bressler NM, Bressler SB, et al. An international classification and grading system for age-related maculopathy and age-related macular degeneration. The International ARM Epidemiological Study Group. Surv Ophthalmol. 1995;39(5):367–74.

2. Ciulla TA, Amador AG, Zinman B. Diabetic retinopathy and diabetic macular edema: pathophysiology, screening, and novel therapies. Diabetes Care. 2003; 26(9):2653–64.

3. Cugati S, Wang JJ, Rochtchina E, Mitchell P. Ten-year incidence of retinal vein occlusion in an older population: the Blue Mountains Eye Study. Arch Ophthalmol. 2006;124(5):726–32.

4. Chakravarthy U, Augood C, Bentham GC, et al. Cigarette smoking and age-related macular degeneration in the EUREYE Study. Ophthalmology. 2007; 114(6):1157–63.

5. Campochiaro PA, Soloway P, Ryan SJ, Miller JW. The pathogenesis of choroidal neovascularization in patients with age-related macular degeneration. Mol Vis. 1999;5:34.

6. Yannuzzi LA, Negrao S, Iida T, et al. Retinal angiomatous proliferation in age-related macular degeneration. Retina. 2001;21(5):416–34.

7. Leung DW, Cachianes G, Kuang WJ, Goeddel DV, Ferrara N. Vascular endothelial growth factor is a secreted angiogenic mitogen. Science. 1989;246(4935): 1306–9.

8. Keck PJ, Hauser SD, Krivi G, et al. Vascular permeability factor, an endothelial cell mitogen related to PDGF. Science. 1989;246(4935):1309–12.

9. Senger DR, Connolly DT, Van de Water L, Feder J, Dvorak HF. Purification and NH2-terminal amino acid sequence of guinea pig tumor-secreted vascular permeability factor. Cancer Res. 1990;50(6):1774–8.

10. Eriksson U, Alitalo K. Structure, expression and receptor-binding properties of novel vascular endothelial growth factors. Curr Top Microbiol Immunol. 1999;237:41–57.

11. Ferrara N, Gerber HP, LeCouter J. The biology of VEGF and its receptors. Nat Med. 2003;9(6): 669–76.

12. Gerhardt H, Ruhrberg C, Abramsson A, Fujisawa H, Shima D, Betsholtz C. Neuropilin-1 is required for endothelial tip cell guidance in the developing central nervous system. Dev Dyn. 2004;231(3):503–9.

13. Kawasaki T, Kitsukawa T, Bekku Y, et al. A requirement for neuropilin-1 in embryonic vessel formation. Development. 1999;126(21):4895–902.

14. Ferrara N. Vascular endothelial growth factor: basic science and clinical progress. Endocr Rev. 2004; 25(4):581–611.

15. Keyt BA, Berleau LT, Nguyen HV, et al. The carboxyl-terminal domain (111–165) of vascular endothelial growth factor is critical for its mitogenic potency. J Biol Chem. 1996;271(13):7788–95.

16. Alon T, Hemo I, Itin A, Pe'er J, Stone J, Keshet E. Vascular endothelial growth factor acts as a survival factor for newly formed retinal vessels and has implications for retinopathy of prematurity. Nat Med. 1995;1(10):1024–8.

17. Csaky KG, Baffi JZ, Byrnes GA, et al. Recruitment of marrow-derived endothelial cells to experimental choroidal neovascularization by local expression of vascular endothelial growth factor. Exp Eye Res. 2004;78(6):1107–16.

18. Lamoreaux WJ, Fitzgerald ME, Reiner A, Hasty KA, Charles ST. Vascular endothelial growth factor increases release of gelatinase A and decreases release of tissue inhibitor of metalloproteinases by microvascular endothelial cells in vitro. Microvasc Res. 1998;55(1):29–42.

19. Pepper MS, Ferrara N, Orci L, Montesano R. Vascular endothelial growth factor (VEGF) induces plasminogen activators and plasminogen activator inhibitor-1 in microvascular endothelial cells. Biochem Biophys Res Commun. 1991;181(2):902–6.

20. Uhlmann S, Friedrichs U, Eichler W, Hoffmann S, Wiedemann P. Direct measurement of VEGF-induced nitric oxide production by choroidal endothelial cells. Microvasc Res. 2001;62(2):179–89.

21. Papapetropoulos A, Garcia-Cardena G, Madri JA, Sessa WC. Nitric oxide production contributes to the angiogenic properties of vascular endothelial growth factor in human endothelial cells. J Clin Invest. 1997;100(12):3131–9.

22. Roberts WG, Palade GE. Neovasculature induced by vascular endothelial growth factor is fenestrated. Cancer Res. 1997;57(4):765–72.

23. Monsky WL, Fukumura D, Gohongi T, et al. Augmentation of transvascular transport of macromolecules and nanoparticles in tumors using vascular endothelial growth factor. Cancer Res. 1999;59(16): 4129–35.

24. Weis S, Shintani S, Weber A, et al. Src blockade stabilizes a Flk/cadherin complex, reducing edema and tissue injury following myocardial infarction. J Clin Invest. 2004;113(6):885–94.

25. Gilbert RE, Vranes D, Berka JL, et al. Vascular endothelial growth factor and its receptors in control and diabetic rat eyes. Lab Invest. 1998;78(8):1017–27.

26. Pe'er J, Shweiki D, Itin A, Hemo I, Gnessin H, Keshet E. Hypoxia-induced expression of vascular endothelial growth factor by retinal cells is a common factor in neovascularizing ocular diseases. Lab Invest. 1995;72(6):638–45.

27. Shima DT, Gougos A, Miller JW, et al. Cloning and mRNA expression of vascular endothelial growth factor in ischemic retinas of *Macaca fascicularis*. Invest Ophthalmol Vis Sci. 1996;37(7):1334–40.

28. Ozaki H, Seo MS, Ozaki K, et al. Blockade of vascular endothelial cell growth factor receptor signaling is sufficient to completely prevent retinal neovascularization. Am J Pathol. 2000;156(2):697–707.

29. Adamis AP, Shima DT, Tolentino MJ, et al. Inhibition of vascular endothelial growth factor prevents retinal ischemia-associated iris neovascularization in a nonhuman primate. Arch Ophthalmol. 1996;114(1):66–71.

30. Krzystolik MG, Afshari MA, Adamis AP, et al. Prevention of experimental choroidal neovascularization with intravitreal anti-vascular endothelial growth factor antibody fragment. Arch Ophthalmol. 2002;120(3):338–46.

31. Kliffen M, Sharma HS, Mooy CM, Kerkvliet S, de Jong PT. Increased expression of angiogenic growth factors in age-related maculopathy. Br J Ophthalmol. 1997;81(2):154–62.

32. Kvanta A, Algvere PV, Berglin L, Seregard S. Subfoveal fibrovascular membranes in age-related macular degeneration express vascular endothelial growth factor. Invest Ophthalmol Vis Sci. 1996;37(9):1929–34.

33. Rakic JM, Lambert V, Devy L, et al. Placental growth factor, a member of the VEGF family, contributes to the development of choroidal neovascularization. Invest Ophthalmol Vis Sci. 2003;44(7):3186–93.

34. Wells JA, Murthy R, Chibber R, et al. Levels of vascular endothelial growth factor are elevated in the vitreous of patients with subretinal neovascularisation. Br J Ophthalmol. 1996;80(4):363–6.

35. Adamis AP, Miller JW, Bernal MT, et al. Increased vascular endothelial growth factor levels in the vitreous of eyes with proliferative diabetic retinopathy. Am J Ophthalmol. 1994;118(4):445–50.

36. Aiello LP, Avery RL, Arrigg PG, et al. Vascular endothelial growth factor in ocular fluid of patients with diabetic retinopathy and other retinal disorders. N Engl J Med. 1994;331(22):1480–7.

37. Noma H, Minamoto A, Funatsu H, et al. Intravitreal levels of vascular endothelial growth factor and interleukin-6 are correlated with macular edema in branch retinal vein occlusion. Graefes Arch Clin Exp Ophthalmol. 2006;244(3):309–15.

38. Pe'er J, Folberg R, Itin A, Gnessin H, Hemo I, Keshet E. Vascular endothelial growth factor upregulation in human central retinal vein occlusion. Ophthalmology. 1998;105(3):412–6.

39. Haines JL, Schnetz-Boutaud N, Schmidt S, et al. Functional candidate genes in age-related macular degeneration: significant association with VEGF, VLDLR, and LRP6. Invest Ophthalmol Vis Sci. 2006;47(1):329–35.

40. Churchill AJ, Carter JG, Lovell HC, et al. VEGF polymorphisms are associated with neovascular age-related macular degeneration. Hum Mol Genet. 2006;15(19):2955–61.

41. Lin JM, Wan L, Tsai YY, et al. Vascular endothelial growth factor gene polymorphisms in age-related macular degeneration. Am J Ophthalmol. 2008;145(6):1045–51.

42. Jayasena SD. Aptamers: an emerging class of molecules that rival antibodies in diagnostics. Clin Chem. 1999;45(9):1628–50.

43. Ishida S, Usui T, Yamashiro K, et al. VEGF164 is proinflammatory in the diabetic retina. Invest Ophthalmol Vis Sci. 2003;44(5):2155–62.

44. Fairbrother WJ, Champe MA, Christinger HW, Keyt BA, Starovasnik MA. Solution structure of the heparin-binding domain of vascular endothelial growth factor. Structure. 1998;6(5):637–48.

45. Lim JI, Spee C, Hangai M, et al. Neuropilin-1 expression by endothelial cells and retinal pigment epithelial cells in choroidal neovascular membranes. Am J Ophthalmol. 2005;140(6):1044–50.

46. Ng EW, Adamis AP. Anti-VEGF aptamer (pegaptanib) therapy for ocular vascular diseases. Ann NY Acad Sci. 2006;1082:151–71.

47. Blaauwgeers HG, Holtkamp GM, Rutten H, et al. Polarized vascular endothelial growth factor secretion by human retinal pigment epithelium and localization of vascular endothelial growth factor receptors on the inner choriocapillaris. Evidence for a trophic paracrine relation. Am J Pathol. 1999;155(2):421–8.

48. Kamba T, McDonald DM. Mechanisms of adverse effects of anti-VEGF therapy for cancer. Br J Cancer. 2007;96(12):1788–95.

49. Nishijima K, Ng YS, Zhong L, et al. Vascular endothelial growth factor-A is a survival factor for retinal neurons and a critical neuroprotectant during the adaptive response to ischemic injury. Am J Pathol. 2007; 171(1):53–67.

50. Starita C, Patel M, Katz B, Adamis AP. Vascular endothelial growth factor and the potential therapeutic use of pegaptanib (macugen) in diabetic retinopathy. Dev Ophthalmol. 2007;39:122–48.

51. Verheul HM, Hammers H, van Erp K, et al. Vascular endothelial growth factor trap blocks tumor growth, metastasis formation, and vascular leakage in an orthotopic murine renal cell cancer model. Clin Cancer Res. 2007;13(14):4201–8.

52. Gonzales CR. Enhanced efficacy associated with early treatment of neovascular age-related macular degeneration with pegaptanib sodium: an exploratory analysis. Retina. 2005;25(7):815–27.

53. Gragoudas ES, Adamis AP, Cunningham Jr ET, Feinsod M, Guyer DR. Pegaptanib for neovascular age-related macular degeneration. N Engl J Med. 2004;351(27):2805–16.

54. Chakravarthy U, Adamis AP, Cunningham Jr ET, et al. Year 2 efficacy results of 2 randomized controlled clinical trials of pegaptanib for neovascular age-related macular degeneration. Ophthalmology. 2006;113(9):1508.e1–25.

55. National Cancer Institute. FDA Approval for Bevacizumab. 08/05/2009; http://www.cancer.gov/cancertopics/druginfo/fda-bevacizumab. Accessed 04/05/2010, 2010.

56. Mordenti J, Thomsen K, Licko V, et al. Intraocular pharmacokinetics and safety of a humanized monoclonal antibody in rabbits after intravitreal administration of a solution or a PLGA microsphere formulation. Toxicol Sci. 1999;52(1):101–6.

57. Mordenti J, Cuthbertson RA, Ferrara N, et al. Comparisons of the intraocular tissue distribution, pharmacokinetics, and safety of 125I-labeled full-length and Fab antibodies in rhesus monkeys following intravitreal administration. Toxicol Pathol. 1999; 27(5):536–44.

58. Bakri SJ, Kitzmann AS. Retinal pigment epithelial tear after intravitreal ranibizumab. Am J Ophthalmol. 2007;143(3):505–7.

59. Miyake T, Sawada O, Kakinoki M, et al. Pharmacokinetics of bevacizumab and its effect on vascular endothelial growth factor after intravitreal injection of bevacizumab in macaque eyes. Invest Ophthalmol Vis Sci. 2010;51(3):1606–8.

60. Nomoto H, Shiraga F, Kuno N, et al. Pharmacokinetics of bevacizumab after topical, subconjunctival, and intravitreal administration in rabbits. Invest Ophthalmol Vis Sci. 2009;50(10):4807–13.

61. Beer PM, Wong SJ, Hammad AM, Falk NS, O'Malley MR, Khan S. Vitreous levels of unbound bevacizumab and unbound vascular endothelial growth factor in two patients. Retina. 2006;26(8):871–6.

62. Krohne TU, Eter N, Holz FG, Meyer CH. Intraocular pharmacokinetics of bevacizumab after a single intravitreal injection in humans. Am J Ophthalmol. 2008;146(4):508–12.

63. Zhu Q, Ziemssen F, Henke-Fahle S, et al. Vitreous levels of bevacizumab and vascular endothelial growth factor-A in patients with choroidal neovascularization. Ophthalmology. 2008;115(10):1750–5. 1755 e1751.

64. Han DP. Intravitreal human immune globulin in a rabbit model of *Staphylococcus aureus* toxin-mediated endophthalmitis: a potential adjunct in the treatment of endophthalmitis. Trans Am Ophthalmol Soc. 2004;102:305–20.

65. Shahar J, Avery RL, Heilweil G, et al. Electrophysiologic and retinal penetration studies following intravitreal injection of bevacizumab (Avastin). Retina. 2006;26(3):262–9.

66. Dib E, Maia M, Longo-Maugeri IM, et al. Subretinal bevacizumab detection after intravitreous injection in rabbits. Invest Ophthalmol Vis Sci. 2008;49(3):1097–100.

67. Geitzenauer W, Michels S, Prager F, et al. Early effects of systemic and intravitreal bevacizumab (avastin) therapy for neovascular age-related macular degeneration. Klin Monbl Augenheilkd. 2006; 223(10):822–7.

68. Geitzenauer W, Michels S, Prager F, et al. Comparison of 2.5 mg/kg and 5 mg/kg systemic bevacizumab in neovascular age-related macular degeneration: twenty-four week results of an uncontrolled, prospective cohort study. Retina. 2008;28(10):1375–86.

69. Michels S, Rosenfeld PJ, Puliafito CA, Marcus EN, Venkatraman AS. Systemic bevacizumab (Avastin) therapy for neovascular age-related macular degeneration twelve-week results of an uncontrolled open-label clinical study. Ophthalmology. 2005;112(6):1035–47.

70. Moshfeghi AA, Rosenfeld PJ, Puliafito CA, et al. Systemic bevacizumab (Avastin) therapy for neovascular age-related macular degeneration: twenty-four-week results of an uncontrolled open-label clinical study. Ophthalmology. 2006;113(11):2002.e1–12.

71. Rosenfeld PJ, Moshfeghi AA, Puliafito CA. Optical coherence tomography findings after an intravitreal injection of bevacizumab (avastin) for neovascular age-related macular degeneration. Ophthalmic Surg Lasers Imaging. 2005;36(4):331–5.

72. Aggio FB, Farah ME, Silva WC, Melo GB. Intravitreal bevacizumab for exudative age-related macular degeneration after multiple treatments. Graefes Arch Clin Exp Ophthalmol. 2007;245(2):215–20.

73. Chen CY, Wong TY, Heriot WJ. Intravitreal bevacizumab (Avastin) for neovascular age-related macular degeneration: a short-term study. Am J Ophthalmol. 2007;143(3):510–2.

74. Cleary CA, Jungkim S, Ravikumar K, Kelliher C, Acheson RW, Hickey-Dwyer M. Intravitreal bevacizumab in the treatment of neovascular age-related macular degeneration, 6- and 9-month results. Eye (Lond). 2008;22(1):82–6.

75. Emerson MV, Lauer AK, Flaxel CJ, et al. Intravitreal bevacizumab (Avastin) treatment of neovascular age-related macular degeneration. Retina. 2007;27(4): 439–44.

76. Ghazi NG, Knape RM, Kirk TQ, Tiedeman JS, Conway BP. Intravitreal bevacizumab (avastin) treatment of retinal angiomatous proliferation. Retina. 2008;28(5):689–95.

77. Goff MJ, Johnson RN, McDonald HR, Ai E, Jumper JM, Fu A. Intravitreal bevacizumab for previously treated choroidal neovascularization from age-related macular degeneration. Retina. 2007;27(4):432–8.

78. Jonas JB, Libondi T, Ihloff AK, et al. Visual acuity change after intravitreal bevacizumab for exudative age-related macular degeneration in relation to subfoveal membrane type. Acta Ophthalmol Scand. 2007;85(5):563–5.

79. Jonas JB, Neumaier M. Vascular endothelial growth factor and basic fibroblast growth factor in exudative age-related macular degeneration and diffuse diabetic macular edema. Ophthalmic Res. 2007;39(3): 139–42.

80. Madhusudhana KC, Hannan SR, Williams CP, et al. Intravitreal bevacizumab (Avastin) for the treatment of choroidal neovascularization in age-related macular degeneration: results from 118 cases. Br J Ophthalmol. 2007;91(12):1716–7.

81. Melamud A, Stinnett S, Fekrat S. Treatment of neovascular age-related macular degeneration with intravitreal bevacizumab: efficacy of three consecutive monthly injections. Am J Ophthalmol. 2008;146(1): 91–5.

82. Pedersen R, Soliman W, Lund-Andersen H, Larsen M. Treatment of choroidal neovascularization using intravitreal bevacizumab. Acta Ophthalmol Scand. 2007;85(5):526–33.

83. Rich RM, Rosenfeld PJ, Puliafito CA, et al. Short-term safety and efficacy of intravitreal bevacizumab (Avastin) for neovascular age-related macular degeneration. Retina. 2006;26(5):495–511.

84. Spaide RF, Laud K, Fine HF, et al. Intravitreal bevacizumab treatment of choroidal neovascularization secondary to age-related macular degeneration. Retina. 2006;26(4):383–90.

85. Wu L, Martinez-Castellanos MA, Quiroz-Mercado H, et al. Twelve-month safety of intravitreal injections of bevacizumab (Avastin): results of the Pan-American Collaborative Retina Study Group (PACORES). Graefes Arch Clin Exp Ophthalmol. 2008;246(1): 81–7.

86. Yoganathan P, Deramo VA, Lai JC, Tibrewala RK, Fastenberg DM. Visual improvement following intravitreal bevacizumab (Avastin) in exudative age-related macular degeneration. Retina. 2006;26(9): 994–8.

87. Aisenbrey S, Ziemssen F, Volker M, et al. Intravitreal bevacizumab (Avastin) for occult choroidal neovascularization in age-related macular degeneration. Graefes Arch Clin Exp Ophthalmol. 2007;245(7):941–8.

88. Algvere PV, Steen B, Seregard S, Kvanta A. A prospective study on intravitreal bevacizumab (Avastin) for neovascular age-related macular degeneration of different durations. Acta Ophthalmol. 2008;86(5): 482–9.

89. Avery RL, Pieramici DJ, Rabena MD, Castellarin AA, Nasir MA, Giust MJ. Intravitreal bevacizumab (Avastin) for neovascular age-related macular degeneration. Ophthalmology. 2006;113(3):363–372.e5.

90. Azad RV, Khan MA, Chanana B, Azad S. Intravitreal bevacizumab for subfoveal choroidal neovascularization secondary to age-related macular degeneration in an Indian population. Jpn J Ophthalmol. 2008; 52(1):52–6.

91. Bashshur ZF, Bazarbachi A, Schakal A, Haddad ZA, El Haibi CP, Noureddin BN. Intravitreal bevacizumab for the management of choroidal neovascularization in age-related macular degeneration. Am J Ophthalmol. 2006;142(1):1–9.

92. Bashshur ZF, Haddad ZA, Schakal A, Jaafar RF, Saab M, Noureddin BN. Intravitreal bevacizumab for treatment of neovascular age-related macular degeneration: a one-year prospective study. Am J Ophthalmol. 2008;145(2):249–56.

93. Bashshur ZF, Haddad ZA, Schakal AR, Jaafar RF, Saad A, Noureddin BN. Intravitreal bevacizumab for treatment of neovascular age-related macular degeneration: the second year of a prospective study. Am J Ophthalmol. 2009;148(1):59–65.e1.

94. Costa RA, Jorge R, Calucci D, Cardillo JA, Melo Jr LA, Scott IU. Intravitreal bevacizumab for choroidal neovascularization caused by AMD (IBeNA Study): results of a phase 1 dose-escalation study. Invest Ophthalmol Vis Sci. 2006;47(10):4569–78.

95. Giansanti F, Virgili G, Bini A, et al. Intravitreal bevacizumab therapy for choroidal neovascularization secondary to age-related macular degeneration: 6-month results of an open-label uncontrolled clinical study. Eur J Ophthalmol. 2007;17(2):230–7.

96. Lazic R, Gabric N. Intravitreally administered bevacizumab (Avastin) in minimally classic and occult choroidal neovascularization secondary to age-related macular degeneration. Graefes Arch Clin Exp Ophthalmol. 2007;245(1):68–73.

97. Weigert G, Michels S, Sacu S, et al. Intravitreal bevacizumab (Avastin) therapy versus photodynamic therapy plus intravitreal triamcinolone for neovascular age-related macular degeneration: 6-month results of a prospective, randomised, controlled clinical study. Br J Ophthalmol. 2008;92(3):356–60.

98. Lazic R, Gabric N. Verteporfin therapy and intravitreal bevacizumab combined and alone in choroidal neovascularization due to age-related macular degeneration. Ophthalmology. 2007;114(6):1179–85.

99. Carneiro AM, Falcao MS, Brandao EM, Falcao-Reis FM. Intravitreal bevacizumab for neovascular age-related macular degeneration with or without prior treatment with photodynamic therapy: one-year results. Retina. 2010;30(1):85–92.

100. Hara R, Kawaji T, Inomata Y, et al. Photodynamic therapy alone versus combined with intravitreal bevacizumab for neovascular age-related macular degeneration without polypoidal choroidal vasculopathy in Japanese patients. Graefes Arch Clin Exp Ophthalmol. 2010;248(7):931–6. Epub 2010 Mar 10.

101. Fung AE, Rosenfeld PJ, Reichel E. The International Intravitreal Bevacizumab Safety Survey: using the internet to assess drug safety worldwide. Br J Ophthalmol. 2006;90(11):1344–9.

102. Ferrara N, Damico L, Shams N, Lowman H, Kim R. Development of ranibizumab, an anti-vascular endothelial growth factor antigen binding fragment, as therapy for neovascular age-related macular degeneration. Retina. 2006;26(8):859–70.

103. Zayit-Soudry S, Alfasi M, Goldstein M, et al. Variability among retina specialists in evaluating fluorescein angiograms of patients with neovascular age-related macular degeneration. Retina. 2007; 27(6):798–803.

104. Rosenfeld PJ, Brown DM, Heier JS, et al. Ranibizumab for neovascular age-related macular degeneration. N Engl J Med. 2006;355(14): 1419–31.

105. Brown DM, Kaiser PK, Michels M, et al. Ranibizumab versus verteporfin for neovascular age-related macular degeneration. N Engl J Med. 2006;355(14):1432–44.

106. Brown DM, Michels M, Kaiser PK, Heier JS, Sy JP, Ianchulev T. Ranibizumab versus verteporfin photodynamic therapy for neovascular age-related macular degeneration: two-year results of the ANCHOR study. Ophthalmology. 2009;116(1):57–65.e5.

107. Boyer DS, Antoszyk AN, Awh CC, Bhisitkul RB, Shapiro H, Acharya NR. Subgroup analysis of the MARINA study of ranibizumab in neovascular age-related macular degeneration. Ophthalmology. 2007;114(2):246–52.

108. Bressler NM. Antiangiogenic approaches to age-related macular degeneration today. Ophthalmology. 2009;116(10 Suppl):S15–23.

109. Cacho I, Dickinson CM, Reeves BC, Harper RA. Visual acuity and fixation characteristics in age-related macular degeneration. Optom Vis Sci. 2007;84(6):487–95.

110. Chang TS, Bressler NM, Fine JT, Dolan CM, Ward J, Klesert TR. Improved vision-related function after ranibizumab treatment of neovascular age-related macular degeneration: results of a randomized clinical trial. Arch Ophthalmol. 2007;125(11): 1460–9.

111. Kaiser PK, Brown DM, Zhang K, et al. Ranibizumab for predominantly classic neovascular age-related macular degeneration: subgroup analysis of first-year ANCHOR results. Am J Ophthalmol. 2007; 144(6):850–7.

112. Regillo CD, Brown DM, Abraham P, et al. Randomized, double-masked, sham-controlled trial of ranibizumab for neovascular age-related macular degeneration: PIER Study year 1. Am J Ophthalmol. 2008;145(2):239–48.

113. Michels M, Francom S, Wilson LJ. Systemic safety and risk factors associated with intravitreal ranibizumab in patients with choroidal neovascularization (CNV) secondary to age-related macular degeneration (AMD). 26th Annual Meeting of the American Society of Retina Specialists. Maui, 2008.

114. Lalwani GA, Rosenfeld PJ, Fung AE, et al. A variable-dosing regimen with intravitreal ranibizumab for neovascular age-related macular degeneration: year 2 of the PrONTO Study. Am J Ophthalmol. 2009;148(1):43–58.e1.

115. Rothenbuehler SP, Waeber D, Brinkmann CK, Wolf S, Wolf-Schnurrbusch UE. Effects of ranibizumab in patients with subfoveal choroidal neovascularization attributable to age-related macular degeneration. Am J Ophthalmol. 2009;147(5):831–7.

116. Kaiser PK, Blodi BA, Shapiro H, Acharya NR. Angiographic and optical coherence tomographic results of the MARINA study of ranibizumab in neovascular age-related macular degeneration. Ophthalmology. 2007;114(10):1868–75.

117. Fung AE, Lalwani GA, Rosenfeld PJ, et al. An optical coherence tomography-guided, variable dosing regimen with intravitreal ranibizumab (Lucentis) for neovascular age-related macular degeneration. Am J Ophthalmol. 2007;143(4):566–83.

118. Engelbert M, Zweifel SA, Freund KB. "Treat and extend" dosing of intravitreal antivascular endothelial growth factor therapy for type 3 neovascularization/retinal angiomatous proliferation. Retina. 2009;29(10):1424–31.

119. Spaide R. Ranibizumab according to need: a treatment for age-related macular degeneration. Am J Ophthalmol. 2007;143(4):679–80.

120. Mitchell P, Korobelnik JF, Lanzetta P, et al. Ranibizumab (Lucentis) in neovascular age-related macular degeneration: evidence from clinical trials. Br J Ophthalmol. 2010;94(1):2–13.

121. Bolz M, Schmidt-Erfurth U. Ranibizumab EXCITE study: exploring the value of optical coherence tomography for the management of ranibizumab therapy in age-related macular degeneration. 8th EURETINA Congress. Vienna, 2008.

122. Holz FG. Flexibly dosed ranibizumab in patients with neovascular AMD: twelve month interim results of the SUSTAIN Trial AAO/SOE Joint Annual Meeting. Atlanta, 2008.

123. Meyer CH, Eter N, Holz FG, Fulano FM. Ranibizumab in patients with subfoveal choroidal neovascularization secondary to age-related macular degeneration. Interim results from the SUSTAIN trial. Invest Ophthalmol Vis Sci. 2008;49:E-Abstract 273.

124. Brown DM, Wang PW, Scott LC. HORIZON extension trial of Ranibizumab for wet AMD: subanalysis of year 1 results. AAO/SOE Joint Annual Meeting. Atlanta, 8–11 Nov 2008.

125. Fong DS, Custis P, Howes J, Hsu JW. Intravitreal bevacizumab and ranibizumab for age-related macular degeneration a multicenter, retrospective study. Ophthalmology. 2010;117(2):298–302.

126. Stepien KE, Rosenfeld PJ, Puliafito CA, et al. Comparison of intravitreal bevacizumab followed by ranibizumab for the treatment of neovascular age-related macular degeneration. Retina. 2009; 29(8):1067–73.

127. Holash J, Davis S, Papadopoulos N, et al. VEGF-Trap: a VEGF blocker with potent antitumor effects. Proc Natl Acad Sci USA. 2002;99(17):11393–8.

128. Cao J, Song H, Renard RA, et al. Systemic or intravitreal administration of VEGF Trap suppresses vascular leak and leukostasis in the retinas of diabetic rats. Invest Ophthalmol Vis Sci. 2006;47: E-abstract 145.

129. Chappelow AV, Kaiser PK. Neovascular age-related macular degeneration: potential therapies. Drugs. 2008;68(8):1029–36.

130. Rudge JS, Thurston G, Davis S, et al. VEGF trap as a novel antiangiogenic treatment currently in clinical trials for cancer and eye diseases, and VelociGene-based discovery of the next generation of angiogenesis targets. Cold Spring Harb Symp Quant Biol. 2005;70:411–8.

131. Nguyen QD, Shah SM, Browning DJ, et al. A phase I study of intravitreal vascular endothelial growth factor trap-eye in patients with neovascular age-related macular degeneration. Ophthalmology. 2009;116(11):2141–8.e1.

132. Benz MS, Nguyen QD, Chu K, et al. Interm results of the phase II, randomized, controlled dose-and interval-ranging study of repeated intravitreal VEGF trap administration in patients with neovascular age-related macular degeneration (AMD). Invest Ophthalmol Vis Sci. 2007;48:E-Abstract 4549.

133. Zhang M, Zhang J, Yan M, Li H, Yang C, Yu D. Recombinant anti-vascular endothelial growth factor fusion protein efficiently suppresses choridal neovasularization in monkeys. Mol Vis. 2008; 14:37–49.

134. Suto K, Yamazaki Y, Morita T, Mizuno H. Crystal structures of novel vascular endothelial growth factors (VEGF) from snake venoms: insight into selective VEGF binding to kinase insert domain-containing receptor but not to fms-like tyrosine kinase-1. J Biol Chem. 2005;280(3):2126–31.

135. Zhang M, Yu D, Yang C, et al. The pharmacology study of a new recombinant human VEGF receptor-fc fusion protein on experimental choroidal neovascularization. Pharm Res. 2009;26(1):204–10.

136. Zhang M, Yan M, Zhang J, Zhu W, Luo D, Yu D. Safety, tolerability, and bioactivity study of intravitreal KH902 in patients with neovascular age-related macular degeneration. Invest Ophthalmol Vis Sci. 2009;50:E-Abstract 5004.

137. Kumar R, Knick VB, Rudolph SK, et al. Pharmacokinetic-pharmacodynamic correlation from mouse to human with pazopanib, a multikinase angiogenesis inhibitor with potent antitumor and antiangiogenic activity. Mol Cancer Ther. 2007;6(7):2012–21.

138. Takahashi K, Saishin Y, King AG, Levin R, Campochiaro PA. Suppression and regression of choroidal neovascularization by the multitargeted kinase inhibitor pazopanib. Arch Ophthalmol. 2009; 127(4):494–9.

139. Yafai Y, Niemeyer M, Yasukawa T, et al. Inhibition of experimental choroidal neovascularization by the VEGF receptor inhibitor pazopanib (GW786034B). Invest Ophthalmol Vis Sci. 2008;49:E-Abstract 534.

140. McLaughlin MM, Bayliffe A, Hunt T, et al. A multi-targeted receptor tyrosine kinase inhibitor for the treatment of neovascular AMD: results of a healthy volunteer safety and tolerability study of pazopanib eye drops. Invest Ophthalmol Vis Sci. 2009;50: E-Abstract 5008.

Combination Therapy with Ocular Photodynamic Therapy for Age-Related Macular Degeneration

7

Nathan Steinle and Peter K. Kaiser

Key Points

- Exudative AMD is the leading cause of blindness in people over 50 years old in the Western world.
- Choroidal neovascularization found in exudative AMD appears to be a multifactoral process involving inflammatory, vascular, and angiogenic components.
- Commercially available treatments for exudative AMD primarily target a solitary component of this multifactoral disease.
- Combining various treatment modalities for exudative AMD targets multiple components of choroidal neovascularization and has the potential for improving efficacy and reducing treatment frequency.

Introduction

Age-related macular degeneration (AMD) is a common degenerative condition that can lead to severe loss of central vision. The most common cause of severe vision loss in AMD is the development of choroidal neovascularization (CNV), a condition termed exudative (also known as wet or neovascular) AMD. Exudative AMD is the leading cause of blindness in people over 50 years of age in the Western world [1–3]. Unfortunately, worldwide prevalence of exudative AMD is predicted to increase as life expectancy continues to improve [4]. A decade ago, patients with exudative AMD faced suboptimal therapeutic options and carried a poor visual prognosis [5]. Fortunately, there have been many recent advances in the management of exudative AMD, including the advent of medical therapies to combat CNV, which has improved the ability to fight this devastating disease.

The traditional model of CNV holds that exudative AMD is solely a vascular disease, with the formation of new blood vessels occurring from the recruitment of pre-existing resident endothelial cells from the adjacent normal choroidal vascular bed [6]. However, this theory has recently undergone revision, with many researchers now suggesting that CNV appears to be a multi-component disease involving neovascular growth, vascular leakage, matrix deposition, remodeling, and inflammation [7, 8]. The complex and multifactorial nature of the pathophysiology of CNV opens the possibility of developing combination therapies aimed at separate aspects of the contributing pathways. Current treatment options can be generally divided into those that target the inflammatory, vascular, or angiogenic component of CNV. Combination therapy with agents that have different modes of action may enable treatments to target multiple components of CNV and could thus have the potential for additive or synergistic effects. Successful combination therapy may reduce

N. Steinle (✉)
Cole Eye Institute, Cleveland Clinic Foundation,
9500 Euclid Ave., Cleveland, OH 44195, USA
e-mail: steinln@ccf.org

A.C. Ho and C.D. Regillo (eds.), *Age-related Macular Degeneration Diagnosis and Treatment*,
DOI 10.1007/978-1-4614-0125-4_7, © Springer Science+Business Media, LLC 2011

99

treatment frequency and/or improve treatment outcomes in exudative AMD. A move towards combination therapy in the treatment of AMD would mirror successful combination treatment regimens currently utilized in other areas of medicine, including oncology [9–13], human immunodeficiency virus [14, 15], and hypertension [16, 17].

Pathogenesis and Development of CNV

CNV secondary to AMD is responsible for 75% of the severe vision loss attributable to AMD [18]. The pathogenesis of the CNV found in exudative AMD has been the subject of widespread research and debate. Zarbin et al. suggested that the pathologic changes that occur at the cellular level during the development of AMD are related to cumulative oxidative stress associated with the aging process and may be initiated by a number of environmental or genetic factors (Fig. 7.1) [8].

> **Pearl**
> The pathogenesis of CNV appears to be mutifactorial and is the subject of significant research interest.

Oxidative stress can cause damage to the retinal pigment epithelium (RPE) and choriocapillaris, resulting in a chronic inflammatory response within Bruch's membrane and the choroid. Injury and inflammation of the choriocapillaris then lead to formation of an abnormal extracellular matrix that impairs diffusion of nutrients to the retina and RPE, leading to further damage. This abnormal extracellular matrix can lead to retinal atrophy. The pathogenic changes within the extracellular matrix also lead to perturbation of the balance between pro- and antiangiogenic substances, especially vascular endothelial growth factor (VEGF) and pigment epithelium-derived factor (PEDF). Ischemia has also been postulated to play a significant role in the pathogenesis of CNV, which initiates the angiogenic cascade by promoting production of angiogenic factors, including VEGF, monocyte colonization protein, and interleukin-8 in the RPE [19–21]. These angiogenic stimuli then promote the activation of vascular endothelial cells and lead to the formation of gaps between the endothelial cells lining the capillary wall [22]. This leads to increased permeability and allows proteins such as fibrinogen to escape, promoting formation of a matrix that supports growth of new blood vessels. It is also possible that hypoxia arises as a consequence of oxidative stress and leads to the subsequent

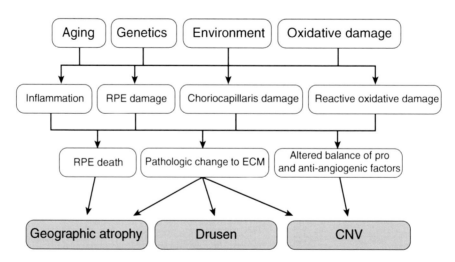

Fig. 7.1 Pathogenesis of AMD and CNV. *AMD* age-related macular degeneration, *CNV* choroidal neovascularization, *ECM* extracellular matrix, *RPE* retinal pigment epithelium

formation of an abnormal extracellular matrix and a thickened Bruch's membrane [8].

It is likely that numerous factors interact to stimulate the initiation of angiogenesis, which is then propagated by various proangiogenic mediators. VEGF is a key mediator involved in the control of angiogenesis and vascular permeability and has been shown to be induced by hypoxia in cultured human RPE [23, 24]. VEGF messenger RNA undergoes alternative splicing events that lead to the production of at least four different proteins with 121, 165, 189, or 206 amino acids ($VEGF_{121}$, $VEGF_{165}$, $VEGF_{189}$, and $VEGF_{206}$, respectively) [25]. $VEGF_{189}$ and $VEGF_{206}$ bind tightly to heparin on cell surfaces and are localized in the extracellular matrix [26]. In contrast, $VEGF_{165}$ is only partially bound and $VEGF_{121}$ diffuses freely; these are the major isoforms involved in angiogenesis and increased permeability [27]. $VEGF_{165}$ is the isoform predominantly associated with pathologic neovascularization, whereas $VEGF_{121}$ is involved in normal physiological neovascularization [28–30]. All isoforms can undergo post-translation cleavage by plasmin to produce a freely soluble isoform, $VEGF_{110}$.

Release of VEGF and several other mediators, including stem cell factor, epidermal growth factor, basic fibroblast growth factor (bFGF), and platelet-derived growth factor, attracts mast cells, which produce enzymes (matrix metalloproteinases) that degrade the surrounding connective tissue and create a space for growth of the new blood vessels [31]. VEGF also induces expression of intercellular adhesion molecule-1 (ICAM-1), which leads to leukocyte adhesion, increased vascular permeability, and capillary nonperfusion, and promotes recruitment of macrophages [32, 33]. Animal models have shown that the presence of VEGF is a prerequisite for the development of neovascularization, and VEGF concentrations in the eye have been shown to increase in parallel with the growth of new vessels [34–37]. Studies in normal animal eyes have also shown that the administration of VEGF results in the development of neovascularization [38–40]. Various other mediators are believed to be involved in angiogenic process, including connective tissue growth factor and transforming factor-beta [41, 42]. In contrast, PEDF is a potent inhibitor of angiogenesis, including that induced by VEGF [43]. PEDF concentrations are reduced in CNV, suggesting that loss of PEDF creates a permissive environment where VEGF-induced angiogenesis can proceed [43].

Overview of Therapeutic Treatment Targets

The pathogenic processes that lead to development, maintenance, and growth of CNV offer several potential targets for treatment (Fig. 7.2). These treatments can be broadly divided into those that target either the inflammatory, vascular, or angiogenic components of CNV. Although this simplistic division of treatment modalities is accurate, it is highly likely that the treatments that are directed primarily at one of these targets will also affect other parts of the process. For example, steroids have antiinflammatory effects, but also upregulate extracellular matrix protein plasminogen activator inhibitor-1 expression, inhibit VEGF, stabilize basement membrane, and downregulate ICAM-1 expression [44]. Similarly, in addition to its angio-occlusive effect, verteporfin PDT has been shown to modify the expression of both proangiogenic and antiangiogenic factors [45]. In order to further enhance the treatment effects seen with monotherapy, the *combination* of therapies offers the potential for even greater efficacy and may offer the possibility of extending the interval between treatments.

Antinflammatory Therapy

Steroids, including triamcinolone and dexamethasone, were some of the first pharmacologic treatments evaluated for the treatment of CNV. In addition to their antiinflammatory effects, corticosteroids also have antifibrotic, antipermeability, and antiangiogenic properties [44, 46]. The beneficial effects of steroids include stabilization of the blood–retinal barrier, resorption of exudation, and down regulation of inflammatory stimuli. Steroids have both direct and indirect angiostatic effects.

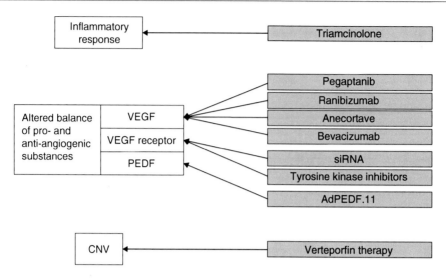

Fig. 7.2 Primary treatment targets of therapeutic agents used, or under investigation, for eyes with CNV due to AMD. *AMD* age-related macular degeneration, *CNV* choroidal neovascularization, *PEDF* pigment epithelium-derived factor, *siRNA* small interfering RNA, *VEGF* vascular endothelial growth factor (Adapted by permission from Informa Healthcare: Kaiser [6]. Copyright 2007)

Corticosteroids are potent inhibitors of neovascularization, and have been shown to impede the neovascular cascade by directly suppressing levels of VEGF [47, 48].

> **Pearl**
> Corticosteroids offer inexpensive and widely available treatment for exudative AMD; however, corticosteroid monotherapy does not represent current standard of care due to efficacy and safety concerns.

A retrospective case series evaluating the early effects of intravitreal triamcinolone acetonide (IVTA) in CNV due to AMD suggested that IVTA may also exert antiangiogenic effects on CNV by enhancing endostatin expression [49]. Further direct angiostatic effects of corticosteroids are mediated through down regulation of extracellular matrix metalloproteinases, dissolution of basement membrane, and the downregulation of ICAM-1 expression [50–54]. The effects of triamcinolone acetonide on ICAM-1 and major histocompatibility complex-1 have been shown to significantly reduce cell permeability in an in-vitro model of the blood–retinal barrier [53, 54]. Reducing the permeability of the blood–retinal barrier may reduce the risk of developing CNV. Indirect effects of steroids include inhibition of migration and activation of inflammatory cells (monocytes, leukocytes, and macrophages) that secrete angiogenic growth factors. Steroids inhibit the synthesis and release of various inflammatory mediators, including prostaglandins and leukotrienes, in addition to their actions on inflammatory cells [55–57].

Preclinical models provided promising evidence of the effects of triamcinolone acetonide on development of CNV. For example, intravitreal triamcinolone acetonide (IVTA) dramatically inhibited development of fibrovascular proliferations in the eyes of rats with laser-induced CNV, and reduced the development of preretinal and optic nerve head neovascularization in pigs with retinal branch vein occlusions generated using photodynamic thrombosis with rose bengal dye and thermal burns from an argon green laser [58, 59]. In rabbit models, IVTA has also been shown to reduce new vessel growth after partial liquefaction of the posterior vitreous with hyaluronidase and injection of dermal fibroblasts and to decrease blood–retinal barrier degradation after laser photocoagulation [60, 61]. These promising preclinical findings are supported by outcomes from a number of small-scale clinical studies in patients with exudative AMD [44]. Importantly, the only large-scale ($n = 151$), randomized, controlled, double-masked study of IVTA 4 mg found that although IVTA significantly reduced the growth of neovascular lesions in eyes with CNV with a classic component, there was no significant reduction in the risk of developing severe vision loss (loss of ≥ 30 letters) between the IVTA and placebo recipients [62]. Although this study showed that IVTA was generally well tolerated, there was an increased incidence of mild or moderate elevation of intraocular pressure, which responded well to treatment, and significant progression of cataract [63]. Other studies have also revealed increases in intraocular pressure as well as an increased risk of endophthalmitis [64–66]. In a retrospective, case series, post-injection endophthalmitis was identified in eight eyes following a total of 922 IVTA treatments [65]. Both bacterial and sterile cases of endophthalmitis have been reported following IVTA treatment [65, 66]. Additional large-scale studies are required to further characterize the safety profile of IVTA. In part due to safety concerns, the current balance of evidence suggests that IVTA cannot be recommended for monotherapy of CNV due to AMD [44]. However, the biological effects warrant further investigation, particularly in combination with other treatment modalities.

Verteporfin Angioocclusive Therapy

Verteporfin photodynamic therapy (VPDT) has a selective mechanism of action based on accumulation of the drug in the target tissue followed by activation with laser light [67]. The vascular component of CNV consists of pericytes, endothelial cell precursors, and vascular endothelial cells, which provide the target for verteporfin. Verteporfin is infused intravenously, accumulates preferentially in proliferating cells such as the endothelium in CNV, and generates short-lived reactive oxygen species when activated by laser

light at a wavelength of 689 nm. The standard-fluence (SF) rate utilized in clinical trials used a treatment of 50 J/cm [2] delivered over 83 s at 600 mW/cm^2 [67, 68]. The reactive oxygen species generated by this photochemical reaction causes highly localized endothelial cell damage leading to rapid and selective occlusion of the CNV without damaging the overlying retina [69, 70]. Specifically, photoactivation of verteporfin generates a reactive oxygen species that causes localized endothelial cell changes. This triggers platelet binding and aggregation, leading to the formation of a stabilized plug and occlusion of the CNV [67, 71]. Although the primary mechanism of action of VPDT involves occlusion of the new vessels, the treatment is also likely to have secondary effects. For example, it has been shown that VPDT induces a response involving increased expression of VEGF, VEGFR-3, and PEDF [45]. However, it is also possible that occlusion of new vessels could directly alter cytokine release or modify angiogenic signals [6].

Verteporfin therapy is currently recommended for patients with subfoveal lesions composed of predominantly classic CNV (regardless of lesion size) and for those with small lesions (≤ 4 disc areas) containing occult with no classic or minimally classic CNV and having evidence of recent disease progression, based on the results of the phase III treatment of age-related macular degeneration with Photodynamic therapy (TAP) Investigation, the phase III Verteporfin In Photodynamic Therapy (VIP) Trial, and the phase II Verteporfin In Minimally Classic CNV (VIM) Trial [72–75]. The ocular and systemic safety of verteporfin was confirmed in phase III studies, and combined safety data have been reported in detail [76]. Acute severe visual acuity decrease (defined as a loss of at least 20 letters of visual acuity within seven days of verteporfin) was a relatively uncommon event, occurring in 0.7% of 402 patients in the TAP Investigation and 4.9% of 225 patients in the VIP Trial [77]. Published data from an extension to the two-year TAP Investigation showed that visual acuity remained stable through five years and that there were no new safety concerns during this period [78].

Antiangiogenic Therapy

Angiogenesis (the growth of new blood vessels from existing vasculature) is associated with loss of visual acuity in a number of ocular diseases, most notably exudative AMD [79]. The rationale for antiangiogenic therapy in the treatment of CNV is based on interrupting the angiogenic cascade involved in the growth of new blood vessels. Antiangiogenic therapies have been shown to inhibit cell proliferation, reduce formation and growth of new blood vessels, as well as minimize vascular leakage [4]. In addition, data indicates that blockade of VEGF can lead to the regression of newly formed vessels if these vessels are targeted before pericyte recruitment and maturation [80]. The first antiangiogenic agent to become clinically available for the treatment of CNV due to AMD was pegaptanib (Macugen, Eyetech, New York, NY), an intravitreally injected ribonucleic acid aptamer linked to two polyethylene glycol moieties [81, 82]. Pegaptanib binds selectively to VEGF165, but not to the smaller VEGF121 or VEGF110 isoforms [82]. In two phase II/III randomized, controlled, double-masked trials, together known as the VEGF Inhibition Study In Ocular Neovascularization (VISION), intravitreal pegaptanib (IVP) monotherapy was shown to reduce the risk of vision loss due to CNV in patients with AMD [81, 83].

Ranibizumab (Lucentis, Genentech, South San Francisco, CA) is an affinity matured, Fab fragment of a humanized monoclonal antibody to VEGF that binds to *all* isoforms of VEGF ("pan-VEGF blockade"), inhibiting vascular permeability and angiogenesis [84]. Intravitreal ranibizumab (IVR) was approved by the FDA for the treatment of exudative AMD in June 2006. Data from the Minimally classic/occult trial of the Anti-VEGF antibody Ranibizumab In the treatment of Neovascular AMD (MARINA) provided promising evidence of efficacy in eyes with minimally classic or occult with no classic CNV [85]. At 12 months, almost 95% of patients receiving IVR 0.3 or 0.5 mg lost less than 15 letters of visual acuity from baseline, compared

with 62% of patients receiving a sham injection, and these results were maintained through two years [85]. In addition, the phase III Anti-VEGF antibody for the treatment of predominantly classic Choroidal neovascularization (ANCHOR) study showed that 94–96% of patients receiving IVR 0.3 or 0.5 mg lost less than 15 letters of visual acuity from baseline, compared with 64% of patients receiving VPDT [86]. Even more exciting was the finding that significantly more patients receiving IVR had improvements in visual acuity of at least 15 letters, versus placebo recipients (34% versus 5%; $P < 0.001$), and visual acuity benefits were maintained at 24 months [85]. A safety study in patients with CNV due to AMD showed that IVR had a good safety profile (transient inflammation and minor injection-site hemorrhages were the most frequent adverse events) [87].

> **Pearl**
> Anti-VEGF therapy offers a greater chance for visual improvement than prior therapeutic modalities.

Bevacizumab (Avastin, Genentech, South San Francisco, CA) is a humanized monoclonal antibody to VEGF that, like ranibizumab, binds to *all* isoforms of VEGF and has been FDA-approved for the treatment of colorectal cancer, breast cancer, lung cancer, and renal cell cancer [88, 89]. Although there is no formulation specifically developed for ocular use, several uncontrolled studies and case series have reported vision improvements similar to IVR when it is used off-label as an intravitreal injection in exudative AMD [90–94]. A study in rabbits found no evidence of retinal toxicity [95]. Several randomized controlled trials are underway worldwide to establish the efficacy and safety of intravitreal bevacizumab (IVB) in treating exudative AMD.

Multiple other antiangiogenic agents are currently under evaluation for the treatment of CNV due to exudative AMD [96–101].

Rationale for Combination Therapy in the Treatment of Exudative AMD

Despite significant advancements made in the understanding and treatment of exudative AMD over the past decade, the need for therapeutic improvement exists. For example, of all the treatments investigated to date, the intravitreal anti-VEGF therapies have been the most clinically successful. However, anti-VEGF monotherapy does not improve vision in all patients, and it appears that frequent treatments are necessary to maintain efficacy [85, 86, 102]. For example, in ANCHOR and MARINA, approximately two-thirds of patients did not gain at least 15 letters at 12 months after treatment with ranibizumab [85, 86]. The extension study of MARINA and ANCHOR, the HORIZON study, reported that when monthly treatments were changed to as needed dosing, visual acuity declined over the next two years. This indicates that long-term and frequent dosing are required to maintain the visual gains with anti-VEGF monotherapy. Furthermore, the PIER Study revealed suboptimal efficacy when quarterly dosing of ranibizumab was compared with monthly treatment regimens in patients with subfoveal CNV due to AMD. In the PIER Study, IVR 0.3 or 0.5 mg (or sham) was administered monthly for three months and quarterly thereafter. Patients receiving 0.5 mg IVR demonstrated vision improvement during the initial monthly dosing with a decline to baseline with subsequent mandated quarterly dosing [103]. This loss was accompanied by an average increase in vascular leakage and mean retinal thickness after initiation of the quarterly dosing regimen, suggesting that some patients need IVR injections more frequently to control the neovascular leakage [103]. And it is important to note that each intravitreal treatment of anti-VEGF therapy carries a risk of endophthalmitis, uveitis, cataract formation, and retinal detachment, not to mention physical, emotional, and financial stress. IVR was associated with a presumed endophthalmitis rate of 0.8–.4% of patients and uveitis in 0.7–1.3% of patients in ANCHOR and MARINA [85, 86, 102].

Evidence suggests that anti-VEGF agents become less effective as neovascularization matures, especially as the vessels become enveloped by pericytes. These pericytes may serve to buffer the neovascularization from the anti-VEGF agents and even secrete VEGF themselves. Thus, anti-VEGF therapy may have a limited effect on the more established vasculature observed in the later stages of exudative AMD [104–106]. Since verteporfin targets the vascular component of CNV by occluding vessels within the CNV lesion, combining the angio-occlusive effect of VPDT with anti-VEGF therapies that inhibit growth and decrease the permeability of new vessels might lead to prolonged reduction of leakage, thus necessitating fewer retreatments. Conversely, studies have demonstrated that VPDT may affect the physiological choriocapillary bed surrounding the pathological CNV lesion, indirectly resulting in upregulation of VEGF that may then further stimulate CNV growth [107, 108]. By combining anti-VEGF agents that target the angiogenic component with VPDT that targets the vascular component, the vicious cycle of VPDT-induced VEGF upregulation may be broken and provide subsequent improvements in visual outcomes and perhaps lead to a less frequent dosing schedule of anti-VEGF agents. In addition, many clinicians also opt for reduced-fluence (RF) VPDT in an attempt to optimize the efficacy by increasing the selectivity of VPDT's angio-occlusive effects (300 mW/cm^2 for 83 s to deliver 25 J/cm^2) [109]. The two-year results of Visudyne in Minimally Classic CNV (VIM) phase II trial have indicated a trend toward better visual acuity (VA) outcomes and a lower incidence of visual disturbance in the RF group compared with the standard-fluence (SF) group at 12 and 24 months [107]. Thus, while evaluating the combination therapies, it would be logical to assess both RF and SF VPDT to help define the most appropriate VPDT combination treatment [109].

The current treatment regimens with intravitreal anti-VEGF injection therapies have no defined endpoint; thus, it is unknown how long these therapies must be continued. Furthermore, the enduring effect on vision is unknown once therapy is halted. It is difficult to predict long-term patient compliance given the high frequency of intravitreal injections in the current anti-VEGF treatment regimens [110]. It is also important to note that VEGF is an important molecule within the normal eye, which is not exclusively expressed by the pathological neovascular tissues. Reducing the number of anti-VEGF injections would lower the risk of potentially disrupting the normal physiological processes mediated by VEGF [111–114]. Sustaining improvements in visual acuity along with angiographic evidence of inactivity with fewer treatments is, therefore, a major goal of combination therapy.

VPDT is also associated with an inflammatory response during the immediate post-treatment period. The combination of VPDT with antiinflammatory agents such as triamcinolone or dexamethasone may further benefit patients. Morphological evaluation using OCT has shown increases in macular edema following VPDT; furthermore, inflammatory cells (such as monocytes, macrophages, platelets, mast cells, and leukocytes) have been observed within treated areas after VPDT [115, 116]. As noted previously, these inflammatory cells release a variety of angiogenic factors, including VEGF and bFGF, as well as releasing cytokines and vasoactive mediators. Thus, corticosteroids (e.g., triamcinolone and dexamethasone) have been used in combination with VPDT and may reduce this inflammatory response [44].

Clinical Data Examining Combination Therapy for Exudative AMD

Verteporfin Therapy in Combination with Triamcinolone

Several studies have investigated the combination of VPDT and IVTA in patients with CNV due to AMD (Table 7.1)[117–132]. For example, Spaide et al. investigated the combination of VPDT and IVTA in both patients who had not previously been treated with VPDT, and patients who had received previous courses of VPDT

[117, 118]. Newly treated patients ($n = 13$) had a mean improvement of +2.5 lines (+13 letters) 12 months after combination therapy, while patients in the prior PDT group ($n = 13$) had a mean improvement of +0.44 lines (+2 letters) [118]. The improvements in visual acuity were associated with cessation of fluorescein leakage on angiography [117]. The number of treatments required in the first year was 1.24 in the newly treated group and 1.2 in the prior VPDT group [118]. The retreatment frequencies reported in this study are lower than those reported in the first year of the TAP Investigation (3.4) [133] and VIP Trial (3.4) [74], although the results of these studies cannot be directly compared because of different entry criteria and sample size considerations. An increase in intraocular pressure occurred in a little over one third of patients (10 of 26, 39%), and was controlled by topical medication in all cases [118]. Although IVTA is associated with increased intraocular pressure and cataract progression, it is still considered a generally well-tolerated option, as long as patients are monitored for elevation of intraocular pressures and treated with pressure-reducing agents as necessary [63]. Similar results have been reported in a retrospective review of case records from 14 patients who received VPDT and IVTA [119]. After a median follow-up of 18 months, 7% of patients gained at least 30 letters and 50% had stable vision (loss or gain of <15 letters) [119]. Another retrospective analysis of eyes with subfoveal CNV treated with VPDT and IVTA showed that visual acuity improved by at least three lines in 21% of 19 eyes that had previously received VPDT and decreased by at least three lines in 26% [120]. In eyes that had not previously received VPDT, visual acuity improved by at least three lines in 6% of 16 eyes, and decreased by at least three lines in 31%. These findings have been supported by other retrospective studies and small-scale, uncontrolled trials [121–123, 126]. Small-scale pilot studies have also indicated that adding triamcinolone to VPDT may have visual acuity benefits in eyes with minimally classic subfoveal CNV, and for juxtafoveal and extrafoveal lesions [124, 125].

Table 7.1 Studies investigating the use of combination intravitreal triamcinolone acetonide and verteporfin therapy in patients with CNV

References	Lesion type	No. of eyes	Treatment	Outcome
Spaide et al. [117, 118]	No restrictions as to lesion type	26	Single 4 mg dose IVTA immediately after VPDT	In 13 treatment-naïve patients, VA improved by 2.5 lines at 12 months. VA was not significantly different from baseline in 13 patients with prior VPDT. An increase in intraocular pressure occurred in 39% of patients, and was controlled with topical medication.
Rechtman et al. [119]	Mix of classic and occult lesion types	14	Single 4 mg dose IVTA within 6 weeks of VPDT. Three patients received additional combined treatment at 6 months	Overall, 57% had improved or stable vision. Mild intraocular pressure elevation occurred in 29%, and cataract progression was seen in 50% of phakic eyes
Moshfeghi et al. [120]	Subfoveal	35	VPDT combined with IVTA	VA improved by 3 or more lines in 21% of 19 patients with prior VPDT and in 6% of patients without prior VPDT
Roth et al. [121]	Subfoveal	72	Single 4 mg dose IVTA 1 week before verteporfin therapy	Decrease in subretinal fluid was seen in 37% of eyes and resolution of leakage in 52% of eyes. VA was stable in 81% of eyes and improved ≥2 lines in 21% of eyes
Augustin et al. [122]	Occult	41	Single 25 mg dose IVTA 12–18 h after verteporfin therapy	VA improved in 22 eyes (54%), stabilized in 16 eyes (39%), and was reduced <3 lines in 3 eyes (7%). A transient increase in intraocular pressure was observed in 9 patients (22%), and was controlled by topical therapy (7 patients) or systemic therapy (2 patients)
El Matri et al. [123]	Not specified	34	Single 4 mg dose IVTA	VA increased in 65% of patients. Intraocular pressure increased temporarily in 1 patient. An increase in the degree of cataract was noted in the majority of patients. Two patients developed endophthalmitis, which resolved with antibiotics
Bhavsar [124]	Minimally classic subfoveal	26	Single 4 mg dose IVTA combined with verteporfin therapy	VA improved or decreased <3 lines in 23 eyes (88%); 17 eyes (65%) required no additional treatment following the initial combined treatment. An earlier report from this study noted that glaucoma requiring topical medication occurred in 5–25 patients (20%) [91]
Spaide et al. [125]	Extrafoveal and juxtafoveal	13 juxtafoveal 2 extrafoveal	Single 4 mg dose IVTA combined with verteporfin therapy	Mean VA improved from 20/50 at baseline to 20/40 at 6 months
Johnson et al. [126]	Subfoveal	24	Single dose IVTA 1 week after VPDT	270 days after treatment, 17 eyes (71%) required no further VPDT, 3 eyes (13%) had VA improvement >2 lines, 2 eyes (8%) had VA decreased >2 lines, and 19 eyes (79%) had stable VA
Augustin et al. [127]	Subfoveal, extrafoveal and Juxtafoveal	148 subfoveal 17 extrafoveal 19 juxtafoveal	Single 25 mg dose IVTA 16 h after verteporfin	VA improved in majority of patients by mean of 1.22 lines. Mean number of treatments was 1.21 over mean of 39 weeks.

(continued)

Table 7.1 (continued)

References	Lesion type	No. of eyes	Treatment	Outcome
Chan et al. [128].	Subfoveal	48	24 eyes received single 4 mg dose IVTA combined with verteporfin therapy, 24 eyes received VPDT alone	Combined therapy stabilized vision more than VPDT alone at 12 months
Ergun et al. [129]	All types	60	Single 4 mg dose IVTA combined with verteporfin therapy	Combination did not prevent decreased vision. The main benefit of this combination treatment was a low number of verteporfin treatments. Baseline VA was the main predictor of the final outcome.
Arias et al. [130]	Classic subfoveal	61	31 eyes received approximately 11 mg dose IVTA combined with verteporfin 30 eyes received verteporfin therapy alone	Improved VA in combination group at 1 year. Reduced in lesion size and foveal thickness in the combination group. Retreatment rate lower in combination group.
Ruiz-Moreno et al. [131]	Subfoveal	30	Verteorfin followed by 19.4 ± 2.1 mg IVTA 5 days later	Two years after combined verteporfin and high dose IVTA, final VA was stable, and the need for retreatment was reduced compared with historical controls
Maberley et al. [132]	Classic subfoveal	100	50 eyes received a same-day 4 mg dose IVTA combined with verteporfin 50 eyes received verteporfin therapy alone	There was no visual benefit to the addition of IVTA to verteporfin at 1 year. Subjects receiving combination IVTA and verteporfin required significantly fewer retreatments.

IVTA intravitreal triamcinolone acetonide, *VPDT* verteporfin photodynamic therapy, *VA* visual acuity

One prospective study of 48 eyes revealed combined VPDT with IVTA was more effective statistically at 12 months for stabilization of vision (<3 logMAR lines change) compared with verteporfin PDT monotherapy [128]. Conversely, a retrospective, interventional case series of 60 eyes of exudative AMD patients treated with combined verteporfin PDT with IVTA revealed that only 23 (38.3%) of 60 eyes had a stable result at 12 months follow-up (loss or gain of less than three lines) and 34 (56.7%) of 60 had a loss of ≥3 lines [129]. Three patients (5%) had an improvement of ≥3 lines. Lesion type, patient age, and lesion size had no influence on the outcome, but baseline VA had a statistically significant effect. One third (20 of 60) of all eyes had an increase in intraocular pressure (IOP) that required therapy. There were no cases of endophthalmitis, but 13 patients (21.6%) developed severe cataract that required surgery. This study concluded that the combination did not prevent a considerable decrease in VA. The main benefit of combination treatment was a low number of verteporfin treatments [129]. Another prospective randomized study of 61 patients with predominantly classic subfoveal CNV secondary to AMD randomized patients to receive VPDT ($n=30$) or VPDT followed by approximately 11 mg IVTA ($n=31$), with retreatment every three months when leakage was documented by fluorescein angiography [130]. At the 12-month follow-up, VA (mean logMAR change from baseline) was significantly better in the group of patients who received combined therapy. Seventy-four percent of patients treated with combined therapy compared with 61% treated with verteporfin alone lost fewer than 15 letters of VA. Reduction in lesion size and in foveal thickness was significantly greater with combined therapy than with verteporfin. The retreatment rate was significantly lower in the combined therapy group. IVTA-related adverse events included glaucoma (25.8%) and cataract progression (32%). Thus, this study concluded that combined VPDT and IVTA therapy seemed to be more effective than VPDT alone for managing predominantly classic subfoveal lesions secondary to AMD [130]. In another prospective, consecutive, comparative, nonrandomized, interventional case series, 30 eyes of 30 consecutive patients with subfoveal CNV associated with AMD were treated by VPDT followed by intravitreal injection of 19.4 ± 2.1 mg triamcinolone [131]. Fifteen eyes were naive to treatment (group 1), and 15 had been treated previously by VPDT alone (group 2). A group of 15 eyes of 15 patients treated by VPDT alone served as controls. The two-year follow-up results revealed that visual acuity did not change significantly in group 1 from baseline; group 2 lost an average -0.6 ± 2.5 line, and the control group lost an average of -2.2 ± 3.4 lines. The average number of VPDT sessions during the 24-month follow-up was 1.9, 1.2, and 3.9 for group 1, group 2, and the control group, respectively. The authors concluded that two years after combined verteporfin PDT with high-dose IVTA to treat AMD-associated CNV, final VA was stable, and the need for retreatment was reduced compared with historical controls [131].

The results of these small pilot studies, while at times indicative of a promising effect of the combination of VPDT and IVTA, should be treated with caution. Large-scale, randomized, controlled studies are required to determine the efficacy and safety of combining VPDT and IVTA and to characterize the patient groups that might have the greatest benefits [44]. Furthermore, examinations into the most effective dose of IVTA as well as the precise sequence of events in dual IVTA and VPDT therapy need to be evaluated.

The largest and most rigorous evaluation to date of combined IVTA and VPDT for predominantly classic CNV in AMD is provided by the Canadian Retinal Trials Group [132]. This multicenter, two-year, double-blind, randomized, sham-controlled trial evaluated 100 individuals with predominantly classic, subfoveal CNV secondary to AMD. Fifty individuals were randomized 1:1 to either VPDT alone versus combined VPDT and 4 mg IVTA. IVTA or sham injections were administered at three-month intervals in conjunction with VPDT when angiographic evidence of leakage was noted. All subjects received VPDT at baseline. The study revealed that combination therapy with VPDT and IVTA when compared to VPDT monotherapy resulted in no significant difference in final visual acuity at one year. Eyes treated with combination therapy lost an average of 17 letters compared with 20 letters for the VPDT group. However, small lesions were found to respond to combination therapy better than VPDT (exploratory analyses). Further, subjects receiving IVTA with VPDT required significantly fewer retreatments over the course of the study than VPDT monotherapy(1.28 vs 1.94, respectively) [132].

Verteporfin PDT Therapy in Combination with Anti-VEGF Agents

To date, combination therapy of VPDT with anti-VEGF agents has been evaluated in several clinical trials (Table 7.2) [81, 134–137]. Patients with all subtypes of subfoveal CNV were enrolled in the phase II/III VISION (VEGF Inhibition Study in Ocular Neovascularization) trials examining pegaptanib, and those with predominantly classic CNV were permitted to receive concomitant VPDT [81]. Among patients with predominantly classic CNV, the difference in the proportion of responders (patients losing less than 15 letters of visual acuity from baseline) at 12 months between IVP 0.3 mg and placebo was statistically significant in the US study (73 vs. 51%, respectively), but not in the European study (63 vs. 62%, respectively) [134]. Notably, a greater percent of patients received verteporfin during the US study (65%) than during the European study (40%), although it is not possible to determine whether this explains the difference in outcomes.

Table 7.2 Significant studies investigating the use of combination VPDT and anti-VEGF agents in CNV due to exudative age-related macular degeneration

Study	Design	Key results
VISION Study [81, 134]	Two phase II/III trials (US and Europe) in patients with all types of subfoveal CNV ($n = 1,186$). Patients received IVP 0.3, 1, or 3 mg or sham every 6 weeks. Eyes with predominantly classic CNV could also receive SF VPDT	In eyes with predominantly classic CNV: in European study there was no significant difference in percent losing < 15 letters of VA between IVP 0.3 mg and sham (40% of IVP group also received VPDT). In US study 73% of IVP 0.3 mg group lost <15 letters of VA compared with 51% with sham (65% of IVP group also received VPDT).
FOCUS Study [135]	Two-year, multicenter, randomized, single-masked, controlled study. Patients with predominantly classic CNV received SF VPDT followed by monthly IVR or sham injections ($n = 162$). VPDT was repeated quarterly as needed.	At 24 months, 88% of eyes receiving combination of VPDT plus IVR lost <15 letters of VA (compared with 75% for VPDT monotherapy), 25% had gained at least 15 letters (compared to VPDT monotherapy), and the two treatment arms differed by 12.4 letters in mean VA change ($P < 0.05$ for all between-group differences).
Lazic and Gabric [136]	Randomized pilot study of minimally classic or occult CNV ($n = 165$). Single session of SF VPDT, vs single dose of 1.25 mg IVB, vs single combination of SF VPDT then IVB one hour later	Significantly ($P < 0.0001$) greater improvement in VA at 3 months in VPDT+IVB vs VPDT vs IVB. Significantly ($P < 0.0005$) greater improvement in central foveal thickness at 3 months in VPDT+IVB vs VPDT vs IVB.
Kaiser [137]	Retrospective, case series registry review ($n = 1,196$). Patients had one or more combination treatments of 1.25 IVB within 14 days of VPDT (SF or RF). No prospective treatments were specified.	After baseline combination treatment, patients received a mean of 0.6 additional VPDT retreatments and 2.0 IVB retreatments over a mean follow-up period of 15.0 months. By 12 months, 82% of patients had stable or improved vision (loss of <3 lines or a gain in VA), 36% improved by ≥3 lines, and 17% improved by ≥6 lines. By 12 months, patients gained approximately 1.2 lines of VA from baseline. Patients who were treatment naïve gained significantly more VA by month 12 compared with those who had been previously treated ($P < 0.01$). The number of retreatments were lower than published reports with either treatment delivered as monotherapy.

CNV choroidal neovascularization, *IVB* intravitreal bevacizumab, *IVP* intravitreal pegaptanib, *IVR* intravitreal ranibizumab, *RF* reduced-fluence, *SF* standard-fluence, *VA* visual acuity, *VPDT* verteporfin photodynamic therapy

The two-year phase I/II study FOCUS (RhuFab V2 Ocular Treatment Combining the Use of Visudyne to Evaluate Safety) was designed to compare the safety, tolerability, and efficacy of IVR treatment in conjunction with VPDT versus VPDT alone in patients with subfoveal, predominantly classic CNV secondary to AMD [135]. Because safety was the primary outcome of interest, patients who had previously been treated with PDT were not excluded. Patients received monthly intravitreal injections of ranibizumab 0.5 mg ($n = 106$) or sham injections ($n = 56$). All patients received VPDT on day zero, then quarterly as needed. Efficacy assessment included changes in visual acuity (VA) and lesion characteristics and VPDT frequency. Through two years, the study has shown IVR plus VPDT was more effective than VPDT alone at maintaining or improving vision. The visual acuity benefits of IVR plus VPDT seen at 12 months were maintained through 24 months. The IVR plus VPDT patients required fewer VPDT retreatments than patients receiving VPDT alone [135].

VPDT and IVB in combination and alone were investigated in a randomized controlled pilot clinical trial by Lazic and Gabric [136]. One hundred sixty-five eyes in 165 subjects were randomly assigned to receive either a single VPDT session (PDT group; $n = 55$), or a single administration of IVB (1.25 mg; IVB group; $n = 55$), or their combination (combination group; $n = 55$). In the combination group, IVB was administered within 1 h of VPDT. At the three-month follow-up, significant improvements in best-corrected VA were observed in the IVB and combination groups ($P < 0.0001$ for both). In the VPDT group, a slight worsening was noted. At the one-month follow-up, 46 subjects (16 IVB, 29 combination, and 1 VPDT) had an improvement >0.2 logMAR in best-corrected VA; at the three-month follow-up, this improvement persisted in 23 subjects (1 IVB, 22 combination, and 0 VPDT). The authors concluded that significant improvements in best-corrected VA after one month and their maintenance over a three-month period were observed after verteporfin PDT combined with intravitreal bevacizumab [136].

A large retrospective registry study examined 1,196 patients with CNV due to AMD who received one or more combination treatments with 1.25 mg IVB within 14 days of VPDT (either standard or reduced-fluence) [137]. No prospective treatments were specified. After their baseline combination treatment, patients received a mean of 0.6 additional VPDT retreatments and 2.0 IVB retreatments over a mean follow-up period of 15 months. By 12 months, 82% of patients (578/701) had stable or improved vision (loss of <3 lines or a gain in VA), 36% (255/701) improved by ≥ 3 lines, and 17% (121/701) improved by ≥ 6 lines. By 12 months, patients gained approximately 1.2 lines (6 letters) of VA from baseline. Patients who were treatment-naïve gained significantly more VA by month 12 (+8.4 letters) compared with those who had been previously treated (+2.4 letters; $P < 0.01$). Thus, the combination therapy with IVB and VPDT led to vision benefit for most patients, particularly those who were treatment-naïve at baseline. Further, the authors noted that the number of retreatments were lower than published reports with either treatment delivered as monotherapy [137].

Randomized clinical trials are underway to confirm the benefits of combination therapy consisting of VPDT and anti-VEGF agents. The ongoing SUMMIT clinical program aims to address clinical questions associated with combination therapy. It comprises the DENALI (the US/Canada, $n = 321$) and MONT BLANC (Europe, $n = 255$) trials (both 12 month, randomized, double-masked, controlled, multicenter trials) that compare the efficacy and safety outcomes of ranibizumab/verteporfin PDT combination treatment with those of IVR monotherapy in patients with any type of subfoveal CNV secondary to AMD [109]. The primary objective of both trials is to demonstrate that combination therapy is noninferior to IVR monotherapy with respect to visual acuity at month 12. In addition (at any time point after month 2), DENALI will assess the proportion of patients with a treatment-free interval of at least three months' duration for the combination therapy. One-year results of the DENALI trial is expected in 2010. The 12-month results of the MONT BLANC study show that combining standard-fluence VPDT with IVR 0.5 mg can deliver visual improvements that are noninferior to a IVR monotherapy regimen with three IVR loading doses followed by injections on a monthly as-needed basis (noninferiority margin of 7 letters) [138]. At 12 months, there was no significant difference between the combination and monotherapy groups with regard to proportion of patients with a treatment-free interval of at least three months duration after month 2. However, additional post hoc analysis showed that 85% of patients in the VPDT combination therapy group, compared with 72% in the IVR monotherapy group, had a treatment-free interval of at least four months duration after month 2. Median time to first retreatment after month 2 was extended by approximately one month in the combination group (month 6) versus the monotherapy group (month 5). Patients in the combination group received, on average, a total of 4.8 IVR injections compared with 5.1 in the monotherapy group and a total of 1.7 VPDT treatments compared with 1.9 sham treatments in the monotherapy group. There were no unexpected safety findings, and adverse event incidence was similar between treatment groups [138].

Triple Therapy for Exudative Age-Related Macular Degeneration

In order to further address the multifactorial pathogenesis of exudative AMD, investigators have begun to examine the combination of corticosteroids, VPDT, and anti-VEGF agents (Table 7.3) [139–143]. This regimen has been referred to by the descriptive term "Triple Therapy" [139]. One of the goals of triple therapy is to improve vision to a level comparable to anti-VEGF monthly monotherapy while reducing the number of treatments in patients with CNV due to AMD. One of the first published reports on triple therapy was a prospective, noncomparative, interventional case series of 104 patients [139]. In contrast to the previous studies with reduced-fluence, VPDT was administered in a reduced–*duration* fashion (42 J/cm², accomplished by light delivery time of 70 s). Approximately 16 h after VPDT, dexamethasone (800 µg) and bevacizumab (1.5 mg) were injected intravitreally. Dexamethasone was selected over IVTA since dexamethasone could be injected as a solution and thus was more rapidly cleared from the vitreous than IVTA suspensions (thereby possibly reducing unwanted corticosteroid side effects) [139]. Patients attended follow-up visits every

six weeks, and fluorescein angiography was performed every three months or earlier if OCT showed significant edema. All 104 patients received one triple therapy cycle (five patients received a second triple treatment due to remaining CNV activity). The triple therapy was complemented in 18 patients (17.3%) by an additional intravitreal injection of bevacizumab. The mean follow-up period was 40 weeks (range, 22–60 weeks). Mean increase in visual acuity was 1.8 lines, which was significant. Mean decrease in retinal thickness was also significant (182 µm). No serious adverse events were observed. Thus, the study concluded that in most patients with CNV due to AMD, triple therapy resulted in significant and sustained visual acuity improvement after only one cycle of treatment. In addition, the therapy was found to be safe and convenient for patients, all at a potentially lower cost compared with therapies that must be administered more frequently [139].

Another study investigating triple therapy examined consecutive patients with subfoveal CNV secondary to AMD [140]. Patients were treated with standard-fluence VPDT using a standard protocol (600 mW/cm² for 83 s to deliver 50 J/cm²) immediately followed by 1.25 mg of bevacizumab and 4 mg of IVTA. Then, 1.25 mg

Table 7.3 Completed studies investigating the use of triple therapy in patients with CNV due to exudative AMD

Investigator	Number of eyes	Initial Regimen	PDT	Steroid	Anti-VEGF	Follow Up
Augustin et al. [139]	104	VPDT then vitrectomy 16 h later with IVD+IVB	Reduced-duration (600 mW/cm² for 70 s to deliver 42 J/cm²)	800 µg IVD (0.2 mL)	1.5 IVB (0.06 mL)	40 weeks
Yip et al. [140]	36	VPDT+immediate IVTA+IVB	Standard-fluence (600 mW/cm² for 83 s to deliver 50 J/cm²)	4 mg IVTA (0.1 mL)	1.25 IVB (0.05 mL)	6 months
Ehmann et al. [141]	32	VPDT+IVD then IVB 1 and 7 week later	Reduced-fluence (300 mW/cm² for 83 s to deliver 25 J/cm²)	800 µg IVD (0.08 mL)	1.25 IVB (0.05 mL)	12 months
Bakri et al. [142]	31	Consecutive VPDT+IVD+IVB	Reduced-fluence (300 mW/cm² for 83 s to deliver 25 J/cm²)	200 µg IVD (0.05 mL)	1.25 IVB (0.05 mL)	12 months
Ahmadieh et al. [143]	17	VPDT then 48 h later IVB+IVTA	Standard-fluence (600 mW/cm² for 83 s to deliver 50 J/cm²)	2 mg IVTA (0.05 mL)	1.25 IVB (0.05 mL)	50 weeks

IVB intravitreal bevacizumab, *IVD* intravitreal dexamethasone, *IVTA* intravitreal triamcinolone acetonidel, *VPDT* verteporfin photodynamic therapy of bevacizumab was given at three months for residual leakage. Thirty-six eyes of 33 patients, with mean follow-up of 14.7 months, were analyzed. At six months,, 61.1% (22/36) showed stable or improved vision, and 27.8% (10/36) gained ≥3 lines. Twenty-eight eyes (77.8%) achieved CNV resolution after this single session of triple therapy. One eye lost more than six lines due to retinal pigment epithelium tear, three eyes showed a significant cataract requiring surgery, and two showed persistent raised IOP at six months. In this study, the short-term results of single session triple therapy suggested that it may be a useful treatment option for neovascular AMD based on its low retreatment rates, sustainable CNV eradication results, and visual gain achievements [140]. Other small studies have also concluded that triple therapy may allow maintenance of visual acuity while reducing the number of necessary treatments [141–143].

> **Pearl**
> Studies evaluating combination AMD therapy are ongoing; within the next few years these studies will hopefully add clarity and allow for optimal treatment protocols.

For a more definitive answer, the RADICAL (Reduced Fluence Visudyne Anti-VEGF-Dexamethasone in Combination for AMD Lesions) study compared the efficacy of reduced-fluence VPDT and ranibizumab combination therapy with or without dexamethasone, with ranibizumab monotherapy in 162 treatment-naive subjects with exudative AMD. The RADICAL study is a Phase II, multicenter, randomized, single-masked study [144]. The unpublished one-year results indicate that triple therapy consisting of half-fluence VPDT with ranibizumab and dexamethasone resulted in a visual improvement of 6.8 letters compared with 6.5 letters in the ranibizumab monotherapy group. In addition, triple therapy with half-fluence VPDT resulted in a mean of three visits at which ranibizumab retreatment was applied compared with 5.4 in the ranibizumab monotherapy group [141].

Combination therapy for age-related macular degeneration (AMD) (verteporfin photodynamic therapy [vPDT] then ranibizumab, with or without dexamethasone) in RADICAL resulted in fewer visits at which retreatments were applied than a ranibizumab monotherapy regimen, with vision outcomes appearing similar to ranibizumab monotherapy (although with wide confidence intervals), at 12 months. Two-year data are pending at this time.

Summary

Exudative AMD is a multifactoral disease with inflammatory, vascular, and angiogenic components. Recent therapeutic advances in the treatment of exudative AMD have been highly successful; however, areas for improvement exist. The currently available exudative AMD treatments primarily target a single component in the pathogenesis of CNV. By combining various treatments, patients may benefit from additive or synergistic effects while reducing the frequency of treatments. Investigations into optimal combination treatment regimens are ongoing.

References

1. Rubin GS, Roche KB, Prasada-Rao P, Fried LP. Visual impairment and disability in older adults. Optom Vis Sci. 1994;71:750–60.
2. Williams RA, Brody BL, Thomas RG, Kaplan RM, Brown SI. The psychosocial impact of macular degeneration. Arch Ophthalmol. 1998;116:514–20.
3. Friedman DS, O'Colmain BJ, Munoz B, et al. Prevalence of age-related macular degeneration in the United States. Arch Ophthalmol. 2004;122: 564–72.
4. Kourlas H, Abrams P. Ranibizumab for the treatment of neovascular age-related macular degeneration: a review. Clin Ther. 2007;29:1850–61.
5. Pauleikhoff D. Neovascular age-related macular degeneration: natural history and treatment outcomes. Retina. 2005;25:1065–84.
6. Kaiser PK. Verteporfin photodynamic therapy and anti-angiogenic drugs: potential for combination therapy in exudative age-related macular degeneration. Cur Med Res Opin. 2007;23:477–87.
7. Kent D, Sheridan C. Choroidal neovascularization: a wound healing perspective. Mol Vis. 2003;9:747–55.

8. Zarbin MA. Current concepts in the pathogenesis of age-related macular degeneration. Arch Ophthalmol. 2004;122:598–614.

9. Gille J. Antiangiogenic cancer therapies get their act together: current developments and future prospects of growth factor- and growth factor receptor-targeted approaches. Exp Dermatol. 2006;15:175–86.

10. Caprioni F, Fornarini G. Bevacizumab in the treatment of metastatic colorectal cancer. Future Oncol. 2007;3:141–8.

11. Giaccone G. The potential of antiangiogenic therapy in non-small cell lung cancer. Clin Cancer Res. 2007;13:1961–70.

12. Mancuso A, Calabro F, Sternberg CN. Current therapies and advances in the treatment of pancreatic cancer. Crit Rev Oncol Hematol. 2006;58:231–41.

13. Han ES, Monk BJ. Bevacizumab in the treatment of ovarian cancer. Expert Rev Anticancer Ther. 2007;7:1339–45.

14. Taiwo BO. Antiretroviral treatment: current approach and future prospects. Afr J Med Med Sci. 2006;35:S1–11.

15. Sturmer M, Staszewski S, Doerr HW. Quadruple nucleoside therapy with zidovudine, lamivudine, abacavir and tenofovir in the treatment of HIV. Antivir Ther. 2007;12:695–703.

16. Weir MR. Risk-based classification of hypertension and the role of combination therapy. J Clin Hypertens (Greenwich). 2008;10:4–12.

17. Elliott WJ. What factors contribute to the inadequate control of elevated blood pressure? J Clin Hypertens (Greenwich). 2008;10:20–6.

18. Klein R, Klein BE, Jensen SC, et al. The five-year incidence and progression of age-related maculopathy: the Beaver Dam Eye Study. Ophthalmology. 1997;104:7–21.

19. Pe'er J, Shweiki D, Itin A, et al. Hypoxia-induced expression of vascular endothelial growth factor by retinal cells is a common factor in neovascularizing ocular diseases. Lab Invest. 1995;72:638–45.

20. Grunwald JE, Metelitsina TI, Dupont JC, et al. Reduced foveolar choroidal blood flow in eyes with increasing AMD severity. Invest Ophthalmol Vis Sci. 2005;46:1033–8.

21. Yoshida S, Yoshida A, Ishibashi T. Induction of IL-8, MCP-1, and bFGF by TNF-alpha in retinal glial cells: implications for retinal neovascularization during post-ischemic inflammation. Graefes Arch Clin Exp Ophthalmol. 2004;242:409–13.

22. Spaide RF. Rationale for combination therapies for choroidal neovascularization. Am J Ophthalmol. 2006;141:149–56.

23. Campochiaro PA. Ocular neovascularisation and excessive vascular permeability. Expert Opin Biol Ther. 2004;4:1395–402.

24. Shima DT, Adamis AP, Ferrara N, et al. Hypoxic induction of endothelial cell growth factors in retinal cells: identification and characterization of vascular endothelial growth factor (VEGF) as the mitogen. Mol Med. 1995;1:182–93.

25. Keyt BA, Berleau LT, Nguyen HV, et al. The carboxyl-terminal domain (111–165) of vascular endothelial growth factor is critical for its mitogenic potency. J Biol Chem. 1996;271:7788–95.

26. Park JE, Keller GA, Ferrara N. The vascular endothelial growth factor (VEGF) isoforms: differential deposition into the subepithelial extracellular matrix and bioactivity of extracellular matrix-bound VEGF. Mol Biol Cell. 1993;4:1317–26.

27. Ng EW, Adamis AP. Targeting angiogenesis, the underlying disorder in neovascular age-related macular degeneration. Can J Ophthalmol. 2005;40:352–68.

28. Shima DT, Kuroki M, Deutsch U, et al. The mouse gene for vascular endothelial growth factor. Genomic structure, definition of the transcriptional unit, and characterization of transcriptional and post-transcriptional regulatory sequences. J Biol Chem. 1996;271:3877–83.

29. Ishida S, Usui T, Yamashiro K, et al. VEGF164-mediated inflammation is required for pathological, but not physiological, ischemia-induced retinal neovascularization. J Exp Med. 2003;198:483–9.

30. McColm JR, Geisen P, Hartnett ME. VEGF isoforms and their expression after a single episode of hypoxia or repeated fluctuations between hyperoxia and hypoxia: relevance to clinical ROP. Mol Vis. 2004;10:512–20.

31. Hiromatsu Y, Toda S. Mast cells and angiogenesis. Microsc Res Tech. 2003;60:64–9.

32. Miyamoto K, Khosrof S, Bursell SE, et al. Vascular endothelial growth factor (VEGF)-induced retinal vascular permeability is mediated by intercellular adhesion molecule-1 (ICAM-1). Am J Pathol. 2000;156:1733–9.

33. Cursiefen C, Chen L, Borges LP, et al. VEGF-A stimulates lymphangiogenesis and hemangiogenesis in inflammatory neovascularization via macrophage recruitment. J Clin Invest. 2004;113:1040–50.

34. Aiello LP, Pierce EA, Foley ED, et al. Suppression of retinal neovascularization in vivo by inhibition of vascular endothelial growth factor (VEGF) using soluble VEGF-receptor chimeric proteins. Proc Natl Acad Sci USA. 1995;92:10457–61.

35. Krzystolik MG, Afshari MA, Adamis AP, et al. Prevention of experimental choroidal neovascularization with intravitreal anti-vascular endothelial growth factor antibody fragment. Arch Ophthalmol. 2002;120:338–46.

36. Aiello LP, Avery RL, Arrigg PG, et al. Vascular endothelial growth factor in ocular fluid of patients with diabetic retinopathy and other retinal disorders. N Engl J Med. 1994;331:1480–7.

37. Malecaze F, Clamens S, Simorre-Pinatel V, et al. Detection of vascular endothelial growth factor messenger RNA and vascular endothelial growth factor-like activity in proliferative diabetic retinopathy. Arch Ophthalmol. 1994;112:1476–82.

38. Schwesinger C, Yee C, Rohan RM, et al. Intrachoroidal neovascularization in transgenic mice over-

expressing vascular endothelial growth factor in the retinal pigment epithelium. Am J Pathol. 2001; 158:1161–72.

39. Tolentino MJ, Miller JW, Gragoudas ES, et al. Vascular endothelial growth factor is sufficient to produce iris neovascularization and neovascular glaucoma in a nonhuman primate. Arch Ophthalmol. 1996;114:964–70.

40. Tolentino MJ, McLeod DS, Taomoto M, et al. Pathologic features of vascular endothelial growth factor-induced retinopathy in the nonhuman primate. Am J Ophthalmol. 2002;133:373–85.

41. He S, Jin ML, Worpel V, Hinton DR. A role for connective tissue growth factor in the pathogenesis of choroidal neovascularization. Arch Ophthalmol. 2003;121:1283–8.

42. Kliffen M, Sharma HS, Mooy CM, et al. Increased expression of angiogenic growth factors in age-related maculopathy. Br J Ophthalmol. 1997;81: 154–62.

43. Holekamp NM, Bouck N, Volpert O. Pigment epithelium derived factor is deficient in the vitreous of patients with choroidal neovascularization due to age-related macular degeneration. Am J Ophthalmol. 2002;134:220–7.

44. Kaiser PK. Verteporfin therapy in combination with triamcinolone: published studies investigating a potential synergistic effect. Curr Med Res Opin. 2005;21:705–13.

45. Schmidt-Erfurth U, Schlotzer-Schrehard U, Cursiefen C, et al. Influence of photodynamic therapy on expression of vascular endothelial growth factor (VEGF), VEGF receptor 3, and pigment epithelium-derived factor. Invest Ophthalmol Vis Sci. 2003;44:4473–80.

46. Kaiser PK. Steroids for choroidal neovascularization. Am J Ophthalmol. 2005;139:533–5.

47. Bandi N, Kompella UB. Budesonide reduces vascular endothelial growth factor secretion and expression in airway (Calu-1) and alveolar (A549) epithelial cells. Eur J Pharmacol. 2001;425:109–16.

48. Folkman J. Ingber DE Angiostatic steroids. Method of discovery and mechanism of action. Ann Surg. 1987;206:374–83.

49. Tatar O, Shinoda K, Kaiserling E, et al. Early effects of triamcinolone on vascular endothelial growth factor and endostatin in human choroidal neovascularization. Arch Ophthalmol. 2008;126:193–9.

50. Wang YS, Friedrichs U, Eichler W, Hoffmann S, Wiedemann P. Inhibitory effects of triamcinolone acetonide on bFGF-induced migration and tube formation in choroidal microvascular endothelial cells. Graefes Arch Clin Exp Ophthalmol. 2002;240:42–8.

51. Fischer S, Renz D, Schaper W, Karliczek GF. In vitro effects of dexamethasone on hypoxia-induced hyperpermeability and expression of vascular endothelial growth factor. Eur J Pharmacol. 2001;411:231–43.

52. Ingber DE, Madri JA, Folkman J. A possible mechanism for inhibition of angiogenesis by angiostatic steroids: induction of capillary basement membrane dissolution. Endocrinology. 1986;119:1768–75.

53. Penfold PL, Wen L, Madigan MC, Gillies MC, King NJ, Provis JM. Triamcinolone acetonide modulates permeability and intercellular adhesion molecule-1 (ICAM-1) expression of the ECV304 cell line: implications for macular degeneration. Clin Exp Immunol. 2000;121:458–65.

54. Penfold PL, Wen L, Madigan MC, King NJ, Provis JM. Modulation of permeability and adhesion molecule expression by human choroidal endothelial cells. Invest Ophthalmol Vis Sci. 2002;43:3125–30.

55. Lewis GD, Campbell WB, Johnson AR. Inhibition of prostaglandin synthesis by glucocorticoids in human endothelial cells. Endocrinology. 1986;119: 62–9.

56. Umland SP, Nahrebne DK, Razac S, et al. The inhibitory effects of topically active glucocorticoids on IL-4, IL-5, and interferon-gamma production by cultured primary CD4+ T cells. J Allergy Clin Immunol. 1997;100:511–9.

57. Bhattacherjee P, Williams RN, Eakins KE. A comparison of the ocular anti-inflammatory activity of steroidal and nonsteroidal compounds in the rat. Invest Ophthalmol Vis Sci. 1983;24:1143–6.

58. Ciulla TA, Criswell MH, Danis RP, Hill TE. Intravitreal triamcinolone acetonide inhibits choroidal neovascularization in a laser-treated rat model. Arch Ophthalmol. 2001;119:399–404.

59. Danis RP, Bingaman DP, Yang Y, Ladd B. Inhibition of preretinal and optic nerve head neovascularization in pigs by intravitreal triamcinolone acetonide. Ophthalmology. 1996;103:2099–104.

60. Antoszyk AN, Gottlieb JL, Machemer R, Hatchell DL. The effects of intravitreal triamcinolone acetonide on experimental preretinal neovascularization. Graefes Arch Clin Exp Ophthalmol. 1993;231:34–40.

61. Wilson CA, Berkowitz BA, Sato Y, Ando N, Handa JT, de Juan Jr E. Treatment with intravitreal steroid reduces blood-retinal barrier breakdown due to retinal photocoagulation. Arch Ophthalmol. 1992;110:1155–9.

62. Gillies MC, Simpson JM, Luo W, et al. A randomized clinical trial of a single dose of intravitreal triamcinolone acetonide for neovascular age-related macular degeneration: one-year results. Arch Ophthalmol. 2003;121:667–73.

63. Gillies MC, Simpson JM, Billson FA, et al. Safety of an intravitreal injection of triamcinolone: results from a randomized clinical trial. Arch Ophthalmol. 2004;122:336–40.

64. Bakri SJ, Beer PM. The effect of intravitreal triamcinolone acetonide on intraocular pressure. Ophthalmic Surg Lasers Imaging. 2003;34:386–90.

65. Moshfeghi DM, Kaiser PK, Scott IU, et al. Acute endophthalmitis following intravitreal triamcinolone acetonide injection. Am J Ophthalmol. 2003;136: 791–6.

66. Nelson ML, Tennant MT, Sivalingam A, Regillo CD, Belmont JB, Martidis A. Infectious and pre-

sumed noninfectious endophthalmitis after intravitreal triamcinolone acetonide injection. Retina. 2003;23:686–91.

67. Schmidt-Erfurth U, Hasan T. Mechanisms of action of photodynamic therapy with verteporfin for the treatment of age-related macular degeneration. Surv Ophthalmol. 2000;45:195–214.

68. Schmidt-Erfurth U, Hasan T, Schomacker K, Flotte T, Birngruber R. In vivo uptake of liposomal benzoporphyrin derivative and photothrombosis in experimental corneal neovascularization. Lasers Surg Med. 1995;17:178–88.

69. Schmidt-Erfurth U, Hasan T, Gragoudas E, Michaud N, Flotte TJ, Birngruber R. Vascular targeting in photodynamic occlusion of subretinal vessels. Ophthalmology. 1994;101:1953–61.

70. Schlotzer-Schrehardt U, Viestenz A, Naumann GO, Laqua H, Michels S, Schmidt-Erfurth U. Dose-related structural effects of photodynamic therapy on choroidal and retinal structures of human eyes. Graefes Arch Clin Exp Ophthalmol. 2002;240:748–57.

71. Debefve E, Pegaz B, van den Bergh H, et al. Video monitoring of neovessel occlusion induced by photodynamic therapy with verteporfin (Visudyne), in the CAM model. Angiogenesis. 2008;11(3):235–43. Epub 2008 Mar 7.

72. Verteporfin Roundtable Participants. Guidelines for using verteporfin (Visudyne) in photodynamic therapy for choroidal neovascularization due to age-related macular degeneration and other causes: update. Retina. 2005;25:119–34.

73. Treatment of Age-Related Macular Degeneration with Photodynamic Therapy (TAP) Study Group. Photodynamic therapy of subfoveal choroidal neovascularization in age-related macular degeneration with verteporfin: two-year results of 2 randomized clinical trials – TAP Report 2. Arch Ophthalmol. 2001;119:198–207.

74. Verteporfin in Photodynamic Therapy (VIP) Study Group. Verteporfin therapy of subfoveal choroidal neovascularization in age-related macular degeneration: two-year results of a randomized clinical trial including lesions with occult with no classic choroidal neovascularization – verteporfin in photodynamic therapy report 2. Am J Ophthalmol. 2001;131:541–60.

75. Visudyne in Minimally Classic CNV (VIM) Study Group. Verteporfin therapy of subfoveal minimally classic choroidal neovascularization in age-related macular degeneration: 2-year results of a randomized clinical trial. Arch Ophthalmol. 2005;123:448–57.

76. Treatment of Age-Related Macular Degeneration with Photodynamic Therapy (TAP) and Verteporfin in Photodynamic Therapy (VIP) Study Groups. Verteporfin therapy of subfoveal choroidal neovascularization in age-related macular degeneration: meta-analysis of 2-year safety results in three randomized clinical trials: treatment of age-related macular degeneration with photodynamic therapy and verteporfin in photodynamic therapy study report no. 4. Retina. 2004;24:1–12.

77. Treatment of Age-Related Macular Degeneration with Photodynamic Therapy (TAP) and Verteporfin in Photodynamic Therapy (VIP) Study Groups. Acute severe visual acuity decrease after photodynamic therapy with verteporfin: case reports from randomized clinical trials – TAP and VIP Report No. 3. Am J Ophthalmol. 2004;137:683–96. Curr Med Res Opin.

78. Kaiser PK, Treatment of Age-Related Macular Degeneration with Photodynamic Therapy (TAP) Study Group. Verteporfin therapy of subfoveal choroidal neovascularization in age-related macular degeneration: 5-year results of two randomized clinical trials with an open-label extension – TAP Report No. 8. Graefes Arch Clin Exp Ophthalmol. 2006;244:1132–42.

79. Michels S, Schmidt-Erfurth U, Rosenfeld PJ. Promising new treatments for neovascular age-related macular degeneration. Expert Opin Investig Drugs. 2006;15:779–93.

80. Adamis AP, Shima DT. The role of vascular endothelial growth factor in ocular health and disease. Retina. 2005;25:111–8.

81. Gragoudas ES, Adamis AP, Cunningham Jr ET, et al. Pegaptanib for neovascular age-related macular degeneration. N Engl J Med. 2004;351:2805–16.

82. Ruckman J, Green LS, Beeson J, et al. 2'-Fluoropyrimidine RNA-based aptamers to the 165-amino acid form of vascular endothelial growth factor (VEGF165). Inhibition of receptor binding and VEGF-induced vascular permeability through interactions requiring the exon 7-encoded domain. J Biol Chem. 1998;273:20556–67.

83. Chakravarthy U, Adamis AP, Cunningham Jr ET, et al. Year 2 efficacy results of 2 randomized controlled clinical trials of pegaptanib for neovascular age-related macular degeneration. Ophthalmology. 2006;113:1508–25.

84. Gaudreault J, Fei D, Rusit J, et al. Preclinical pharmacokinetics of Ranibizumab (rhuFabV2) after a single intravitreal administration. Invest Ophthalmol Vis Sci. 2005;46:726–33.

85. Rosenfeld PJ, Brown DM, Heier JS, et al. Ranibizumab for neovascular age-related macular degeneration. N Engl J Med. 2006;355:1419–31.

86. Brown DM, Kaiser PK, Michels M, et al. Ranibizumab versus verteporfin for neovascular age-related macular degeneration. N Engl J Med. 2006;355:1432–44.

87. Heier JS, Antoszyk AN, Pavan PR, et al. Ranibizumab for treatment of neovascular age-related macular degeneration: a phase I/II multicenter, controlled, multidose study. Ophthalmology. 2006;113(4):642.e1–4.

88. Hurwitz H, Fehrenbacher L, Novotny W, et al. Bevacizumab plus irinotecan, fluorouracil, and leucovorin for metastatic colorectal cancer. N Engl J Med. 2004;350:2335–42.

89. Waisbourd M, Loewenstein A, Goldstein M, Leibovitch I. Targeting vascular endothelial growth factor: a promising strategy for treating age-related macular degeneration. Drugs Aging. 2007;24:643–62.

90. Avery RL, Pieramici DJ, Rabena MD, et al. Intravitreal bevacizumab (Avastin) for neovascular age-related macular degeneration. Ophthalmology. 2006;113:363–72.

91. Bashshur ZF, Bazarbachi A, Schakal A, et al. Intravitreal bevacizumab for the management of choroidal neovascularization in age-related macular degeneration. Am J Ophthalmol. 2006;142:1–9.

92. Costa RA, Jorge R, Calucci D, et al. Intravitreal bevacizumab for choroidal neovascularization caused by AMD (IBeNA Study): results of a phase I dose-escalation study. Invest Ophthalmol Vis Sci. 2006;47:4569–78.

93. Spaide RF, Laud K, Fine HF, et al. Intravitreal bevacizumab treatment of choroidal neovascularization secondary to age-related macular degeneration. Retina. 2006;26:383–90.

94. Rich RM, Rosenfeld PJ, Puliafito CA, et al. Short-term safety and efficacy of intravitreal bevacizumab (Avastin) for neovascular age-related macular degeneration. Retina. 2006;26:495–511.

95. Manzano RP, Peyman GA, Khan P, Kivilcim M. Testing intravitreal toxicity of bevacizumab (Avastin). Retina. 2006;26:257–61.

96. Slakter JS, Bochow TW, D'Amico DJ, et al. Anecortave acetate (15 milligrams) versus photodynamic therapy for treatment of subfoveal neovascularization in age-related macular degeneration. Ophthalmology. 2006;113:3–13.

97. Clark AF. AL-3789: a novel ophthalmic angiostatic steroid. Expert Opin Investig Drugs. 1997;6:1867–77.

98. Kwak N, Okamoto N, Wood JM, Campochiaro PA. VEGF is major stimulator in model of choroidal neovascularization. Invest Ophthalmol Vis Sci. 2000;41:3158–64.

99. Shen J, Samul R, Silva RL, et al. Suppression of ocular neovascularization with siRNA targeting VEGF receptor 1. Gene Ther. 2006;13:225–34.

100. Ciulla TA, Criswell MH, Danis RP, et al. Squalamine lactate reduces choroidal neovascularization in a laser-injury model in the rat. Retina. 2003;23:808–14.

101. Campochiaro PA, Dong NQ, Mahmood SS, et al. Adenoviral vector-delivered pigment epithelium-derived factor for neovascular age-related macular degeneration: results of a phase I clinical trial. Hum Gene Ther. 2006;17:177–9.

102. Rosenfeld PJ, Rich RM, Lalwani GA. Ranibizumab: phase III clinical trial results. Ophthalmol Clin North Am. 2006;19:361–72.

103. Regillo CD, Brown DM, Abraham P, et al. Randomized, double-masked, sham-controlled trial of ranibizumab for neovascular age-related macular degeneration: PIER Study Year 1. Am J Ophthalmol. 2008;145:239–48.

104. Bergers G, Song S, Meyer-Morse N, et al. Benefits of targeting both pericytes and endothelial cells in the tumor vasculature with kinase inhibitors. J Clin Invest. 2003;111:1287–95.

105. Bradley J, Ju M, Robinson GS. Combination therapy for the treatment of ocular neovascularization. Angiogenesis. 2007;10:141–8.

106. Jo N, Mailhos C, Ju M, et al. Inhibition of platelet-derived growth factor B signaling enhances the efficacy of anti-vascular endothelial growth factor therapy in multiple models of ocular neovascularization. Am J Pathol. 2006;168:2036–53.

107. Azab M, Boyer DS, Bressler NM, et al. Verteporfin therapy of subfoveal minimally classic choroidal neovascularization in age-related macular degeneration: 2-year results of a randomized clinical trial. Arch Ophthalmol. 2005;123:448e57.

108. Schmidt-Erfurth U, Schlotzer-Schrehard U, Cursiefen C, et al. Influence of photodynamic therapy on expression of vascular endothelial growth factor (VEGF), VEGF receptor 3, and pigment epithelium-derived factor. Invest Ophthalmol Vis Sci. 2003;44:4473e80.

109. Kaiser PK. Combination therapy with verteporfin and anti-VEGF agents in neovascular age-related macular degeneration: where do we stand? Br J Ophthalmol. 2010;94(2):143–5.

110. Shah GK, Sang DN, Hughes MS. Verteporfin combination regimens in the treatment of neovascular AMD. Retina. 2009;29(2):133–48.

111. Alon T, Hemo I, Itin A, Pe'er J, Stone J, Keshet E. Vascular endothelial growth factor acts as a survival factor for newly formed retinal vessels and has implications for retinopathy of prematurity. Nat Med. 1995;1:1024–8.

112. Emerson MV, Lauer AK. Emerging therapies for the treatment of neovascular age-related macular degeneration and diabetic macular edema. BioDrugs. 2007;21:245–57.

113. Nishijima K, Ng YS, Zhong L, et al. Vascular endothelial growth factor-A is a survival factor for retinal neurons and a critical neuroprotectant during the adaptive response to ischemic injury. Am J Pathol. 2007;171:53–67.

114. Schlingemann RO. Role of growth factors and the wound healing response in age-related macular degeneration. Graefes Arch Clin Exp Ophthalmol. 2004;242:91–101.

115. Rogers AH, Martidis A, Greenberg PB, Puliafito CA. OCT findings following PDT of CNV. Am J Ophthalmol. 2002;240:748–57.

116. Schmidt-Erfurth U, Laqua H, Schlotzer-Schrehard U, et al. Histopathological changes following photodynamic therapy in human eyes. Arch Ophthalmol. 2002;120:835–44.

117. Spaide RF, Sorenson J, Maranan L. Combined photodynamic therapy with verteporfin and intravitreal triamcinolone acetonide for choroidal neovascularization. Ophthalmology. 2003;110:1517–25.

118. Spaide RF, Sorenson J, Maranan L. Photodynamic therapy with verteporfin combined with intravitreal injection of triamcinolone acetonide for choroidal neovascularization. Ophthalmology. 2005;112:301–4.

119. Rechtman E, Danis RP, Pratt LM, Harris A. Intravitreal triamcinolone with photodynamic therapy for subfoveal choroidal neovascularisation in age related macular degeneration. Br J Ophthalmol. 2004;88:344–7.

120. Moshfeghi A, Puliafito C, Rosenfeld P. Combination verteporfin therapy and intravitreal triamcinolone n neovascular age-related macular degeneration. Presented at the 2004 Meeting of the Retina Society, Baltimore, 30 Sept–3 Oct 2004.

121. Roth DB, Walsman S, Modi A, et al. Intravitreal triamcinolone combined with photodynamic therapy for exudative macular degeneration. Presented at the American Academy of Ophthalmology and European Society of Ophthalmology 2004 Joint Meeting; New Orleans, 23–26 Oct 2004.

122. Augustin AJ, Schmidt-Erfurth U. PDT and triamcinolone for the treatment of occult CNV in AMD. Presented at the 27th Annual Macula Society Meeting, Las Vegas, 26 Feb–1 Mar 2004.

123. El Matri L, Baklouti K, Mghaieth F, et al. Photodynamic therapy and intravitreal triamcinolone for exudative [sic] age related macular degeneration. Invest Ophthalmol Vis Sci. 2004;45:EAbstract 3162.

124. Bhavsar AR. Combined verteporfin therapy and intravitreal triamcinolone in the treatment of minimally classic subfoveal CNV with or without RAP lesions. Presented at the American Academy of Ophthalmology and European Society of Ophthalmology 2004 Joint Meeting, New Orleans, 23–26 Oct 2004.

125. Spaide RF, Sorenson J, Maranan L. Combined photodynamic therapy with verteporfin and intravitreal triamcinolone for juxtafoveal and extrafoveal choroidal neovascularization. Presented at the American Academy of Ophthalmology and European Society of Ophthalmology 2004 Joint Meeting, New Orleans, 23–26 Oct 2004.

126. Johnson RN, Yang S, McDonald HR, Ai E, Jumper JM. Combined photodynamic therapy and intravitreal triamcinolone acetonide for AMD. Presented at the American Academy of Ophthalmology and European Society of Ophthalmology 2004 Joint Meeting, New Orleans, 23–26 Oct 2004.

127. Augustin AJ, Schmidt-Erfurth U. Verteporfin therapy combined with intravitreal triamcinolone in all types of CNV due to AMD. Ophthalmology. 2006;113(1):14–22.

128. Chan WM, Lai TY, Wong AL, Tong JP, Liu DT, Lam DS. Combined photodynamic therapy and intravitreal triamcinolone injection for the treatment of subfoveal choroidal neovascularisation in age related macular degeneration: a comparative study. Br J Ophthalmol. 2006;90:337–41.

129. Ergun E, Maar N, Ansari-Shahrezaei S, Wimpissinger B, Krepler K, Wedrich A, et al. Photodynamic therapy with verteporfin and intravitreal triamcinolone acetonide in the treatment of neovascular age-related macular degeneration. Am J Ophthalmol. 2006;142:10–6.

130. Arias L, Garcia-Arumi J, Ramon JM, Badia M, Rubio M, Pujol O. Photodynamic therapy with intravitreal triamcinolone in predominantly classic choroidal neovascularization: one-year results of a randomized study. Ophthalmology. 2006;113:2243–50.

131. Ruiz-Moreno JM, Montero JA, Barile S, Zarbin MA. Photodynamic therapy and high-dose intravitreal triamcinolone to treat exudative age-related macular degeneration: 2-year outcome. Retina. 2007;27:458–61.

132. Maberley D et al. Photodynamic therapy and intravitreal triamcinolone for neovascular age-related macular degeneration a randomized clinical trial. Ophthalmology. 2009;116(11):2149–57.

133. Treatment of Age-Related Macular Degeneration with Photodynamic Therapy (TAP) Study Group. Photodynamic therapy of subfoveal choroidal neovascularization in age-related macular degeneration with verteporfin: one-year results of 2 randomized clinical trials — TAP report 1. Arch Ophthalmol. 1999;117:1329–45.

134. Eyetech Pharma. Division of Anti-inflammatory, Analgesic and Ophthalmic Drug Products Advisory Committee Meeting Briefing Package for Macugen 2004. Available at http://www.fda.gov/ohrms/dockets/ac/04/briefing/2004-053B1_02_FDA Backgrounder.pdf. Accessed January 23, 2010.

135. Antoszyk AN et al. Ranibizumab combined with verteporfin photodynamic therapy in neovascular age-related macular degeneration (FOCUS): year 2 results. Am J Ophthalmol. 2008;145(5):862–74.

136. Lazic R, Gabric N. Veteporfin therapy and intravitreal bevacizumab combined and alone in CNV due to AMD. Ophthalmology. 2007;114(6):1179–85.

137. Kaiser PK et al. Verteporfin photodynamic therapy combined with intravitreal bevacizumab for neovascular age-related macular degeneration. Ophthalmology. 2009;116:747–55.

138. QLT Annouces 12-Month Results From Novartis Sponsored MONT BLANC Study. Available at http://www.qltinc.com/newsCenter/2009/090615.htm. Accessed June 9, 2011

139. Augustin AJ, Puls S, Offermann I. Triple therapy for CNV due to AMD. Retina. 2007;27(2):133–40.

140. Yip PP, Woo CF, Tang HHY, Ho CK. Triple therapy for neovascular AMD using single-session PDT combined with intravitreal bevacizumab and triamcinolone. Br J Ophthalmol. 2009;93(6):754–8.

141. Ehmann D, García R. Triple therapy for neovascular age-related macular degeneration (verteporfin photodynamic therapy, intravitreal dexamethasone, and intravitreal bevacizumab). Can J Ophthalmol. 2010;45(1):36–40.

142. Bakri SJ, Couch SM, McCannel CA, Edwards AO. Same-day triple therapy with photodynamic therapy, intravitreal dexamethasone, and bevacizumab in wet age-related macular degeneration. Retina. 2009;29(5):573–8.

143. Ahmadieh H et al. Single-session photodynamic therapy combined with intravitreal bevacizumab and triamcinolone for neovascular AMD. BMC Ophthalmol. 2007;7:10.

144. Reduced Fluence Visudyne-Anti-VEGF-Dexamethasone In Combination for AMD Lesions (RADICAL). Available at http://www.clinicaltrials.gov/ct2/show/NCT00492284. Accessed June 9, 2011.

The Future of Non-neovascular Age-Related Macular Degeneration

8

Ketan Laud, Sri Krishna Mukkamala, Claudia Brue, and Jason S. Slakter

Key Points

- Age-related macular degeneration (AMD) is broadly subdivided into the exudative (wet) and nonexudative (dry) subtypes.
- Hard and soft varieties of drusen can be clinically differentiated based on morphological appearance. Hard drusen are small discrete nodules that appear flat and have sharp borders. Soft drusen tend to be larger and more amorphous with borders that are less well defined. They frequently exhibit confluence with surrounding drusen and have a more notable elevation on biomicroscopic evaluation.
- Geographic atrophy (GA) of the retinal pigment epithelium is the advanced form of atrophic dry AMD and is responsible for approximately 20% of legal blindness. Patients with GA tend to be older than those with neovascular forms of AMD at presentation. GA may appear primarily or subsequent to other forms of AMD.
- Fundus photography is commonly used for baseline documentation and for close monitoring of progression in dry AMD. Fundus autofluorescence (FAF) best demonstrates alterations of the retinal pigment epithelium (RPE), including identification of GA. Optical coherence tomography (OCT) can be used to assess drusen size and overall presence, attenuation of the RPE, and integrity of vital structures in the outer retina. Fourier domain/spectral domain OCT (SD-OCT) provides better anatomical detail, has a shorter image acquisition time, and reduces motion artifacts. It is preferred in comparison to time domain technology in dry AMD patients in assessing drusen size and volume and the integrity of vital structures.
- Several clinical trials are studying a variety of pathways with various methods of drug delivery, including surgical implantation.
- Age-related macular degeneration (AMD) is the leading cause of irreversible vision loss in the United States in patients 60 years of age and older. It is estimated that over 8 million people throughout the United States are affected by AMD [1, 2]. The visual impairment caused by AMD results in frequent visits to a retinal specialist for close clinical monitoring. With the aging of the population and with overall longer life expectancies, AMD will become more prevalent in the future. Overall, the disease leads to an extensive decline in quality of life (QOL) and increased need for daily living assistance resulting in a loss of independence in the later years of life of those affected.

AMD is broadly subdivided into the exudative and nonexudative subtypes. In the exudative (wet) form of AMD, novel abnormal blood vessels of fine capillary networks develop from

J.S. Slakter (✉)
Vitreous-Retina-Macula Consultants of New York,
460 Park Ave., 5th Fl.,
New York, NY 10022, USA
e-mail: jslakter@aol.com

A.C. Ho and C.D. Regillo (eds.), *Age-related Macular Degeneration Diagnosis and Treatment*,
DOI 10.1007/978-1-4614-0125-4_8, © Springer Science+Business Media, LLC 2011

the choriocapillaris and invade the macula either in the sub-RPE space (type 1 choroidal neovascularization (CNV)) or through the retinal pigment epithelium (RPE) in the subretinal space (type 2 CNV) [3]. Leakage of serosanguinous fluid and hemorrhage can ensue leading to significant visual loss. Although a minority of patients with AMD manifest the exudative form of the disease, the majority of patients with severe central visual loss (20/200 or worse) from AMD have the exudative form. In contrast, nonexudative (dry) AMD constitutes the majority of cases and typically leads to a gradual and progressive diminution of central vision.

There are a myriad of clinical findings in patients with dry AMD. The hallmark clinical feature is the presence of drusen, metabolic waste products of the RPE which deposit between the RPE and the underlying Bruch's membrane. Other features include alteration in the pigmentation of the RPE, including both hypopigmentation and hyperpigmentation and degenerative changes to the RPE. Ultimately, these alterations can result in a confluent atrophy of the RPE referred to as geographic atrophy (GA). These areas of cell loss can gradually expand and coalesce resulting in visual decline and the formation of an absolute central scotoma.

Drusen

Drusen can be broadly classified into hard and soft varieties, which can be differentiated clinically based on their morphological appearance. They can be recognized by their yellow

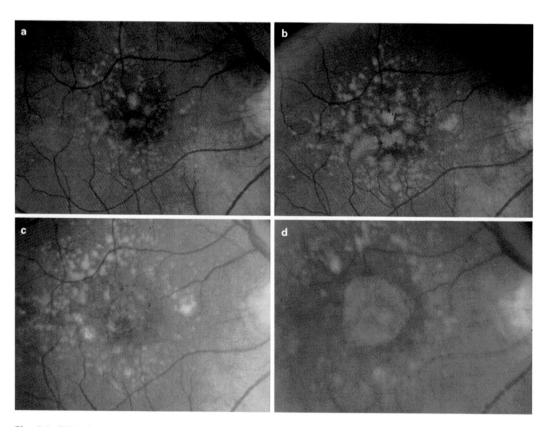

Fig. 8.1 Clinical progression of dry AMD over an 11 year time interval. (**a**) Fundus photograph of the right eye showing a collection of small, intermediate and large sized drusen within the macula. (**b**) With time, there is some progression of the maculopathy with additional drusen formation and pigment deposition. (**c**) On subsequent follow-up 8 years after baseline there is resorbtion of central drusen and a central area of GA. (**d**) At last follow-up 11 years after presentation, there is progression of the central GA, with well defined margins

appearance and sub-RPE location. Their overall prevalence increases with age as they represent metabolic waste products of an aging cell monolayer, the RPE. Hard drusen are small discrete nodules that appear flat and have sharp borders. Soft drusen tend to be larger (>63 μm) and more amorphous with borders that are less well defined. They frequently exhibit confluence with surrounding drusen and have a more notable elevation on biomicroscopic evaluation (Fig. 8.1). At times, large confluent drusen can coalesce to form a focal elevation of the RPE referred to as a drusenoid pigment epithelial detachment (PED), which can masquerade as a neovascular complex. Exudative drusen are important as clinical markers for dry forms of the disease, in its earliest stages. More importantly, their characteristics may serve as predictors of future risk in the development of exudative forms of AMD. Specifically, large confluent drusen (defined as greater than or equal to 125 μm in diameter with indistinct margins) and significant pigmentary changes within the retina are the major risk factors for the progression to more advanced forms of both dry and wet AMD [4–8]. Discussion of the increased risk for progression, need for close clinical monitoring, and role of nutrition and antioxidant supplementation is therefore imperative in this subset of patients.

> **Pearl**
> Large, confluent drusen (≥125 μm) and pigmentary alterations are risk factors for progression to advanced disease

Geographic Atrophy

GA of the RPE is the advanced form of atrophic dry AMD, and is responsible for approximately 20% of legal blindness. Patients with GA tend to be older than those with neovascular forms of AMD at the time of initial presentation. GA may appear primarily or subsequent to other forms of AMD. Development of atrophy in AMD is seen in association with pigmentary alterations and drusen in the macula. The regression of large, soft drusen can lead to GA if the distinct areas of focal atrophy enlarge and coalesce. The clinical appearance of GA varies considerably; it may appear as a single patch or as multiple zones of atrophy (Fig. 8.2). In the early phase of the disease, atrophy is limited to the perifoveal region, then it expands, old atrophic areas may coalesce and new areas appear, with a resulting horseshoe configuration of atrophy. In more severe cases, atrophic areas may spare the fovea, forming a ring-like configuration around it. Complete foveal involvement

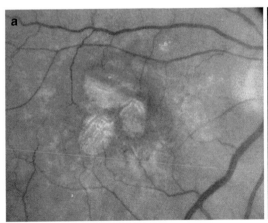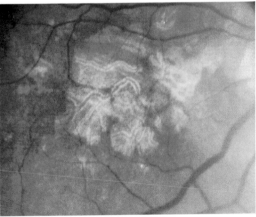

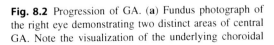

Fig. 8.2 Progression of GA. (**a**) Fundus photograph of the right eye demonstrating two distinct areas of central GA. Note the visualization of the underlying choroidal vessels through the attenuated RPE. (**b**) Follow-up examination 8 years later shows marked progression of the central GA

occurs in the later stages of this process even in cases when there is some partial initial foveal involvement. There is a high degree of symmetry between fellow eyes in total size of atrophy and atrophy morphology. Of note, peripapillary atrophy is observed very commonly in eyes with GA. In very advanced stages, extensive contiguous atrophy may ensue and progress to the temporal arcade vessels or to the nasal retina. The pathophysiologic mechanisms underlying the atrophic process, which involve not only the RPE but also the outer neurosensory retina and choriocapillaris, are poorly understood at present.

> **Pearl**
> Clinical appearance of GA may vary significantly. The optimal imaging modality to monitor progression of GA is fundus autofluorescence.

Imaging Modalities in Dry AMD

A variety of imaging techniques and modalities are utilized in the diagnosis and management of patients with dry AMD. Patients with funduscopic findings of dry AMD such as drusen and RPE alterations can be monitored with serial fundus photography. Fundus photography is commonly utilized for baseline documentation and for close monitoring of progression of dry AMD. The use of fundus photography is also invaluable in educating patients on their condition. Alterations of the RPE including the identification of GA are best demonstrated with the use of fundus autofluorescence (FAF).

FAF imaging is a quick, noninvasive imaging tool for evaluating patients with nonexudative AMD. FAF demonstrates the topographic distribution of lipofuscin throughout the fundus, thereby providing a map of RPE integrity. A localized increase in FAF is observed in AMD patients with PED and within areas of focal hyperpigmentation [9, 10]. GA results in a well-demarcated area of decreased FAF corresponding to the atrophic lesion on fundus examination (Fig. 8.3). Increased FAF is often present along the margins of areas of GA [9, 11]. This increase in FAF along the margins of GA represents areas of oxidative stress or defective or altered metabolism affecting RPE integrity and might serve as markers of atrophic progression. FAF is useful for mapping an expansile creep of GA which may not be clinically apparent. This is important in reconciling the patient's symptoms and the clinical exam.

Optical coherence tomography (OCT) is a noninvasive imaging technique that has proven to be invaluable to diagnose and monitor a variety of retinal diseases that affect the macula. Time-domain OCT relies upon differential reflections of light to produce two-dimensional cross sections of the retina. OCT images are obtained rapidly and have a spatial resolution of approximately 8 mcm. OCT is particularly useful for quantifying retinal thickness and monitoring treatment efficacy [12]. In neovascular AMD, OCT can be useful for identifying intraretinal, subretinal, or sub-RPE fluid. OCT serves as an adjunct to fluorescein angiography, but is increasingly used preferentially to assess presence of intraretinal and/or subretinal fluid in guiding the decision to retreat patients using anti-vascular endothelial growth factor agents. OCT can be utilized in non-neovascular AMD to assess drusen size and overall presence, attenuation of the RPE, and the integrity of vital structures in the outer retina that may become compromised with disease progression.

Fourier domain OCT (SD-OCT) has been recently utilized to better image retinal pathology. Advances in the reduction of image acquisition times and greater resolution provide better anatomical detail and to diagnose subtle pathology. Furthermore, motion artifacts can be reduced with eye tracking capability and better alignment and reproducibility of images is possible with tracking of corresponding retinal vessels. It is preferred in comparison to time-domain technology in dry AMD patients in assessing drusen size and volume using segmentation software as well as the integrity of vital structures for photoreceptor function in the outer retina. It is essential in monitoring shallow areas of subretinal and

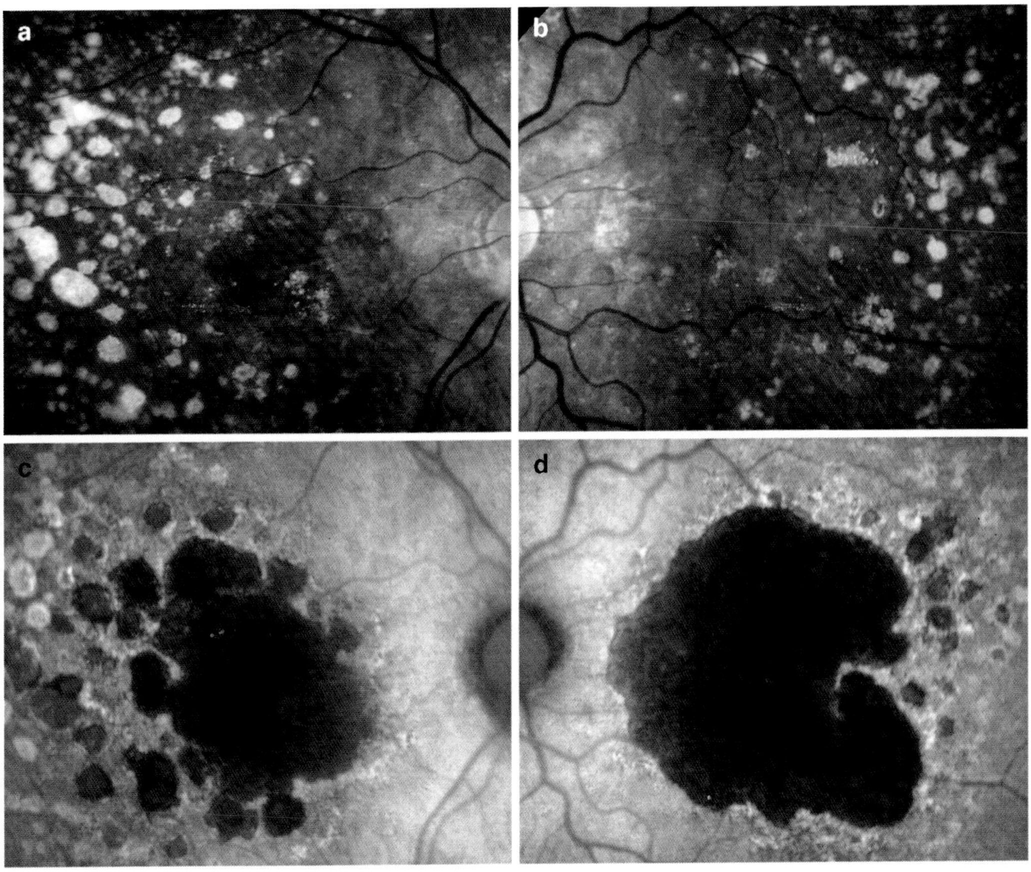

Fig. 8.3 Fundus photographs of the right (**a**) and left (**b**) eye in a patient with dry AMD shows deposition of variably sized drusen in the perifoveal and temporal paramacular region. Note that there is evidence of early RPE alterations and atrophy. Fundus AF of the right (**c**) and left (**d**) eyes shows that there is a large area of well-defined central GA in both eyes. There is a faint, irregular rim of hyperfluorescence along the margins of the GA at the border of preserved and attenuated RPE

intraretinal fluid collection in neovascular AMD patients [13, 14].

Pearl

FAF is a noninvasive measure of lipofuscin distribution and RPE integrity throughout the fundus. FAF can be utilized to monitor progression of patients with dry AMD. OCT is a noninvasive imaging modality that can be used to sequentially monitor the response to therapy. Fourier domain/spectral domain OCT provides greater image resolution and can be used to assess drusen volume using segmentation software.

Clinical Trials for Dry AMD

Study Design

Although there is no proven Food and Drug Administration (FDA)-approved drug treatment for GA, smoking cessation [15] and treatment based on oral supplements as outlined in the Age-Related Eye Disease Study (AREDS) trial [16] may slow the disease progression. Numerous therapeutic strategies have been postulated with three main endpoints: preservation of photoreceptors and RPE (neuroprotection), prevention of oxidative damage, and suppression of inflammation. The most important endpoint to assess efficacy for dry AMD is obviously the preservation of visual acuity, but this endpoint would take many years to assess. To shorten the time period, other surrogate endpoints have been developed to assess efficacy of drugs in trials involving dry AMD.

Some trials have evaluated the change in drusen area by fundus photography, while others aim to determine a drug's effects on the growth of GA, since GA is a feature of dry AMD that directly correlates with the loss of photoreceptors and RPE. Although there is uncertainty surrounding the best molecular pathway to target for the treatment of dry AMD, several different strategies have evolved. The utilization and development of novel imaging modalities combined with the results of clinical trials will translate new insights into future study design and appropriate clinical endpoints.

Risk Reduction in Dry AMD

AREDS

The most significant trial on modulation of risk of AMD and nutrition was the AREDS clinical trial [17]. Patients were enrolled in the AREDS clinical trial if they had extensive small drusen, intermediate drusen, large drusen, noncentral GA, or pigment abnormalities in one or both eyes, or advanced AMD or vision loss due to AMD in one eye. The 3640 participants in the trial were randomly assigned to receive either: (1) antioxidants (vitamin C, 500 mg; vitamin E, 400 IU; and beta-carotene, 15 mg); (2) zinc, 80 mg, as zinc oxide and copper, 2 mg, as cupric oxide; (3) antioxidants plus zinc; or (4) placebo. The primary outcome measures were photographic documentation of progression to or treatment for advanced AMD or at least moderate visual acuity loss from baseline (≥ 15 letters). Those participants with extensive small drusen, nonextensive intermediate size drusen, or pigment abnormalities had only a 1.3% five-year probability of progression to advanced AMD [17]. Upon exclusion of these participants, it was determined that those receiving zinc and antioxidants plus zinc significantly reduced the odds of developing advanced AMD in the higher-risk group. There was a statisti-

cally significant reduction in the rates of moderate visual acuity loss in those participants receiving antioxidants plus zinc [17]. The study concluded therefore that patients with extensive intermediate size drusen, at least one large druse, noncentral GA in one or both eyes, or advanced AMD or vision loss due to AMD in one eye, and without contraindications such as smoking should consider supplementation with antioxidants plus zinc. The effect of supplementation with lutein, zeaxanthine, and omega-3 fatty acids is under investigation in the AREDS 2 trial.

> **Pearl**
>
> **AREDS – Vitamin and Antioxidant Composition**
> - Vitamin C 500 mg
> - Vitamin E 400 International Units (IU)
> - Beta-carotene 15 milligrams (mg)
> - Zinc 80 milligrams (mg)
> - Copper 2 milligrams (mg)

Laser/CAPT

Drusen, as risk factors for progression of AMD, have been the target of laser therapy. Gass first reported on the disappearance of drusen adjacent to sites of laser photocoagulation. He proposed that laser may promote improved approximation of RPE to Bruch's membrane thereby preventing visual loss in the area of drusen. Gass also commented on the possible complications including stimulation of CNV and RPE atrophy at the site of laser [18].

There are several speculations about the mechanism of laser-induced drusen regression and visual acuity stabilization. Photocoagulation may decrease drusen debris production by damaging overlying RPE. Alternatively, it may stimulate RPE metabolic and phagocytic activity clearing debris. Animal models have shown than laser induces an increased number of choriocapillaris endothelial cell processes and choroidal pericyte activity that may contribute to debris digestion on Bruch's membrane [19].

The 1990s were the backdrop for many anecdotal and small series studies on the efficacy of laser photocoagulation on the disappearance of drusen, the progression of dry to exudative forms, and visual outcomes in dry AMD patients. Abdelsalam reviewed many of these controlled and uncontrolled studies, which showed promise in decreasing drusen volume and stabilization or improvement in vision compared to control eyes [20]. Though most smaller studies showed no significant complications, he noted that the larger Choroidal Neovascularization Prevention Trial (CNVPT) was suspended prematurely due to the higher short-term risk of choroidal neovascularizations (CNVMs) in the treated eyes.

The current role of laser in dry AMD has been guided by a National Eye Institute (NEI)-sponsored multicenter randomized clinical trial, the Complications of Age-Related Macular Degeneration Prevention Trial (CAPT) [21]. The study, with 1,052 participants, aimed to evaluate the efficacy of low-intensity laser on outcome measures including vision loss (≥ 3 lines) and development of CNV and GA. Patients with ≥ 10 drusen larger than 125 μm were treated with 60 barely visible burns in a grid pattern between 1,500 and 2,500 μm from the foveal center. At 12 months, some patients received a further 30 laser burns targeting drusen. No significant adverse effects, such as CNV, were reported as a direct result of the laser application technique. However, the CAPT trial concluded that at five years, low-intensity laser did not affect visual outcomes including visual acuity, contrast threshold, or critical print size. It also did not decrease progression to GA or CNV [21].

Anecortave Acetate

The largest of these risk reduction trials was the Anecortave Acetate Risk Reduction Trial, which evaluated the steroid derivative anecortave acetate (Retaane, Alcon) and which was designed to determine if this drug therapy was able to reduce the rate of disease progression from dry to wet AMD. Although the drug failed to meet its primary endpoint in prevention of choroidal

neovascular development, it was a landmark trial in establishing the feasibility of this type of study design and will serve as a template for future clinical trials of dry AMD.

Control of Disease Progression

Mediators to modify disease progression in dry AMD can be designed to target the photoreceptors and by-products of their continuous turnover, the functioning of the RPE cells, and the choroidal circulation. Studies aimed at controlling disease progression in dry AMD have focused on the anti-oxidant, antiinflammatory, and anti-angiogenic properties of various compounds. There has been significant interest in clinical trials in controlling disease progression in GA. Clinical trials centered on altering the rates of progression in GA remain a logical target as it represents an advanced form of the disease with significant visual loss and can be readily quantified. Results garnered from current trials and their application to future studies will aid in elucidating, more precisely, the molecular pathways that can be modulated in controlling disease progression.

Visual Cycle Inhibition: Antioxidants

The recent tide of focus on autofluorescence (AF) imaging has led to the recognition that in dry AMD, hyper-AF in areas of drusen is followed by the development of zones of hypo-AF, likely representing RPE and photoreceptor death. Clinically, these areas may ultimately be seen as GA. Searching for the cause of the initial hyper-AF, by compounds such as lipofuscin and vitamin A metabolites, might provide insight into the patho-physiology of AMD [22].

One of these vitamin A metabolites is bis-retinoid pyridinium salt, A2E. The effect of this retinal fluorophore can be seen by studying its accumulation in other tapetoretinal degenerative conditions such as Stargardt macular degeneration, ABCA4 mutation-related autosomal recessive retinitis pigmentosa, and recessive cone-rod dystrophies. These conditions have mutations in the ABCA4 (or ABCR) gene that codes for an

ATP-binding cassette transporter that removes all-trans-retinaldehyde (RAL) from cone and rod outer segment discs after light exposure. Inability to do so results in accumulation of RPE lipofuscin pigments, yellow-brown pigment granules containing residues of lysosomal digestion [23].

A2E has many documented cytotoxic effects, including sensitization of RPE to blue-light damage, impairment of phospholipid degradation in phagocytosed outer segments, induction of mitochondrial proapoptotic protein release, and the destabilization of cellular membranes. Further oxidation of A2E results in epoxides that induce DNA fragmentation [23]. The combination of these A2E cytotoxic effects may explain the patho-physiology of photoreceptor destruction in ABCA4 mutation-related retinal degenerations. With a similar initial hyper-AF as seen in the above conditions, perhaps AMD is mediated by A2E related RPE and photoreceptor destruction.

In an effort to reduce the amount of toxic A2E and lipofuscin in AMD patients, fenretinide (4-hydroxy (phenyl) retinamide) is in trials for visual cycle inhibition. As a synthetic retinoid, it competes with retinol for binding to retinol-binding protein (RBP) and transthyretin. The decreased metabolism of retinol results in less A2E buildup in mouse models [23]. Sirion Theraputics (Tampa, FL) recently completed enrollment of a 245-patient phase two fenretinide trials. It was double-masked and involved two doses of oral fenretinide (100 and 300 mg) and a placebo. As the per the company's press release, a subgroup of 78 patients in the 300 mg group at the 18-month follow-up visit showed a GA area growth rate of 22.7% compared to 41.6% in the placebo group, a 45% reduction in median lesion growth rate [24].

Fenretinide's safety profile has been documented in clinical trials for other uses, including cancer, rheumatoid arthritis, acne, and cystic fibrosis. In a large series of 2,867 women using fenretinide for prevention of secondary breast malignancy, common adverse effects included diminished dark adaptation (19%), dermatologic disorders (18.6%), and ocular surface disorders (10.9%) [25]. Given the competitive inhibition of the visual cycle, the dark adaption difficulty is not unexpected and is likely well tolerated given the alterative of progressive vision loss in AMD.

In the new class of visual cycle modulator is ACU-4429 (Acucela Inc., Bothell, WA). It is a nonretinoid molecule that slows regeneration of 11-cis-retinal in rods. A single-center, randomized, double-masked, placebo-controlled, dose-escalation study has shown that oral administration was well tolerated up to 20 mg [26]. The study showed a prolonged course of electroretinogram (ERG) dark adaptation that might indicate a slowing of the rod visual cycle, which will likely result in decreased A2E and lipofuscin accumulation.

Pearl
A2E is a retinal fluorophore with cytotoxic effects and its inhibition is an integral target for various clinical trials.

Antioxidants

The above discussion of visual cycle modulators focuses on decreased production of lipofuscin and A2E. However, the discovery that antioxidants reversed A2E cytotoxic effects has led to a host of other potential treatment options [27]. Recently, OT-551 (Othera Pharmaceuticals Inc., Exton, PA) was studied in phase 2 clinical trials for its topical use in dry AMD and in prevention of post-vitrectomy cataract progression. OT-551 is a cornea permeable topical precursor molecule that is converted by an ocular esterase into TEMPOL-H (OT-674), a cell-permeable hydrophilic nitroxide. It is a stable, free radical compound that protects against reactive oxygen species toxicity, likely through a reaction with hydroxyl (−OH) radicals [28].

Albino rat models injected with OT-551 showed functional (by ERG), morphologic (by histologic evaluation of outer nuclear layer thickness), and laboratory (by Western blot analysis of oxidative end products) evidence of photoreceptor cell protection against light induced damage [29]. Tanito et al. the authors of the above study, propose inhibition of lipid peroxidation as the mechanism of protection [29]. Since lipid peroxidation has been explored as an etiologic process leading to drusen development, OT-551 may have a role in dry AMD. Another possible mechanism involves OT-551's ability to down-regulate intracellular tumor necrosis factor alpha (TNF-α and nuclear factor kappa B (NF-kB), a protein that controls DNA transcription and is often found to be overly expressed in autoimmune and inflammatory conditions [30]. The compound's antioxidative stress, antiinflammatory, and antiangiogenic effects seen in animal models were thought to make it useful for both dry and wet AMD. Although the studies have been halted, future trials utilizing antioxidative approaches for AMD are likely.

Complement

The current clinical approach to dry AMD management is directed toward modifiable risk factors including sun exposure, diet, and smoking. The future focus may be mitigating the effect of less modifiable genetic risk factors. To this extent, complement factor H (CFH) polymorphisms are the most studied genetic association. These polymorphisms may have a role in the development of drusen, the hallmark of dry AMD, as well as in the risk for developing more advanced forms of the disease.

Drusen are extracellular deposits between the inner layer of Bruch's membrane and the basal lamina of the RPE [31]. They may be the result of poor RPE function leading to impaired metabolism of photoreceptor outer segments and accumulation of their byproducts. The histological characteristics of these deposits in AMD include a variety of proteins and inflammatory components such as complement factors, amyloid, and human leukocyte antigen (HLA) and major histocompatibility complex (MHC) Class II antigens. The presence of these immune-modulatory components has led to an investigation into the role of the immune system, in particular the complement system, in the development of drusen [31].

After the physical barrier of the skin, the innate immune system involving complement factors is the second human defense mechanism. It is termed innate because it is inborn and not modifiable, unlike the third defense, an adaptive

immune system that helps create immunity to new pathogens and maintains memory. The innate immune system is a collection of liver-synthesized circulating inactive proteins that are activated in a cascade to form a membrane attack complex (MAC) which lead to pathogen destruction.

There are three pathways involved in the innate complement system: the classical, alternative, and lectin pathways. The classical pathway is triggered by antigen-antibody complexes, the alternative pathway is activated by nonspecific antigens on microbial surfaces, and the lectin pathway involves binding to mannose residues. The three pathways share a common biochemical activation of component C3 by cleavage to C3a and C3b. The second product, C3b, is deposited on both host and pathogens and results in cell destruction. CFH regulates the activity of C3b by binding to glycosaminoglycans (GAGs), heparin, or sialic acid that are present on the host but not on pathogen cell surfaces [31]. On the host surface, in conjunction with Factor I, it inactivates C3b, protecting host cells and allowing for selective C3b destruction of pathogens. CFH also binds directly to C3b resulting in the decay of an alternative pathway enzyme C3-convertase (Fig. 8.4).

Domain 7 on the CFH is responsible for its binding to normal host cells. A single nucleotide polymorphism (SNP) in this domain may reduce CFH's affinity to host cells and its ability to inactivate C3b. One of these SNPs involves a substitution of tyrosine to histidine at codon 402 of the CFH gene, also referred to as an Y402H polymorphism [32]. The polymorphism purportedly decreases its ability to bind to the host heparin site and C-reactive protein (CRP). This may make RPE and choroid susceptible to alternative pathway complement attacks, resulting in their dysfunction, and ultimately to drusen formation. The presence of elevated CRP that has been associated with AMD and the immuno-histo-chemical confirmation of MAC and CFH in drusen may support this hypothesis.

To further establish the genotype-phenotype relationship between a CFH mutations and drusen, membranoproliferative glomerulonephritis type II (MPGN2) can be studied. This condition,

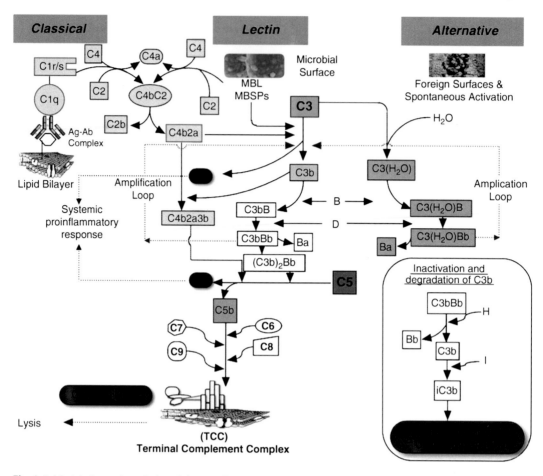

Fig. 8.4 Modulation and regulation of the complement system (Courtesy of Potentia Pharmaceuticals)

like AMD, has been associated with CFH mutations resulting in attenuated function. Immuno-
histo-chemistry shows deposition of complement
factor C3c onto glomerular basement membranes
similar to AMD in which complement debris is
seen below RPE in the form of drusen. Sub-RPE
drusen seen in patients with MPGNII are clinically and histologically similar to those seen in
AMD [31, 33, 34].

Modifiable risk factors may also play a role in
the complement mediated immune destruction of
RPE and choroid. Studies have shown that cigarette smoking can cause activation of the alternate complement pathway. This activation along
with the attenuation of CFH activity in a patient
with an Y402H polymorphism may contribute to
pathologic destruction of host cells [35].

Large population studies have been performed
to determine the genetic effect of the Y402H
polymorphism on developing an AMD phenotype. These studies termed allele T as the normal
CFH and allele C as one with the Y402H SNP. A
meta-analysis of eight of these studies, with a
total of about 4,800 patients, indicates that
heterozygotes for the SNP (i.e., TC) are 2.5 times
more likely to have AMD than patients with a TT
genotype [32]. Patients with a CC genotype were
six times more likely to have AMD. The authors
conclude that each C genotype results in an incremental increase in AMD risk. Thakkinstian et al.
concluded that the combined TC and CC genotypes have a population-attributable risk (PAR),
or contribute to 58.9% of AMD. In addition to the
1q31 locus of the CFH gene, an SNP at the 10q26

locus responsible for possible lymphocyte activation has also been found to have an AMD-attributable risk as high as 57% [31, 36].

Translating this knowledge about the genetics of complement dysregulation into a therapeutic approach for dry AMD is in its nascent stages. POT-4 (Potentia Pharmaceuticals, Louisville, KY), a derivative of Compstatin, is known to inhibit the complement system by binding to C3 and inhibiting its cleavage by C3 convertase, thereby preventing downstream complement activation and inhibiting the complement amplification cycle. In preclinical testing, the molecule was found to form gel deposits in the eye after intravitreal injection. These deposits slowly dissolved over a period of six months or more, releasing active drug into the vitreous cavity over time. A recently completed phase I trial in patients with exudative AMD demonstrated that these gel deposits were formed at higher doses and persisted for at least three months. In addition to an excellent safety profile, there was some evidence of reduced exudation in patients with active CNV. Phase II studies in both dry and wet AMD are planned.

Eculizumab (Alexion Pharmaceuticals Inc., Cheshire, CT) is a complement inhibitor currently in Phase II clinical trials. The COMPLETE (Complement Inhibition with Eculizumab for the Treatment of NonExudative Age-Related Macular Degeneration) study is evaluating the safety and efficacy of an intravenous (IV) infusion of eculizumab versus a saline placebo on drusen volume and GA area. The humanized monoclonal antibody targets complement component, C5, a common component of all three innate pathways and of the membrane attack complex (MAC). As a component of the MAC, the final common pathway of the complement system, C5b-9 could all be potential target.

ARC-1905 (Ophthotech, Princeton, NJ) is a pegylated aptamer, or nucleic acid molecule, which selectively inhibits C5. This drug is in phase I trials for both dry and wet AMD and with and without combination intravitreal Lucentis (Genentech, Inc., San Francisco, CA). Complement inhibitors may prevent pathologic development of drusen; however, there is a concern that these therapies may also alter the body's natural response to

pathogens: both intraocular and systemic. For intravitreal pathogens, this is not a great concern because the complement system does not play a large role in defense in this space. For intravenous infusions, the safety profile will continue to be monitored. ARC-1905, as a C5 inhibitor, spares upstream complement enzymes such as C3 which have MAC-independent defense roles such as promoting opsonization of pathogens.

Potential future anti-complement therapies can target any component of the complement cascade. They can also include a variety of modalities such as antibodies, nucleotides, peptides and proteins, peptidomimetics, and recombinant human factors including CFH. These can be used in combination with existing anti-vascular endothelial growth factor (VEGF) therapies for dry and wet AMD.

As mentioned above, any component of the complement cascade is a potential target for the treatment of dry AMD. Currently, Genentech, Inc. (San Francisco, CA) is conducting phase 1 trials on humanized murine anti-Factor D antibodies (FCFD4514S). Factor D has a role in the alternative pathway by cleaving factor B bound to C3b, generating a C3bBb enzyme which plays an important role as a C3-convertase. Factor D is the only known enzyme able to catalyze this reaction and it has a serum concentration of $1.8\pm.4\ \mu g/mL$, the lowest of any complement protein. These two factors make it the rate-limiting step and absolutely essential to the alternative pathway and a promising target for anti-complement therapy [37–39]. Tanox, Inc. (Houston, TX) will also be assessing the utility of anti-Factor D antibodies (MAb 166–32) during cardiopulmonary bypass surgery, in which the circulation of blood outside the body through mechanical devices can activate the complement system resulting in inflammation (Fig. 8.4).

> **Pearl**
> Complement Factor H polymorphisms have been linked with a risk for developing AMD. Immune system modification through complement factor H inhibition is a key target for future clinical trials in AMD.

Neuroprotective Agents

Prevention of apoptosis by using neuroprotective agents, such as ciliary neurotrophic factor (CNTF), has been another adopted strategy. CNTF inhibits photoreceptor apoptosis in an animal model of retinal degeneration and is being evaluated as a treatment for dry AMD. Neurotech Pharmaceuticals (Lincoln, RI) has developed a sustained release platform that produces CNTF for a year or longer, using encapsulated cell technology that permits CNTF-producing transfected cells to be implanted in the vitreous cavity. The phase 2 study is complete and the collected data are under analysis. Brimonidine tartrate intravitreal implant (Allergan, Irvine, CA) and topical tandospirone (Alcon, Fort Worth, TX) are other neuroprotective agents in evaluation for dry AMD.

Modulators of Choroidal Circulation

Two studies are examining the effect of preventing ischemia by improving choroidal circulation in patients with dry AMD. A multicenter, randomized, placebo-controlled study, ongoing in Europe, is investigating the vasodilatory effect of Alprostadil, also known as prostaglandin E1 (PGE1). A second, ongoing multicenter, randomized, placebo-controlled study in Europe is investigating the use of an off-label, generic drug, Trimetazidine (Vastarel MR, 35 mg tablet), a drug currently in use for angina pectoris. It is believed to have cytoprotective effects in ischemic conditions.

Recovery

Gene Therapy

Advancements in the field of molecular genetics have improved our understanding of the genetic basis of AMD. When developing gene-based therapy, there are several potential targets. One approach is gene replacement therapy in conditions where a defective gene is not producing a protein essential for normal function. For example, genetic variants of the complement system including cofactor H, factor B, and complement component 2 have been shown to be responsible for up to 74% of AMD phenotypes [40]. Transferring normal copies of these genes may help the body regain normal complement function. This approach may supplement or replace the use of anti-complement therapies, which target the effect and not the underlying cause of a poorly regulated immune system.

Another potential target of gene therapy is the angiogenesis seen in wet AMD. Current therapy consists of periodic anti-VEGF intravitreal injections. However, transferring genes responsible for antiangiogenic factors could yield a less invasive, more effective approach. Campochiaro and Rasmussen have reported on their PEDF (pigment epithelium-derived factor)-based gene therapy [41, 42]. Using an adenovirus vector, they transfer the cDNA of this potent human antiangiogenic protein via an intravitreal injection directly to the retina. They report on murine models that showed a significant, up to 85%, reduction in neo-vascularization. Phase 1 trials of the same adenovirus based PEDF therapy on 28 patients with wet AMD showed mild intraocular inflammation. This adenoviral vector-based therapy may be useful for further gene products in the prevention of GA progression or CNV management [41, 42].

Though the above therapies show unlimited possibilities, the near future in FDA-approved clinical options will likely be dominated by RNA interference (RNAi)-based gene therapy. RNA interference involves two types of small RNA molecules, mircoRNA (miRNA) and small interfering RNA (siRNA), which bind and regulate the activity of messenger RNA (mRNA). These molecules can be injected intravitreally to induce destruction of VEGF mRNA. Since they downregulate future VEGF production and do not affect already existing VEGF, they can be used synergistically with FDA-approved anti-VEGF monoclonal antibody therapies such as ranibizumab [43]. RTP-801i (Pfizer, New York, NY), an RNAi-based therapy, is currently in a phase 1 clinical trial and seeks to inhibit RTP-801, a hypoxia-inducible gene involved in exudative AMD.

> **Pearl**
> Alterations in essential protein compounds through gene-based therapy are being evaluated in both dry and wet AMD.

Stem Cell Therapy

A controversial therapeutic option is the use of human embryonic stem cells (ESCs) for AMD therapy. In 2009, the FDA approved the phase 1 trial of a stem-cell-based therapy, GRNOPC1 (Geron Corp., Menlo Park, CA), for patients with acute spinal cord injury. The Institute of Ophthalmology at University College London and Moorfields Eye Hospital are on the forefront of ECSs use for patients with AMD. Embryonic transcription factors are first used to endow pluripotent properties to somatic cells, which are referred to as induced pluripotent stem (iPS) cells. Carr, et al., showed that these iPS cells could be differentiated into RPE cells [44]. In vitro and in vivo rat models reveal that these cells are morphologically and functionally similar to RPE cells and can aid in phagocytosis of photoreceptors outer segments. Preservation of RPE, and therefore photoreceptor function, in AMD holds the hope of preventing disease progression.

If RPE cells cannot be transferred in whole through ESC therapy, there is a possibility of transferring genes that promote RPE function. Chaum discusses his in vitro study transfecting human RPE cells with an insulin-like growth factor (IGF)-1 tagged plasmid vector. IGF-1 is known to have antiangiogenic and antiapoptotic features among other qualities that can enhance RPE survival [45].

In summary, gene therapies offer a limitless variety of AMD therapies. For dry AMD, the focus is on transferring genes that preserve RPE function and on using ESCs for transferring new RPE cells to diseased retina. Therapies for wet AMD aim to transfer antiangiogenic factors to the host genome and directly block genes responsible for the production of vascular growth factor genes. These therapies, in various stages of laboratory and clinical testing, may prove to be the mainstay of AMD management in the future, offering individualized treatment based on patient genetic makeup.

Retinal Prostheses

The potential to reverse severe visual loss in patients with severe dry AMD and retinitis pigmentosa by targeting impaired retinal photoreceptors exists with a retinal prosthetic device. To replace photoreceptor cell function, an electronic prosthetic device can be used such that retinal secondary neurons receive a signal that simulates an external visual image [46]. The composite device has a miniature video camera mounted on the patient's eyeglasses, which captures images and passes them to a microprocessor that converts the data to an electronic signal. This signal, in turn, is transmitted to an array of electrodes placed on the retinal surface, which transmits the patterned signal to the remaining viable secondary neurons. Electrode microarrays have been located in the epiretinal, subretinal, or suprachoroidal locations of the eye globe or in the intracranial position. With subretinal implantation, the prosthesis is aimed at substituting photoreceptor cells that generate a potential shift proportional to the light intensity they receive. Alternatively, epiretinal devices would stimulate ganglion cells that generate action potentials more typical for neural tissues. Neuronal transmission (ganglion, bipolar cells, etc.) then processes the signal and is transmitted via the optic nerve to the visual cortex for final integration into a visual image.

The photoelectric dye-coupled polyethylene film as a retinal prosthesis consists of two components, polyethylene and photoelectric dye 2-[2-[4-(dibutylamino)phenyl]ethenyl]-3-carboxymethylbenzothiazolium bromide. Polyethylene has long been implanted in patients as part of vascular grafts or artificial joints, and has been proven safe and stable in the body. The photoelectric dye as part of the retinal prosthesis has been recently tested for safety and efficacy.

Photoelectric dye-coupled extrusion-blown polyethylene film and photoelectric dye-coupled recrystallized film were implanted in the subretinal space of normal adult rats [46]. At one week and one month after implantation, retinal tissue deterioration was exiguous with no inflammatory cells and few apoptotic cells. An inconsequential tissue reaction to polyethylene film implantation is the basic requirement for biological safety of medical devices, including retinal prostheses.

Glial fibrillary acidic protein (GFAP) was significantly upregulated in Muller cells in the area where dye-coupled polyethylene films were implanted, compared with the adjacent areas of the retina. Such GFAP upregulation would be attributed to the foreign body reaction of Muller cells to the dye-coupled polyethylene films. GFAP in retinal Muller cells is known to be upregulated in a pathological condition, anyway no evidence exists as to whether the upregulation would be good or bad for the function of Muller cells [47].

The efficacy of this prosthesis implanted in the subretinal space of the eye of blind rats was tested by means of assessing behavioral functional tests. Rats were located in a round cage with a transparent wall and a drum with black-and-white stripes was rotated in the forward or reverse direction around the cage at a slow speed (2 or 4 rpm). Rats with implanted photoelectric dye-coupled polyethylene film showed a positive visual response compared with sham-operated rats or rats that underwent no surgery.

The Kelvin probe measurements conferred some evidence that photoelectric dye-coupled polyethylene films could function to generate electric potentials in response to light. Moreover, the quality of the dye-coupled films could be assessed by the Kelvin probe as a means of quality control for possible medical devices.

In the near future, these retinal prostheses would be implanted subretinally into patients with AMD, via a standard three-port vitrectomy procedure. The device is inserted into the vitreous cavity through a 20-gauge pars plana port and then to the subretinal space. Thorough preoperative evaluation to select patients with potential for visual improvement is imperative.

OCT could be used as a preoperative tool to assess the function of the degenerated retina in AMD, which is correlated with the preserved structured of retinal layers around the macula. However, evaluation of the device's efficacy is limited as patients admitted into the trial have little or no vision. Thus, methods must be developed that accurately and reproducibly record small improvements in visual function after implantation. Standard tests such as visual acuity, visual field, electroretinography, or even contrast sensitivity may not adequately record some aspects of improvement that relate to a quality of life (QOL). As a result, some tests are now relying more on measures of functional capacity that better assesses possible improvement in activities of daily living. Moreover, a new battery of tests have been suggested that include standard psychophysical testing, performance in tasks that are used in real-life situations such as object discrimination, mobility, etc., and well-crafted questionnaires that assess the patient's own feelings as to the usefulness of the device. In the Phase 1 trial of the SSMP 16-electrode device, six subjects with severe retinitis pigmantosa were implanted with ongoing testing and monitoring. Although light perception was restored in all six patients, it was evident that even limited sight restoration remains a slow, learning process that takes months for improvement to become evident. All subjects ultimately saw discrete phosphenes and could perform simple visual spatial and motion tasks. The device furthest along in development is an epiretinal implant sponsored by Second Sight Medical Products (SSMP). This first-generation device had 16 electrodes with human testing in a Phase 1 clinical trial beginning in 2002. Currently, the second-generation devices are in Phase 2/3 clinical trials, consistent with 60+ electrodes, a 250+ device, and one with over 1,000 electrodes. Increased numbers of electrodes are planned for future versions of the device [47].

Each has the possibility of significantly improving a patient's vision and QOL, being smaller and safer in design and lasting for the lifetime of the patient. From theoretical modeling, it is estimated that a device with approximately 1,000 electrodes could give good functional vision, that is, face recognition and reading ability. Though not currently optimized, regular use of these devices could potentially be available within a 5 to 10-year horizon. In summary, no retinal prostheses are currently available for severely affected patients with dry AMD. An electrical prosthetic device seems to offer hope in restoring the function of degenerating or dead photoreceptor neurons. Devices with new, sophisticated designs and increasing numbers of electrodes could allow for long-term restoration of functional sight in patients with improvement in object recognition, mobility, independent living, and general QOL.

Pearl

Implantation of retinal prosthesis holds promise to restore ambulatory vision for AMD and other degenerative retinal disorders.

Summary

AMD is the leading cause of significant visual loss to affect the elderly population within the United States. The nonexudative subtype is the most commonly seen type, and can lead to overall visual diminution significantly affecting QOL functions in the patient population. The spectrum of non exudative can vary widely from drusen subtype, pigmentary alterations, and with the degree of subsequent atrophy of the RPE and choriocapillaris. Although modifiable risk factors such as cigarette smoking and the utilization of vitamin and antioxidant supplementation have been clearly delineated, pharmacologic intervention in the management of nonexudative AMD currently has not. However, with the plethora of clinical trials targeting a variety of downstream pathways and with various methods of drug delivery including surgical implantation, there will be a greater arsenal to modify and potentially reverse further vision loss in the near future for patients with nonexudative AMD.

References

1. Age-Related Eye Disease Study Research Group. Potential public health impact of of Age-Related Eye Disease Study results: AREDS report no. 11. Arch Ophthalmol. 2003;121:1621–4.
2. National Society to Prevent Blindness. Visual problems in the United States: Definitions, Data Sources, Detailed Data Tables, Analyses, Interpretation. New York: National Society to Prevent Blindness; 1980. p. 1–46.
3. Gass JDM. Stereoscopic atlas of macular diseases: diagnosis and treatment. 4th ed. St. Louis: Mosby; 1997. p. 52–70.
4. Klein R, Klein R, Davis M, Magli Y, Segal P, Klein B, et al. The Wisconsin age-related maculopathy grading system. Ophthalmology. 1991;98:1128–34.

5. Klein ML, Ferris III FL, Armstrong J, AREDS Research Group, et al. Retinal precursors and the development of geographic atrophy in age-related macular degeneration. Ophthalmology. 2008;115:1026–31.
6. Bressler NM, Bressler SB, Seddon JM, Gragoudas ES, Jacobson LP. Drusen characteristics in patients with exudative versus nonexudative age-related macular degeneration. Retina. 1988;8:109–14.
7. Sarks JP, Sarks SH, Killingsworth MC. Evolution of soft drusen in age-related macular degeneration. Eye. 1994;8(pt 3):269–83.
8. Holz FG, Wolfensberger TJ, Piguet B, et al. Bilateral macular drusen in agerelated macular degeneration: prognosis and risk factors. Ophthalmology. 1994;101: 1522–8.
9. von Rückmann A, Fitzke FW, Bird AC. Fundus autofluorescence in age-related macular disease imaged with a laser scanning ophthalmoscope. Invest Ophthalmol Vis Sci. 1997;38:478–86.
10. Solbach U, Keilhauer C, Knabben H, Wolf S. Imaging of retinal autofluorescence in patients with age-related macular degeneration. Retina. 1997;17:385–9.
11. Holz FG, Bellmann C, Margaritidis M, Otto TP, Völcker HE. Pattern of increased in vivo fundus autofluorescence in the junctional zone of geographic atrophy of the retinal pigment epithelium associated with age-related macular degeneration. Graefes Arch Clin Exp Ophthalmol. 1999;237:145–52.
12. Jaffe GJ, Caprioli J. Optical coherence tomography to detect and manage retinal disease and glaucoma. Am J Ophthalmol. 2004;137:156–69.
13. Sayanagi K, Sharma S, Yamamoto T, Kaiser PK. Comparison of spectral-domain versus time-domain optical coherence tomography in management of age-related macular degeneration with ranibizumab. Ophthalmology. 2009;116(5):947–55. Epub 2009 Feb 20.
14. Witkin AJ, Vuong LN, Srinivasan VJ, Gorczynska I, Reichel E, Baumal CR, et al. High-speed ultrahigh resolution optical coherence tomography before and after ranibizumab for age-related macular degeneration. Ophthalmology. 2009;116(5):956–63.
15. Seddon JM, Willett WC, Speizer FE, Hankinson SE. A prospective study of cigarette smoking and age-related macular degeneration in women. JAMA. 1996;276(14):1141–6.
16. Clemons TE, Milton RC, Klein R, Seddon JM, Ferris FL 3rd; Age-Related Eye Disease Study Research Group. Risk factors for the incidence of Advanced Age-Related Macular Degeneration in the Age-Related Eye Disease Study (AREDS) AREDS report no. 19. Ophthalmology. 2005;112(4):533–9.
17. Age-Related Eye Disease Study Research Group. A randomized, placebo-controlled, clinical trial of high-dose supplementation with vitamins C and E, beta carotene, and zinc for age-related macular degeneration and vision loss AREDS Report No. 8. Arch Ophthalmol. 2001;119:1417–36.
18. Gass JD. Photocoagulation of macular lesions. Trans Am Acad Ophthalmol Otolaryngol. 1971;75:580–608.

19. Guymer RH, Hageman GS, Bird AC. Choroidal endothelial cell processes into Bruch's membrane. Invest Ophthalmol Vis Sci. 1997;38:S353.
20. Abdelsalam A, Zarbin MA. Drusen in age-related macular degeneration: pathogenesis, natural course, and laser photocoagulation-induced regression. Surv Ophthalmol. 1999;44(1):1–29.
21. Complications of Age-Related Macular Degeneration Prevention Trial Research Group. Laser treatment in patients with bilateral large drusen: the complications of age-related macular degeneration prevention trial. Ophthalmology. 2006;113:1974–86.
22. Schmitz-Valckenberg S, Fleckenstein M, Scholl HP, Holz FG. Fundus autofluorescence and progression of age-related macular degeneration. Surv Ophthalmol. 2009;54:96–117.
23. Radu RA, Yuan Q, Hu J, Peng JH, et al. Accelerated accumulation of lipofuscin pigments in the RPE of a mouse model for ABCA4-mediated retinal dystrophies following Vitamin A supplementation. Invest Ophthalmol Vis Sci. 2008;49(9):3821–9.
24. Sirion therapeutics announces positive results from interim analysis of phase II trial and receives FDA fast track designation for denretinide. Available at: http://www.siriontherapeutics.com/investmed/09pr/4–15–09Sirion Positive Phase II Results and FDA Fast Track for Fenretinide.pdf. Accessed on 10 Jan 2010.
25. Camerini T, Mariani L, De Palo G, Marubini E, et al. Safety of the synthetic retinoid fenretinide: long-term results from a controlled clinical trial for the prevention of contralateral breast cancer. J Clin Oncol. 2001;19(6):1664–70.
26. Kubota R, Birch D, David R. Phase 1, dose-escalating study of the safety, tolerability, and pharmacokinetics of ACU-4429 in healthy volunteers. Poster presentation at the Association for Research in Vision and Ophthalmology (ARV O) annual conference 2009, Ft. Lauderdale, 2009.
27. Vives-Bauza C, Anand M, Shirazi AK, Magrane J, et al. The age lipid A2E and mitochondrial dysfunction synergistically impair phagocytosis by retinal pigment epithelial cells. J Biol Chem. 2008;283(36):24770–80.
28. Kudo W, Yamato M, Yamada K, Kinoshita Y, et al. Formation of TEMPOL-hydroxylamine during reaction between TEMPOL and hydroxyl radical: HPLC/ECD study. Free Radic Res. 2008;42(5):505–12.
29. Tanito M, Li F, Elliott MH, Dittmar M, Anderson RE. Protective effect of TEMPOL derivatives against light-induced retinal damage in rats. Invest Ophthalmol Vis Sci. 2007;48(4):1900–5.
30. Mousa SA, Dier E, Kannanayakal T, Patil G. Anti-angiogenesis efficacy of the novel NF-κB and oxidative stress inhibitor, OT-551. Poster presentation at ARVO annual conference 2008, Ft. Lauderdale, 2008.
31. Donoso LA, Kim D, Frost A, Callahan A, Hageman G. The role of inflammation in the pathogenesis of age-related macular degeneration. Surv Ophthalmol. 2006;51(2):137–52.
32. Thakkinstian A, Han P, McEvoy M, Smith W, et al. Systematic review and meta-analysis of the association between complement factor H Y402H polymorphisms and age-related macular degeneration. Hum Mol Genet. 2006;15(18):2784–90.
33. Mullins RF, Aptsiauri N, Hageman GS. Structure and composition of drusen associated with glomerulonephritis: implications for the role of complement activation in drusen biogenesis. Eye. 2001;15:390–5.
34. Huang SJ, Costa DL, Gross NE, Yannuzzi LA. Peripheral drusen in membranoproliferative glomerulonephritis type II. Retina. 2003;23(3):429–31.
35. Kew RR, Ghebrehiwet B, Janoff A. Cigarette smoke can activate the alternative pathway of complement in vitro by modifying the third component of complement. J Clin Invest. 1985;75(3):1000–7.
36. de Córdoba SR, de Jorge EG. Translational mini-review series on complement factor H: genetics and disease associations of human complement factor H. Clin Exp Immunol. 2008;151(1):1–13.
37. Barnum SR, Niemann MA, Kearney JF, Volanakis JE. Quantitation of complement factor D in human serum by a solid-phase radioimmunoassay. J Immunol Meth. 1984;67:303–9.
38. Lesavre PH, Muller-Eberhard HJ. Mechanism of action of factor D of the alternative complement pathway. J Exp Med. 1978;148:1498–509.
39. Volanakis JE, Narayana SV. Complement factor D, a novel serine protease. Protein Sci. 1996;5(4):553–64.
40. Gold B, Merriam JE, Zernant J, et al. Variation in factor B (BF) and complement component 2 (C2) genes is associated with age-related macular degeneration. Nat Genet. 2006;38(4):458–62.
41. Campochiaro PA, Nguyen QD, Shah SM, et al. Adenoviral vector-delivered pigment epithelium-derived factor for neovascular age-related macular degeneration: results of a phase I clinical trial. Hum Gene Ther. 2006;17(2):167–76.
42. Rasmussen H, Chu KW, Campochiaro P, et al. Clinical protocol. An open-label, phase I, single administration, dose-escalation study of ADGVPEDF.11D (ADPEDF) in neovascular age-related macular degeneration (AMD). Hum Gene Ther. 2001;12(16):2029–32.
43. Singerman L. Combination therapy using the small interfering RNA bevasiranib. Retina. 2009;29:S49–50.
44. Carr AJ, Vugler AA, Hikita ST, et al. Protective effects of human iPS-derived retinal pigment epithelium cell transplantation in the retinal dystrophic rat. PLoS ONE. 2009;4(12):e8152.
45. Chaum E, Yang H. Transgenic expression of IGF-1 modifies the proliferative potential of human retinal pigment epithelial cells. Invest Ophthalmol Vis Sci. 2002;43(12):3758–64.
46. Yanai D, Weiland JD, Mahadevappa M, Greenberg RJ, Fine I, Humayun MS. Visual performance using a retinal prosthesis in three subjects with retinitis pigmentosa. Am J Ophthalmol. 2007;143:820–7.
47. Chader GJ, Weiland J, Humayun MS. Artificial vision: needs, functioning, and testing of a retinal electronic prosthesis. Prog Brain Res. 2009;175:317–32.

The Future of Neovascular Age-Related Macular Degeneration

Chirag P. Shah and Jeffrey S. Heier

Key Points

- The treatment of neovascular age-related macular degeneration (AMD) will continue to evolve dramatically.
- Researchers are working to find new therapeutics targeting important pathways involved in angiogenesis, including:
  - Vascular endothelial growth factor (VEGF) inhibition
  - Vascular endothelial growth factor receptor (VEGFR) and platelet-derived growth factor receptor inhibition (PDGFR), including tyrosine kinase inhibitors, RNA interference, and vaccine therapy
  - Radiation therapy utilizing novel local approaches of delivery
  - Antiinflammatory and immunosuppressive pathways, including inhibition of complement, tumor necrosis factor alpha (TNFα), and mammalian target of rapamycin (mTOR)
  - Gene therapy, transferring genes for pigment epithelial-derived growth factor (PEDF) and potent VEGF binders
  - Other pathways, including the nicotinic acetylcholine receptor pathway antagonism, blockade of cell membrane ion trans-

port, disruption of microtubule formation, integrin inhibition, neuroprotection, and inhibition of sphingosine-1-phosphate
- Combining existing and future therapies that affect distinctly separate pathways in the pathogenesis of neovascular AMD, coupled with enhanced drug delivery technologies, may continue to enhance visual outcomes while reducing treatment burdens.

Introduction

The only thing certain about the future of neovascular age-related macular degeneration (AMD) is its evolution. Ophthalmologists have witnessed dramatic and accelerated growth in the management of this disease since the Macular Photocoagulation Study began enrolling patients in 1979. Treatment options have evolved from laser photocoagulation to photodynamic therapy to intravitreal anti-vascular endothelial growth factor (VEGF) agents, with a commensurate improvement in efficacy. The short- and long-term future is sure to hold many new therapeutic options with even better outcomes.

At the time of this writing, monotherapy with intravitreal anti-VEGF agents, namely ranibizumab and bevacizumab, remained the standard of care for neovascular AMD. Future therapies will likely target different pathways in the pathogenesis of choroidal neovascularization (CNV). Combination treatments will affect multiple

C.P. Shah (✉)
Ophthalmic Consultants of Boston, 50 Staniford Street, Suite 600, Boston, MA 02114, USA
e-mail: cpshah@eyeboston.com

A.C. Ho and C.D. Regillo (eds.), *Age-related Macular Degeneration Diagnosis and Treatment*, DOI 10.1007/978-1-4614-0125-4_9, © Springer Science+Business Media, LLC 2011 pathways simultaneously, and may prove more efficacious than monotherapy. Further, anticipated improvements in drug delivery will likely decrease treatment burden. The effect on the cost of treatment remains to be seen – a decrease in treatment burden could reduce the cost of AMD treatment, but the development of new agents, and their use either as monotherapy, or more likely, in combination with other agents, could result in increased costs of therapy.

Emerging and Future Therapies

Anti-vascular Endothelial Growth Factor Agents

VEGF plays a key role in normal and pathologic angiogenesis. The VEGF family consists of VEGF A through F and placental growth factor

(PlGF), which share structural domains but have different biological properties [1]. VEGF has multiple isoforms formed through alternative splicing and named based on the number of amino acids [1].

Multiple pharmacologic agents target VEGF along various pathways in an effort to inhibit CNV (see Fig. 9.1). Pegaptanib, ranibizumab, bevacizumab, and VEGF Trap-Eye bind and inhibit VEGF, preventing it from activating VEGF receptor. VEGF receptor tyrosine kinase inhibitors prevent transduction of the VEGF-binding signal. Small interfering RNA molecules, or siRNAs, silence mRNA to prevent the translation of VEGF (bevasiranib) or VEGF receptor-1 (Sirna-027).

Ranibizumab

Ranibizumab (Lucentis®, Genentech, Inc., South San Francisco, CA, USA) is a recombinant,

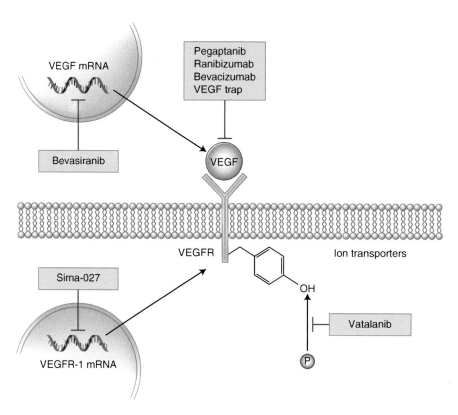

Fig. 9.1 Mechanisms of inhibition of vascular endothelial growth factor-A (VEGFR). Pegaptanib, ranibizumab, bevacizumab and VEGFR-Trap all bind VEGFR, inhibiting it from binding and activating VEGFR receptor. Bevasiranib is a small interfering RNA (siRNA) that prevents translation of VEGFR. Likewise, Sirna-027 is a siRNA that prevents the translation of VEGFR receptor. VEGFR receptor tyrosine kinase inhibitors, like Vatalanib, prevent transduction of the VEGFR binding signal (Vascular Endothelial Growth Factor Receptor).

humanized, monoclonal antibody Fab fragment against VEGF-A, capable of binding and inhibiting all isoforms. Ranibizumab's VEGF binding site was affinity-matured, allowing the drug to be five–to twenty-fold more potent in binding VEGF-A than bevacizumab on a molar basis [2].

Intravitreal ranibizumab revolutionized the treatment paradigm of neovascular AMD by actually improving visual acuity on average, as demonstrated in two phase III studies. The MARINA (Minimally Classic/Occult Trial of the Anti-VEGF Antibody Ranibizumab in the Treatment of Neovascular AMD) Study Group evaluated 716 patients with minimally classic or occult neovascular AMD. The study reported a mean gain of 6.6 letters at two years in the group receiving 0.5 mg of ranibizumab monthly, compared to a mean loss of 14.9 letters in the group receiving sham injections [3]. Likewise, ANCHOR (Anti-VEGF Antibody for the Treatment of Predominantly Classic CNV in AMD) evaluated 423 patients with predominantly classic neovascular AMD. The trial demonstrated a mean gain of 10.7 letters in the 0.5 mg ranibizumab group at two years compared to a mean loss of 9.8 letters in the verteporfin photodynamic therapy group [4, 5]. Please refer to Chapter 6 for more details regarding ranibizumab.

Though ranibizumab represented a major breakthrough for neovascular AMD when compared to all previous therapies – including the first approved anti-VEGF medication, pegaptanib – the success of regular intravitreal injections is coupled with several disadvantages. These include the burden of monthly office visits of patients and their caregivers, the direct and indirect costs of treatment, and the risks and discomfort associated with frequent intravitreal injections. Anti-VEGF therapy will likely continue to be part of the neovascular AMD arsenal in the future, if it is not replaced by more potent, longer acting, and/or less expensive alternatives.

Bevacizumab

Bevacizumab (Avastin®, Genentech, Inc., South San Francisco, CA, USA) is a full-length anti-VEGF monoclonal antibody that binds and inhibits all VEGF-A isoforms. Intravitreally, the half-life of bevacizumab is roughly twice that of ranibizumab, thought due to bevacizumab's greater size (149 kDa vs. 48 kDa) and presence of the Fc portion.

The Comparison of Age-Related Macular Degeneration Treatments Trials [6] (CATT) is a phase III trial assessing the efficacy of bevacizumab versus ranibizumab. The trial will also evaluate an as-needed dosing regimen. If noninferior to ranibizumab, bevacizumab would be a proven and far cheaper anti-VEGF agent in our armamentarium against neovascular AMD. Please refer to Chapter 6 for more details regarding bevacizumab.

VEGF Trap-Eye

Aflibercept (VEGF Trap-Eye or Eyelea Regeneron, Terrytown, NY, USA, and Bayer HealthCare, Leverkusen, Germany) is an antagonist that binds and inactivates VEGF. It is comprised of portions of the extracellular domains of two different VEGF receptors (VEGFR). Specifically, it is a 110 kDa recombinant protein with binding portions of VEGFR-1 and VEGFR-2 fused to the Fc region of human IgG. VEGF Trap-Eye has a much higher affinity for VEGF than humanized monoclonal antibodies, about 140 times that of ranibizumab, and thus has the potential for greater efficacy and duration. Furthermore, VEGF Trap-Eye binds all isoforms of VEGF-A, as well as placental growth factor 1 and 2 (PlGF1 and PlGF2), which may be helpful in treating CNV [7].

Intravenous VEGF Trap was evaluated in a phase I study (CLEAR) [8]. It demonstrated a dose-dependent improvement in retinal thickness, as well as a dose-dependent increase in systemic blood pressure with a maximum tolerated dose of 1 mg/kg. Subsequently, efforts were directed towards intravitreal drug delivery. A phase I study (CLEAR IT-1) [9] evaluated

> **Pearl**
> Anti-VEGF agents will likely continue to be part of the neovascular AMD arsenal in the future, if it is not replaced by more potent, longer acting, and/or less expensive alternative.

intravitreal VEGF Trap-Eye, finding injections up to 4 mg were well tolerated. A phase II trial (CLEAR IT-2) [10] randomized 157 patients to various doses on fixed monthly or quarterly regimens for the first 12 weeks, followed by as-needed dosing for the following 40 weeks. At one year, patients receiving four monthly injections of 2 mg VEGF Trap-Eye followed by as-needed dosing improved an average of nine letters from baseline ($p < 0.0001$), correlating with a decrease in retinal thickness of 143 μm ($p < 0.0001$). During the as-needed phase, patients required an average of only 1.6 additional VEGF Trap-Eye injections. The results for the 2 mg group were more favorable than those for the 0.5 mg group. Patients initially receiving four monthly doses boasted better visual acuity gains than those receiving quarterly injections, suggesting the value of a loading dose. Overall, the medication was well tolerated without any serious adverse events.

These promising results prompted two large phase III trials. VIEW 1 [11], conducted in the United States and Canada, and VIEW 2 [12], conducted in Europe, Asia, Japan, Australia, and South America, have each enrolled over 1,200 patients. The trials compare 2 and 0.5 mg of VEGF Trap-Eye dosed monthly, as well as 2 mg dose every other month following a loading dose, with ranibizumab. Results are expected in late 2010 or early 2011. See Chapter 6 for preliminary one year results.

Bevasiranib

Small interfering RNA (siRNA) molecules work upstream from VEGF. They inactivate specific messenger RNAs and thus inhibit translation of particular proteins, such as VEGF. Clinically, siRNA drugs are delivered as double stranded RNA molecules that are transported across cellular membrane. An enzyme, Dicer, shortens the siRNA to 21–24 nucleotides, which is then incorporated into a RNA-induced silencing complex (RISC). When activated, RISC binds and digests complementary mRNA, allowing a single molecule of siRNA to degrade multiple copies of mRNA.

Bevasiranib [13] (formerly Cand5, OPKO Health, Inc., Miami, FL, USA) was the first siRNA

directed towards intraocular VEGF production. It has no effect on existing VEGF in the eye, and thus may have synergy when used in combination with conventional anti-VEGF agents to impact the disease in the short term. The phase II Cand5 Anti-VEGF RNA Evaluation (CARE) study evaluated three doses of intravitreal bevasiranib (0.2, 1.5, and 3.0 mg) administered every six weeks ($n = 127$ eyes). At 12 weeks, all groups lost vision, with a mean letter loss of 4.1, 6.9, and 5.8 in each group, respectively [14, 15]. Given these lackluster results compared to the visual improvement experienced with anti-VEGF antibody treatment, researchers hypothesized that bevasiranib may have a delayed benefit because it works upstream from existing VEGF. Monotherapy with bevasiranib was abandoned. Subsequently, a phase III trial evaluated the combination of 2.5 mg bevasiranib and ranibizumab. The COBALT trail (Combining Bevasiranib And Lucentis Therapy) completed enrollment, but was terminated in March 2009 because the Independent Data Monitoring Committee felt the combination was unlikely to reduce vision loss [16, 17].

Bevasiranib may be considered as part of the neovascular AMD treatment regimen in the future, but with a different approach. Possibilities include different dosing protocols, other combinations with complementary medications, and enhanced drug delivery vehicles [17]. The CARBON trial is underway, a phase III trial evaluating three doses of bevasiranib (1.0, 2.0, and 2.5 mg) used in combination with ranibizumab [18].

VEGF Receptor, Platelet-Derived Growth Factor, and PDGR Receptor Inhibition

VEGF must bind to VEGF receptor (VEGFR) to perform its biologic functions. The VEGFR family consists of protein-tyrosine kinases (VEGFR-1, VEGFR-2, and VEGFR-3) and two nonprotein kinase coreceptors (neuropilin-1 and neuropilin-2) [19]. VEGFR-2 mediates almost all of VEGF's cellular responses, allowing transduction of the VEGF-binding signal. The role of VEGFR-1 is less clear; it may be a decoy receptor, evolved to trap free VEGF-A and prevent VEGFR-2 activation [20].

Platelet-derived growth factor (PDGF) stimulates angiogenesis, as well as pericyte recruitment and maturation [21]. Pericytes play an important role in angiogenesis because they protect endothelial cells against VEGF inhibition [22]. Thus, inhibition of PDGF increases endothelial cell sensitivity to anti-VEGF agents [22]. PDGF binds to PDGF receptor (PDGFR), which is found in two isoforms: PDGFRα and PDGFRβ(beta). Inhibition of PDGFR, as well as VEGFR, may be a mechanism to treat CNV in AMD.

Pearl
Platelet-derived growth factor (PDGF) stimulates angiogenesis, as well as pericyte recruitment and maturation. Blockade of PDGF or its receptors can decrease pericyte density in neovascular vessels and improve the effect of anti-VEGF agents. Lesion regression may be possible.

Vatalanib

Vatalanib (formerly PTK-787, Novartis, Basel Switzerland) is a potent tyrosine kinase inhibitor that binds and inhibits all known VEGF receptor tyrosine kinases (VEGFR-1, VEGFR-2, and VEGFR-3), PDGFRβ(beta), and c-Kit receptor kinases. C-kit is a proto-oncogene that is a member of the receptor tyrosine kinase family; it is closely related to PDGFR. Preclinical models suggest vatalanib causes dose-dependent regression of VEGF-induced angiogenesis [23]. Vatalanib boasts good oral availability. Oral vatalanib was evaluated in a phase I/II clinical trial in combination with photodynamic therapy (ADVANCE study [24]). This study of 50 patients was completed in November 2007, but not published. Vatalanib demonstrated some biologic activity, but had safety issues. It may reemerge if revised.

TG100801

TG100801 (TargeGen, San Diego, CA), another tyrosine kinase inhibitor, is a prodrug of TG100572, which binds and inhibits VEGFR and PDGFR [25]. In a murine model, systemic delivery of TG100572 induced regression of CNV, but with associated weight loss suggestive of systemic toxicity. Thus, researchers developed a topical inactive prodrug, TG100801, achieving good retinal and choroidal concentrations of TG100572 without detection in plasma [25]. A phase I trial demonstrated safety and tolerability of two concentrations in 42 patients twice a day for 14 days [26, 27]. Unfortunately, toxicity led to discontinuation of the trial although it demonstrated biologic activity [28]. Patients receiving topical TG100801 developed corneal toxicity with deposits in all layers. The corneal changes remained largely irreversible. If refined, the topical route of administration would be a very favorable alternative or adjunct to intravitreal injections.

Pazopanib

Pazopanib (GW786034, GlaxoSmithKline, Middlesex, UK) is a second-generation multitargeted tyrosine kinase inhibitor against all VEGFRs, both PDGFRα and PDGRFβ, and c-kit [29]. Pazopanib, administered topically, was evaluated in a phase II trial [30], which was extended with results currently pending [31].

Sirna-027

Sirna-027 (Sirna Therapeutics, San Francisco, CA, USA) is a small interfering RNA (siRNA) structured to silence the gene for VEGFR-1 [32]. A phase I trial of 26 patients exhibited safety of doses ranging from 100 to 1,600 μg. Each patient received one intravitreal injection, with 24 of 26 showing visual acuity stabilization at three months. Four of 26 (15%) experienced clinically significant improvement in visual acuity [33]. A phase II trial, however, was terminated because it failed to show visual improvement [34]. The trial contained four arms, three of which evaluated different doses of monthly Sirna-027 versus the control arm of monthly ranibizumab [35]. Sirna-027 may reemerge in the future as part of a combination protocol or, possibly, researchers may alter

Sirna-027 to silence other contributory genes, such as that for VEGFR-2.

Anti-VEGFR Vaccine Therapy

A study showed CD8+ cytotoxic T-lymphocyte mediated regression of physiologic and pathologic new vessels [36]. An animal model demonstrated CNV regression by inducing cellular immunity specific for VEGFR-2 [37]. Currently, a phase 1 study is recruiting patients [38]. Patients will be vaccinated weekly for 12 weeks with subcutaneous VEGFR-1 peptide (1 mg) and VEGFR-2 (1 mg) mixed with Montanide ISA 51 [39].

> **Pearl**
> Tyrosine kinase inhibitors, siRNAs, and vaccine therapy can inhibit VEGF receptors to block the angiogenic effects of VEGF.

E10030

E10030 (Ophthotech Corporation, Princeton, NJ, USA) is an aptamer directed against PDGF-B. Pericytes, which are recruited and matured by PDGF, protect endothelial cells from anti-VEGF agents and thus promote resistance to therapy [22]. E10030 decreases pericyte density in neovascular vessels, and therefore improves the effect of anti-VEGF agents [22]. A phase I study of 22 patients evaluated intravitreal E10030 as monotherapy and in combination with ranibizumab [40]. The results in the combination group were promising, with 59% of patients experiencing at least a three-line visual acuity gain at 12 weeks. Further, there was an 86% mean decrease in CNV area at 12 weeks with a progressive decrease in macular thickness. E10030 was well tolerated without drug-related adverse effects [41, 42]. Of note, the choroidal neovascular lesions had to have evidence of classic CNV, and had to be less than five disc areas.

Radiation

Radiation therapy has antiangiogenic, antiinflammatory, and antifibrotic characteristics; it is not new to the treatment of neovascular AMD. However, prior studies evaluating monotherapy with either external beam [43–45] or proton beam irradiation [46] failed to show a treatment benefit [43–46]. The external delivery of radiation, and subsequent exposure to nonpathologic tissues, limited its efficacy. Localized radiation may provide a novel treatment modality with a distinct mechanism of action compared to current anti-VEGF therapies. Localized radiation has been shown to inhibit neovascularization and fibroblast proliferation [47, 48], affording it the potential to induce choroidal neovascular regression and inhibit scar formation in neovascular AMD. Moreover, targeted radiation, which may induce CNV regression, theoretically does not affect the overlying retina when delivered below threshold levels.

Radiation therapy may have an additive effect when combined with anti-VEGF treatment. Adjunctive bevacizumab with standard chemoradiotherapy proved efficacious in a phase II study treating advanced colorectal carcinoma [49]. Researchers feel that in addition to its antivascular effect, VEGF-targeted therapy may sensitize tumors to radiation through two mechanisms: by normalizing the tumor vasculature, leading to greater tumor oxygenation and thereby increasing the cytotoxicity of radiation to cancer cells, and by increasing the radiosensitivity of tumor-associated endothelial cells [50]. This same additive response may prove beneficial in the treatment of neovascular AMD.

> **Pearl**
> Radiation therapy has antiangiogenic, antiinflammatory, and antifibrotic characteristics; localized therapy holds promise in the treatment of neovascular AMD.

Epi-Rad90™ Ophthalmic System

The Epi-Rad90™ Ophthalmic System (NeoVista, Fremont, CA, USA) delivers strontium 90 directly to the neovascular complex during a vitrectomy, thereby delivering localized radiation (brachytherapy) while minimizing collateral exposure to surrounding tissues. The device is a handheld intraocular instrument with a retractable tip. The tip contains the radiation source, which remains protected and insulated until engaged over the fovea. The target dose is 24 Gy to the fovea, a level that decreases dramatically (10% every 0.1 mm) as a function of distance from the radiation source.

Preclinical studies in animal models demonstrated safety of this device, with no reported cases of radiation-induced optic neuropathy or retinopathy. A feasibility trial of 34 patients, NVI-068, evaluated the safety and effectiveness of delivering a single treatment of either 15 Gy (8 patients) or 24 Gy (26 patients) beta radiation using the Epi-Rad90™ Ophthalmic System [51]. During the course of the study, the investigators altered eligibility requirements and excluded 11 patients from the analysis (five were diabetic, two had lesions greater than 5.4 mm, two had baseline visual acuity outside the inclusion criteria parameters, one displayed Alzheimer-like symptoms, and one was treated outside of the establish protocol, having received an initial 24 Gy dose and an additional 24 Gy dose after the six-month visit). Twelve-month data were available for 21 patients. All lost fewer than three lines of vision. In the 24 Gy group, 5 of 17 (29%) gained three or more lines of vision. There were no adverse events attributed to radiation exposure.

Another prospective feasibility study, protocol NVI-111, treated 34 patients with 24 Gy by the Epi-Rad90™ Ophthalmic System with concomitant intravitreal bevacizumab [52, 53]. Patients were randomized to two groups. Group I ($n = 12$) received bevacizumab prior to surgery (10 ± 4 days) and at one month after surgery. Group II ($n = 22$) received bevacizumab intraoperatively and at one month post surgery. After the two mandatory intravitreal bevacizumab injections, 25 patients (74%) did not require further injections at 24 months of follow-up. Retreatment was entirely based upon investigator evaluation, not on strict retreatment criteria [52]. As a result, patients may have been undertreated based on current practices. Patients achieved visual gains despite this possible undertreatment. Seven patients (20.6%) gained at least three lines of

vision at two years, while 22 patients (64.7%) maintained vision, losing less than or equal to three lines. Visual outcomes appeared confounded by cataract formation; half of phakic patients (12 of 24) developed cataract. Though all patients lost a mean of 2.4 letters, phakic patients lost 4.8 letters while pseudophakes gained 3.8. Researchers felt cataract formation was due to vitrectomy and not radiation, as the lens only receives 0.6 mGy during the procedure. Two patients developed subretinal fibrosis. Most importantly, there were no cases of radiation retinopathy.

The results of these pilot studies prompted the CNV Secondary to AMD Treated with Beta Radiation Epiretinal Therapy (CABERNET) trial, a phase III study that completed enrollment in September 2009. A total of 450 patients were randomized to either the experimental arm of the 24 Gy Epi-Rad90™ Ophthalmic System and two injections of ranibizumab, one at the time of surgery and another at one month, or the control arm of monthly ranibizumab for the first three months followed by quarterly injections for two years. Retreatment injections are possible in both arms at monthly intervals per specific retreatment criteria. If proven efficacious and safe, the Epi-Rad90™ Ophthalmic System would add a surgical option for neovascular AMD and has the potential to decrease the treatment burden of monthly injections.

Preliminary successes with the Epi-Rad90™ Ophthalmic System have spawned additional trials. MERITAGE I is a phase I/II study evaluating the Epi-Rad90™ Ophthalmic System for patients with neovascular AMD who require relatively frequent anti-VEGF therapy for adequate response [54]. ROSE is a phase II feasibility study evaluating epiretinal beta radiation in suboptimal responders to anti-VEGF therapy [55]. MERLOT is a phase IV study in the United Kingdom comparing epiretinal beta radiation to monthly ranibizumab [56].

IRay

IRay (Oraya Therapeutics, Inc., Newark, CA, USA) is an externally-applied stereotactic orthovoltage irradiation device. This office-based procedure allows noninvasive application of ionizing radiation to the submacular choroidal neovascular membrane. The device uses three sequential beams, which pass through the pars plana and overlap at the macula. Phase I data of 16 Gy IRay demonstrated safety with no retinal, choroidal, retinal pigment epithelium, or optic nerve toxicity, and no cataract progression. All patients developed mild, self-limited punctate keratopathy secondary to the superficial corneal guidance device. The trial suggested therapeutic effect, with improvement of fluid on OCT and shrinkage of lesion size on fluorescein angiography [57]. Researchers are designing a phase II study in Europe [58], as well as a second study for the United States. If proven efficacious, IRay's noninvasive, office-based delivery system would be an attractive means of applying ionizing radiation directly to choroidal neovascular membranes.

Antiinflammatory/Antiimmune Pathways

Studies have suggested an inflammatory component in the pathogenesis of neovascular AMD [59–61]. A histologic study found macrophages in choroidal neovascular membranes; these macrophages secrete tissue factor, which is involved in fibrinogenesis [61]. Further, several genes in the complement pathway are implicated in neovascular AMD [60]. The bioactive forms of complement 3 and 5 (C3a and C5a) are present in AMD drusen, and they induce VEGF expression in vivo and in vitro [62]. Overexpression of the pleiotropic cytokine tumor necrosis factor (TNF), which is mainly produced by T cells and monocytes, has been found in neovascular membranes of eyes with AMD [63]. Thus, inhibition of inflammatory and immune pathways may play a therapeutic role in neovascular AMD.

> **Pearl**
> Inhibition of inflammatory and immune pathways may play a therapeutic role in neovascular AMD.

POT-4

Complement 3 (C3) is a central component of all known complement activation pathways. Thus, inhibition of C3 disables all downstream complement cascade activation that could lead to local inflammation, tissue damage, and upregulation of VEGF [39, 64]. POT-4 (Potentia Pharmaceuticals, Louisville, KY, USA) binds and inhibits C3. A phase I, dose-escalating trial of intravitreal POT-4 exhibited safety in all doses tested. POT-4 demonstrated signs of activity in a few end-stage wet AMD patients. Researchers measured sustained serum levels of POT-4 in patients receiving the highest dose, and expect a single intravitreal POT-4 injection to provide sustained therapeutic levels for several months. A phase II study to further define the safety, efficacy, and pharmacokinetic profile of POT-4 is under design [64, 65].

ARC1905

ARC1905 (Ophthotech Corporation, Princeton, NY, USA) inhibits complement factor 5 (C5), preventing the formation of key terminal fragments C5a and C5b-9. C5a induces vascular permeability, and recruitment and activation of phagocytes. C5b-9 is involved in membrane attack complex formation, which initiates cell lysis [39, 62]. A phase I study is evaluating intravitreal ARC1905 with either an induction dose or multiple doses of ranibizumab for neovascular AMD [66]. In addition, another phase I study is evaluating intravitreal ARC1905 for dry AMD [67].

Infliximab

The anti-TNF-α monoclonal antibody infliximab (Remicade®, Centocor, Inc., Horsham, PA, USA) is used for various inflammatory conditions, such as rheumatoid arthritis, inflammatory bowel disease, psoriasis, and noninfectious uveitis. Researchers observed regression of CNV and improvement of visual acuity in three neovascular AMD patients treated with intravenous infliximab for inflammatory arthritis [63]. Intravitreal infliximab has regressed laser-induced CNV in rats [68]. Subsequent experiments of intravitreal infliximab found doses up to 2 mg were safe in the rabbit eye [69]. Intravitreal infliximab was administered to three patients with neovascular

AMD, resulting in improved visual acuity and central foveal thickness on OCT [70]. A phase I study is underway, evaluating intravitreal infliximab for neovascular AMD, as well as for refractory diabetic macular edema [71].

Sirolimus

Sirolimus (Rapamycin, MacuSight, Inc., Union City, CA) was originally developed as a macrolide antifungal agent, but was found to possess potent immunosuppressive and antiproliferative properties. It is used to prevent rejection after organ transplantation, particularly after renal transplant. Sirolimus-eluting coronary stents are used for treatment of coronary artery disease.

Sirolimus inhibits the mammalian target of rapamycin, or mTOR, which effects cell growth and proliferation via the regulation of protein synthesis [72]. Sirolimus's anti-angiogenic properties are linked to a decrease in VEGF production and to a markedly inhibited response of vascular endothelial cells to stimulation by VEGF [73]. Further, sirolimus downregulates hypoxia-inducible factor-1α, a major upstream regulator of VEGF [74].

In a murine model, systemic sirolimus inhibited both choroidal and retinal neovascularization [75]. A phase I study [76] of 30 patients found intravitreal and subconjunctival sirolimus to be safe and well tolerated in all doses. A single administration of sirolimus was associated with improvement in visual acuity and retinal thickness. Preliminary findings suggested that subconjunctival administration was as effective, if not more so, that intravitreal sirolimus [77]. The phase II trial, known as EMERALD, is currently evaluating subconjunctival sirolimus in combination with intravitreal ranibizumab [78]. If proven effective, sirolimus's subconjunctival delivery would be less invasive and potentially safer and better tolerated than intravitreal alternatives.

Gene Therapy

Gene therapy could possibly treat and prevent angiogenesis by blocking stimulatory proteins or increasing expression of endogenous inhibitors.

Ocular gene transfer is an appealing treatment approach because of its potential to provide a sustained therapeutic response within the eye with little systemic impact.

Pearl
Gene therapy could possibly treat and prevent angiogenesis by blocking stimulatory proteins or increasing expression of endogenous inhibitors. Ocular gene transfer is an appealing treatment approach because of its potential to provide a sustained therapeutic response within the eye with little systemic impact.

Successful gene therapy technology hinges on a detailed understanding of the molecular pathogenesis of retinal and subretinal neovascularization, along with a safe and effective vector for gene transfer. Adenoviral (Ad) vectors are relatively easy to produce, have good capacity, and can mediate good expression levels in many cells types with an appropriate promoter. One concern with adenoviral vectors is that they induce an inflammatory response, which could destroy transduced cells and prevent repeat injections. Adeno-associated viral (AAV) vectors are more difficult to produce than adenoviral vectors, with a capacity limited to less than 5 kb. However, adeno-associated viral vectors beget little to no immune response, mediating prolonged transgene expression with little toxicity [79].

AdPEDF.11

Pigment epithelial-derived growth factor (PEDF) has neurotrophic, neuroprotective, and anti-angiogenic properties [80–82]. Researchers have shown that an adenoviral vector containing complementary DNA encoding human PEDF, known as AdPEDF.11 (GenVec, Inc., Gaithersburg, MD, USA) or Ad$_{GV}$PEDF.11D, inhibits ocular neovascularization in two murine models [82]. AdPEDF.11 induces apoptosis of endothelial cells in new blood vessels, but not in normal vasculature [82]. Intriguingly, subconjunctival

AdPEDF.11 in a murine model resulted in transduction of episcleral cells that produced PEDF [83]. The PEDF penetrated the sclera with high choroidal levels that induce regression of CNV.

A phase I trial of AdPEDF.11 in 28 patients failed to identify any dose-related toxicities and suggested a sustained anti-angiogenic effect for several months after a single intravitreal injection of at least 10^8 particle units [84–86]. Moreover, repeated adenovector administration into the eye does not appear to incite a systemic immune response [87], affording the possibility of repeat injections. This study demonstrates the viability of ocular gene transfer via an adenoviral vector. Further study is warranted to fully appreciate AdPEDF.11's potential as a therapy in this disease.

AAV2-sFLT01

The high-affinity VEGF receptor Flt-1 is one of the most potent naturally occurring VEGF binders. sFLT01 is a novel chimeric VEGF-binding molecule that consists of one Flt-1 domain linked to the human IgG1 heavy-chain Fc region, resulting in a forced homodimer with high affinity for VEGF. Pechan and colleagues integrated sFLT01 into an adeno-associated virus serotype 2 (AAV2) vector, so called AAV2-sFLT01 (Genzyme, Cambridge, MA, USA). AAV2-mediated intravitreal gene delivery of sFLT01 inhibited angiogenesis in the mouse oxygen-induced retinopathy model [88].

A phase 1 trial to evaluate the safety and feasibility of AAV2-sFLT01 in treating patients with neovascular AMD is underway [89].

Other Pathways

ATG-3

ATG-3 (CoMentis, formerly Athenagen, South San Francisco, CA, USA) is the proprietary eye drop formulation of mecamylamine, which antagonizes the nicotinic acetylcholine receptor pathway that mediates angiogenesis and downregulates VEGF. Mecamylamine suppressed CNV in a murine model, both by subcutaneous and topical application [90]. A phase I trial treated 80 patients with ATG-3 eye drops twice daily up to 14 days. ATG-3 was well tolerated and safe, with very low levels of the compound found in the blood following application. However, a phase II trial examining two doses of ATG-3 in 343 patients was terminated [91]. Another phase II trial is evaluating the safety and efficacy of ATG-3 drops in patients receiving maintenance intravitreal injections of ranibizumab or bevacizumab. This trial is currently ongoing, but not recruiting [92].

Squalamine Lactate

Squalamine lactate (Evizon®, Genaera Corporation, Plymouth Meeting, PA) is an anti-angiogenic amino sterol derived from dogfish shark (*Squalus acanthus*) cartilage. It blocks cell membrane ion transport that controls pH and cell metabolism. It also blocks VEGF action and integrin expression when bound to calmodulin. Squalamine must be administered intravenously, as it is ineffective intravitreally [15, 93]. Systemically administered squalamine lactate partially reduced choroidal neovascular membrane development induced by laser trauma in a rat model [94]. In a phase I/II trial of 40 patients receiving 25 or 50 mg/m² weekly for four weeks, no patients lost vision and 26% gained three or more lines [15]. Despite these results, Genaera abandoned this product. Phase II [95–97] and III [98] trials have been terminated.

Combretastatin A4 Phosphate/CA4P

Combretastatin A4 Phosphate, or CA4P (Zybrestat, OXiGENE, South San Francisco, CA, USA), is a microtubule-disrupting agent that rapidly shuts off blood flow in new vessels and induces regression [99, 100]. In a murine model of tumor angiogenesis, CA4P selectively targeted endothelial cells, but not smooth muscle cells, and induced regression of unstable nascent tumor neovessels by rapidly disrupting the molecular engagement of vascular endothelial-cadherin, an endothelial cell-specific junctional molecule. CA4P increased endothelial cell permeability, while inhibiting endothelial cell migration and capillary tube formation, thereby leading to rapid vascular collapse and tumor necrosis [100]. Interestingly, however, CA4P failed to induce regression of diabetes-like retinal neovascularization in a canine model [101].

A phase I/II trial in patients with neovascular AMD treated with intravenous CA4P demonstrated side effects, namely hypertension and increased QTc interval [102]. A phase II study in patients with myopic CNV showed weakly positive results [103, 104]. OXiGENE is currently testing a topical application that achieved good retinal and choroidal concentrations in a rabbit model [105].

JSM6427

Integrin $\alpha 5\beta 1$ is the principal fibronectin receptor and plays a key role in angiogenesis [106]. Inhibition of $\alpha 5\beta 1$ integrin function induces apoptosis of actively proliferating but not quiescent cells [106]. JSM6427 (Jerini AG, Berlin, Germany) is a potent $\alpha 5\beta 1$ integrin antagonist that has been shown to modulate hypoxia-induced neovascularization in mice [107]. Preclinical work was done in rabbit and monkey models of CNV. Intravitreal JSM6427 inhibited CNV in a dose-dependent manner without any ocular adverse effects or systemic safety signals [108]. Interestingly, JSM6427 may also prove beneficial in proliferative retinopathies. It has a strong inhibitory effect on human retinal pigment epithelial cell attachment, proliferation, and migration [109].

A phase I dose-escalation trial [110] demonstrated safety and some degree of biologic activity in end-stage lesions. However, the relatively short half life led to concerns regarding treatment duration. Further study is on hold until researchers develop extended delivery of the drug.

Volociximab

Volociximab (Ophthotech Corporation, Princeton, NY, USA) is a monoclonal antibody that targets $\alpha 5\beta 1$ integrin. It appears to inhibit neovascularization independent of the growth factor stimulation, either by VEGF or other angiogenic factors

[106]. A phase I study evaluated the safety of intravitreal volociximab combined with ranibizumab for neovascular AMD [111]. Volociximab was used in combination with ranibizumab because the integrin antagonist likely needs anti-VEGF cotreatment due to the lack of a significant antipermeability effect. Preliminary results from 10 subjects receiving two doses of volociximab in combination with ranibizumab revealed a visual acuity improvement of 10.8 letters at nine weeks, with a mean decrease in central macular thickness of 136 μm. These results do not separate the independent contributions from ranibizumab and volociximab. Dose escalation of volociximab has been completed without evidence of dose-limiting toxicity or drug-related adverse events [112].

NT-501, Ciliary Neurotrophic Factor

Ciliary neurotrophic factor (CNTF) (Neurotech Pharmaceuticals, Lincoln, RI) is a potent neuroprotective agent capable of protecting photoreceptors in animal models of retinal degeneration [113]. The definitive neuroprotective mechanism of CNTF in the degenerating retina remains unknown [114]. Indirect rescue of photoreceptors by CNTF is a function of reversible biochemical and morphological changes in rod photoreceptors that lead to reduced photoresponsiveness [115].

Researchers have adapted encapsulated cell technology to permit CNTF-producing transfected cells to release CNTF for a year or longer after implantation into the vitreous cavity. The intravitreal implant, known as NT-501, requires surgical implantation through the pars plana with scleral fixation. NT-501 is being evaluated in patients with dry AMD or retinitis pigmentosa, but may someday hold promise in protecting photoreceptors of neovascular AMD patients.

NT-501 was safe and well tolerated in a phase II study of geographic atrophy [116], with stability of visual acuity and improvement in macular volume. There was evidence that implants continued to elute CNTF for up to 18 months [117]. Both CNTF and encapsulated cell technology have potential to help patients with neovascular AMD in the future.

Sonepcizumab

Sphingosine-1-phosphate (S1P) is a lipid molecule that stimulates endothelial cell migration, proliferation, and survival in vitro, and tumor angiogenesis in vivo [118]. Local S1P is elevated by hypoxia, inflammation, and injury. Sonepcizumab (iSONEP™, Lpath, Inc., San Diego, CA) is a humanized monoclonal antibody against S1P. A murine model showed intraocular injection of sonepcizumab strongly suppressed retinal and CNV [118]. Another murine model found it to inhibit subretinal fibrosis [119]. A phase I trial [120] evaluating intravitreal sonepcizumab in 15 patients found it to be well tolerated with evidence of biologic activity [121]. Four of the seven patients with large choroidal neovascular membranes actually had reduction in lesion size after a single sonepcizumab injection. Sonepcizumab holds promise for neovascular AMD as it affects a novel pathway in angiogenesis. A phase II trial is in design.

> **Pearl**
> Other pathways affecting the nicotinic acetylcholine receptor pathway, integrin expression and function, microtubule integrity, and photoreceptor neuroprotection may prove effective.

Summary

There are a myriad of new treatments for neovascular AMD currently under development, targeting various arms of the angiogenic pathway (Table 9.1). Numerous treatment modalities block VEGF or its several receptors. Platelet-derived growth factor (PDGF) and its receptor represent other angiogenic targets. Tyrosine kinase inhibition blocks receptors for VEGF and PDGF. Small interfering RNA technology may someday prove

effective in silencing important genes involved in angiogenesis. Localized radiation treatment provides antiangiogenic, antiinflammatory, and antifibrotic activity directly to choroidal neovascular membranes. Complement inhibition and potent immunosuppressive agents may impact the inflammatory component of AMD. Gene therapy offers the potential for sustained rebalancing of angiogenic and anti-angiogenic factors. Targeting other pathways, like the nicotinic acetylcholine receptor pathway or α5β1 integrin function, may prove effective, especially when combined with other therapies. Neuroprotection, with agents such as CNTF, may help preserve photoreceptors during inhibition of angiogenesis in neovascular AMD patients.

As new treatments evolve, so will combination therapies. Combining different treatments with disparate modes of action can have an additive or synergistic effect.

> **Pearl**
> Combining disparate treatments can have an additive or synergistic effect.

For instance, an anti-PDGF agent can strip pericytes from neovascular vessels, allowing better effect of anti-VEGF agents. An additional neuroprotective agent, like CNTF, may help protect photoreceptors and thereby prevent atrophy during antiangiogenic treatment. (Please refer to Chapter 7 for a detailed discussion regarding combination therapies for neovascular AMD.) Advancements in the delivery of potent medications, with longer-acting formulations to minimize treatment burden while improving compliance, will likely add to our armamentarium.

The future of neovascular AMD will utilize several technologies to target multiple angiogenic pathways, allowing better visual outcomes for this sight-threatening disease.

Table 9.1 Summary of neovascular AMD therapeutic agents, mechanisms of action, and phase of development

Classification	Agent	Mechanism	Route	Phase	Notes
Anti-VEGF	Ranibizumab	Monoclonal antibody Fab fragment (48 kDa) against VEGF-A	Intravitreal	IV	
	Bevacizumab	Full-length monoclonal antibody (149 kDa) against VEGF-A	Intravitreal	III	
	VEGF Trap-Eye	Recombinant protein with binding portion of two VEGF receptors fused to Fc region of human IgG (110 kDa)	Intravitreal	III	
	Bevasiranib	siRNA silencing VEGF production	Intravitreal	III	
Inhibition of VEGF receptor, platelet-derived growth factor (PDGR), and PDGR receptor	Vatalanib	Tyrosine kinase inhibitor that inhibits all known VEGF receptor tyrosine kinases (VEGFR-1, VEGFR-2, VEGFR-3), PDGFRβ, & c-kit receptor kinases	Oral	I/II	Some biologic activity but problems with safety
	TG100801	Tyrosine kinase inhibitor that inhibits VEGFR and PDGFR	Topical	II	Corneal toxicity, trial discontinued
	Pazopanib	Second-generation multi-targeted tyrosine kinase inhibitor against all VEGFR's, both PDGFRα and PDGRF β, and c-kit	Topical	II	
	Sirna-027	siRNA silencing VEGFR-1	Intravitreal	II	Trial discontinued; failed to improve vision
	Anti-VEGFR vaccine	Induces cytotoxic T-lymphocyte response	Subcutaneous	I	
	E10030	Aptamer against PDGF-B, decreases pericyte density	Intravitreal	I	
Radiation	Epi-Rad90™	Anti-angiogenic, anti-inflammatory, and anti-fibrotic	Localized radiation during vitrectomy	III	
	IRay	Anti-angiogenic, anti-inflammatory, and anti-fibrotic	Externally-applied stereotactic orthovoltage device	II	
Anti-inflammatory and anti-immune pathways	POT-4	Binds and inhibits complement 3	Intravitreal	II	
	ARC1905	Binds and inhibits complement 5	Intravitreal	I	
	Infliximab	Anti-TNF-alpha monoclonal antibody	Intravitreal	I	
	Sirolimus	Inhibits mammalian target of rapamycin	Subconjunctival	II	

(continued)

Table 9.1 (continued)

Classification	Agent	Mechanism	Route	Phase	Notes
Gene therapy	AdPEDF.11	Adenoviral vector transferring gene for pigment epithelial-derived growth factor	Intravitreal	I	
	AAV2-sFLT01	Adeno-associated virus vector transferring gene for a potent VEGF-binding molecule	Intravitreal	I	
Other pathways	ATG-3 (mecamylamine)	Antagonizes the nicotinic acetylcholine receptor pathway	Topical	II	
	Squalamine lactate	Blocks cell membrane ion transport	Intravenous	III	Trial discontinued
	Combretastatin A4 phosphate	Microtubule disrupting agent	Intravenous	II	Intravenous route discontinued due to safety; topical route currently being tested
	JSM6427	α(alpha)5β(beta)1-integrin antagonist	Intravitreal	I	Project on hold
	Volociximab	Monoclonal antibody targeting α(alpha)5β(beta)1-integrin	Intravitreal	I	
	NT-501 (ciliary neurotrophic factor)	Neuroprotective agent protecting photoreceptors	Encapsulated cell technology, intravitreal implant with scleral fixation	II	
	Sonepcizumab	Humanized monoclonal antibody against sphingosine-1-phosphate	Intravitreal	I	

References

1. Ferrara N. Vascular endothelial growth factor: basic science and clinical progress. Endocr Rev. 2004;25(4):581–611.

2. Ferrara N, Damico L, Shams N, et al. Development of ranibizumab, an anti-vascular endothelial growth factor antigen binding fragment, as therapy for neovascular age-related macular degeneration. Retina. 2006;26(8):859–70.

3. Rosenfeld PJ, Brown DM, Heier JS, et al. Ranibizumab for neovascular age-related macular degeneration. N Engl J Med. 2006;355(14):1419–31.

4. Brown DM, Kaiser PK, Michels M, et al. Ranibizumab versus verteporfin for neovascular age-related macular degeneration. N Engl J Med. 2006;355(14):1432–44.

5. Brown DM, Michels M, Kaiser PK, et al. Ranibizumab versus verteporfin photodynamic therapy for neovascular age-related macular degeneration: two-year results of the ANCHOR study. Ophthalmology. 2009;116(1):57–65.e5.

6. Comparison of age-related macular degeneration treatments trials: lucentis-avastin trial [ClinicalTrials. gov identifier: NCT00593450]. ClinicalTrials.gov online. http://www.clinicaltrials.gov/ct2/show/ NCT00593450. Accessed 16 Dec 2009.

7. Rakic JM, Lambert V, Devy L, et al. Placental growth factor, a member of the VEGF family, contributes to the development of choroidal neovascularization. Invest Ophthalmol Vis Sci. 2003;44(7):3186–93.

8. Nguyen QD, Shah SM, Hafiz G, et al. A phase I trial of an IV-administered vascular endothelial growth factor trap for treatment in patients with choroidal neovascularization due to age-related macular degeneration. Ophthalmology. 2006;113(9):1522.e1–14.

9. Nguyen QD, Shah SM, Browning DJ, et al. A phase I study of intravitreal vascular endothelial growth factor trap-eye in patients with neovascular age-related macular degeneration. Ophthalmology. 2009;116(11):2141–8.e1.

10. Bayer HealthCare and Regeneron Announce VEGF trap-eye achieved durable improvement in vision over 52 weeks in a phase 2. http://www.medicalnewstoday.com/articles/119267.php. Accessed 4 Dec 2009.

11. Vascular Endothelial Growth Factor (VEGF) trap-eye: investigation of efficacy and safety in wet age-related macular degeneration (AMD) (VIEW 1). ClinicalTrials.gov identifier: NCT00509795. ClinicalTrials.gov online. http://www.clinicaltrials. gov/ct2/show/NCT00509795. Accessed 4 Dec 2009.

12. Vascular Endothelial Growth Factor (VEGF) trap-eye: investigation of efficacy and safety in wet age-related macular degeneration (AMD) (VIEW 2). ClinicalTrials.gov identifier: NCT00637377. ClinicalTrials.gov online. http://www.clinicaltrials. gov/ct2/show/NCT00637377. Accessed 4 Dec 2009.

13. Singerman L. Combination therapy using the small interfering RNA bevasiranib. Retina. 2009;29 (6 Suppl):S49–50.

14. Singerman LJ. VEGF small interfering (si) RNA, for treatment of wet age-related macular degeneration (AMD). Presented at American Society of Retina Specialists, Cannes, 2006.

15. Emerson MV, Lauer AK. Current and emerging therapies for the treatment of age-related macular degeneration. Clin Ophthalmol. 2008;2(2):377–88.

16. Safety & Efficacy Study Evaluating the Combination of Bevasiranib & Lucentis Therapy in Wet AMD (COBALT). ClinicalTrials.gov identifier: NCT00499590. ClinicalTrials.gov online. http:// www.clinicaltrials.gov/ct2/show/NCT00499590. Accessed 5 Dec 2009.

17. Bevasiranib, an siRNA targeting Vascular Endothelial Growth Factor (VEGF) for the treatment of age-related macular degeneration (AMD), is the most advanced siRNA at OPKO and the first siRNA in the industry to enter a Phase III clinical trial. OPKO's website. http:// www.opko.com/research/?doc=ophthalmics. Accessed 5 Dec 2009.

18. Safety & Efficacy Study Evaluating the Combination of Bevasiranib & Lucentis Therapy in Wet AMD (CARBON). ClinicalTrials.gov identifier: NCT00557791. ClinicalTrials.gov online. http:// www.clinicaltrials.gov/ct2/show/NCT00557791. Accessed 5 Dec 2009.

19. Ferrara N, Gerber HP, LeCouter J. The biology of VEGF and its receptors. Nat Med. 2003;9(6):669–76.

20. Zeng H, Dvorak HF, Mukhopadhyay D. Vascular permeability factor (VPF)/vascular endothelial growth factor (VEGF) peceptor-1 down-modulates VPF/ VEGF receptor-2-mediated endothelial cell proliferation, but not migration, through phosphatidylinositol 3-kinase-dependent pathways. J Biol Chem. 2001;276(29):26969–79.

21. Hellstrom M, Gerhardt H, Kalen M, et al. Lack of pericytes leads to endothelial hyperplasia and abnormal vascular morphogenesis. J Cell Biol. 2001;153(3):543–53.

22. Hellberg C, Ostman A, Heldin CH. PDGF and vessel maturation. Recent Results Cancer Res. 2010;180:103–14.

23. Kaiser PK. Antivascular endothelial growth factor agents and their development: therapeutic implications in ocular diseases. Am J Ophthalmol. 2006; 142(4):660–8.

24. Safety and efficacy of oral PTK787 in patients with subfoveal choroidal neovascularization secondary to age-related macular degeneration (AMD) (ADVANCE). ClinicalTrials.gov identifier: NCT00138632. ClinicalTrials.gov online. http:// clinicaltrials.gov/ct2/show/NCT00138632. Accessed 20 Nov 2009.

25. Doukas J, Mahesh S, Umeda N, et al. Topical administration of a multi-targeted kinase inhibitor suppresses choroidal neovascularization and retinal edema. J Cell Physiol. 2008;216(1):29–37.

26. Roberts D. Antiangiogenic drugs are stopping neovascularization in wet macular degeneration. http://www.mdsupport.org/library/anti-angio.html. Accessed 6 Dec 2009.

27. A phase 1 safety study of TG100801 eye drops in healthy volunteers. http://www.clinicaltrials.gov/ct2/show/NCT00414999. Accessed 6 Dec 2009.

28. Open-label, pilot study of TG100801 in patients with choroidal neovascularization due to AMD. ClinicalTrials.gov identifier: NCT00509548. ClinicalTrials.gov online. http://clinicaltrials.gov/ct2/show/NCT00509548. Accessed 20 Nov 2009.

29. Sonpavde G, Hutson TE. Pazopanib: a novel multitargeted tyrosine kinase inhibitor. Curr Oncol Rep. 2007;9(2):115–9.

30. A study to evaluate the pharmacodynamics, safety, and pharmacokinetics of pazopanib drops in adult subjects with neovascular AMD. ClinicalTrials.gov identifier: NCT00612456. http://www.clinicaltrials.gov/ct2/show/NCT00612456. Accessed 6 Dec 2009.

31. An extension to study MD7108240. ClinicalTrials.gov identifier: NCT00733304. http://www.clinicaltrials.gov/ct2/show/NCT00733304. Accessed 6 Dec 2009.

32. Shen J, Samul R, Silva RL, et al. Suppression of ocular neovascularization with siRNA targeting VEGF receptor 1. Gene Ther. 2006;13(3):225–34.

33. Sirna therapeutics reports final results from phase 1 study in its RNAi-based therapeutic for age-related macular degeneration. http://www.medicalnewstoday.com/articles/49334.php. Accessed 6 December 2009.

34. Allergan drops development of siRNA Rx for AMD on poor phase II data. http://www.genomeweb.com/rnai/allergan-drops-development-sirna-rx-amd-poorphase-ii-data. Accessed 2 Jan 2010.

35. A study using intravitreal injections of a small interfering RNA in patients with age-related macular degeneration. ClinicalTrials.gov identifier: NCT00395057. ClinicalTrials.gov online. http://www.clinicaltrials.gov/ct2/show/NCT00395057. Accessed 6 Dec 2009.

36. Wigginton JM, Gruys E, Geiselhart L, et al. IFN-gamma and Fas/FasL are required for the antitumor and antiangiogenic effects of IL-12/pulse IL-2 therapy. J Clin Invest. 2001;108(1):51–62.

37. Mochimaru H, Nagai N, Hasegawa G, et al. Suppression of choroidal neovascularization by dendritic cell vaccination targeting VEGFR2. Invest Ophthalmol Vis Sci. 2007;48(10):4795–801.

38. Anti-VEGFR vaccine therapy in treating patients with neovascular maculopathy. ClinicalTrials.gov identifier: NCT00791570. ClinicalTrials.gov online. http://www.clinicaltrials.gov/ct2/show/NCT00791570. Accessed 6 Dec 2009.

39. Ni Z, Hui P. Emerging pharmacologic therapies for wet age-related macular degeneration. Ophthalmologica. 2009;223(6):401–10.

40. A phase 1, safety, tolerability and pharmacokinetic profile of intravitreous injections of E10030 (Anti-PDGF Pegylated Aptamer) in subjects with neovascular age-related macular degeneration. ClinicalTrials.gov identifier: NCT00569140. ClinicalTrials.gov online. http://www.clinicaltrials.gov/ct2/show/NCT00569140. Accessed 27 Dec 2009.

41. Kuppermann B. Combined inhibition of platelet-derived growth factor (PDGF) and VEGF for treatment of neovascular AMD – Results of a phase 1 study. Retina Congress, NYC, NY 2009.

42. Study of Anti-PDGF and Anti-VEGF therapy shows significant neovascular regression and enhanced visual outcome. http://www.medicalnewstoday.com/articles/148727.php. Accessed 27 Dec 2009.

43. The Radiation Therapy for Age-related Macular Degeneration (RAD) Study Group. A prospective, randomized, double-masked trial on radiation therapy for neovascular age-related macular degeneration (RAD Study). Ophthalmology. 1999;106(12):2239–47.

44. Marcus DM, Sheils W, Johnson MH, et al. External beam irradiation of subfoveal choroidal neovascularization complicating age-related macular degeneration: one-year results of a prospective, double-masked, randomized clinical trial. Arch Ophthalmol. 2001;119(2):171–80.

45. Hart PM, Chakravarthy U, Mackenzie G, et al. Visual outcomes in the subfoveal radiotherapy study: a randomized controlled trial of teletherapy for age-related macular degeneration. Arch Ophthalmol. 2002;120(8):1029–38.

46. Zambarakji HJ, Lane AM, Ezra E, et al. Proton beam irradiation for neovascular age-related macular degeneration. Ophthalmology. 2006;113(11):2012–9.

47. Krishnan L, Krishnan EC, Jewell WR. Immediate effect of irradiation on microvasculature. Int J Radiat Oncol Biol Phys. 1988;15(1):147–50.

48. Chakravarthy U, Gardiner TA, Archer DB, Maguire CJ. A light microscopic and autoradiographic study of non-irradiated and irradiated ocular wounds. Curr Eye Res. 1989;8(4):337–48.

49. Willett CG, Duda DG, di Tomaso E, et al. Efficacy, safety, and biomarkers of neoadjuvant bevacizumab, radiation therapy, and fluorouracil in rectal cancer: a multidisciplinary phase II study. J Clin Oncol. 2009;27(18):3020–6.

50. Willett CG, Kozin SV, Duda DG, et al. Combined vascular endothelial growth factor-targeted therapy and radiotherapy for rectal cancer: theory and clinical practice. Semin Oncol. 2006;33(5 Suppl 10):S35–40.

51. Avila MP, Farah ME, Santos A, et al. Twelve-month safety and visual acuity results from a feasibility study of intraocular, epiretinal radiation therapy for the treatment of subfoveal CNV secondary to AMD. Retina. 2009;29(2):157–69.

52. Dugel P. Epimacular brachytherapy for the treatment of neovascular AMD: NVI-111 24 Month VA outcomes. Presented at retina congress 2009, New York City, 2009. http://www.neovistainc.com/docs/press/Final-24-Month-Review-of-NVI-111-Study.pdf. Accessed 7 Dec 2009.

53. Avila MP, Farah ME, Santos A, et al. Twelve-month short-term safety and visual-acuity results from a multicentre prospective study of epiretinal strontium-90 brachytherapy with bevacizumab for the treatment of subfoveal choroidal neovascularisation

secondary to age-related macular degeneration. Br J Ophthalmol. 2009;93(3):305–9.

54. A study of the NeoVista ophthalmic system for the treatment of subfoveal CNV associated with wet AMD in patients that require persistent anti-VEGF therapy (MERITAGE). ClinicalTrials.gov identifier: NCT00809419. ClinicalTrials.gov online. http://clinicaltrials.gov/ct2/show/NCT00809419. Accessed 7 Dec 2009.

55. A study to evaluate the Neovista ophthalmic system for the treatment of subfoveal CNV in patients with AMD that have failed primary anti-VEGF therapy (ROSE). ClinicalTrials.gov identifier: NCT00679445. ClinicalTrials.gov online. http://clinicaltrials.gov/ct2/show/NCT00679445. Accessed 22 Dec 2009.

56. Macular EpiRetinal Brachytherapy Versus Lucentis® Only Treatment (MERLOT). ClinicalTrials.gov identifier: NCT01006538. ClinicalTrials.gov online. http://clinicaltrials.gov/ct2/show/NCT01006538. Accessed 22 Dec 2009.

57. Kaiser P. Externally-applied stereotactic orthovoltage irradiation for age-related macular degeneration: case presentations from a phase I clinical trial. Retina Congress, NYC, NY, 2009.

58. Safety & efficacy study of the IRay system in patients with choroidal neovascularization (CNV) secondary to age-related macular degeneration (AMD). ClinicalTrials.gov identifier: NCT01016873. ClinicalTrials.gov online. http://clinicaltrials.gov/ct2/show/NCT01016873. Accessed 22 Dec 2009.

59. Kijlstra A, La Heij E, Hendrikse F. Immunological factors in the pathogenesis and treatment of age-related macular degeneration. Ocul Immunol Inflamm. 2005;13(1):3–11.

60. Reynolds R, Hartnett ME, Atkinson JP, et al. Plasma complement components and activation fragments: associations with age-related macular degeneration genotypes and phenotypes. Invest Ophthalmol Vis Sci. 2009;50(12):5818–27.

61. Grossniklaus HE, Ling JX, Wallace TM, et al. Macrophage and retinal pigment epithelium expression of angiogenic cytokines in choroidal neovascularization. Mol Vis. 2002;8:119–26.

62. Nozaki M, Raisler BJ, Sakurai E, et al. Drusen complement components C3a and C5a promote choroidal neovascularization. Proc Natl Acad Sci USA. 2006;103(7):2328–33.

63. Oh H, Takagi H, Takagi C, et al. The potential angiogenic role of macrophages in the formation of choroidal neovascular membranes. Invest Ophthalmol Vis Sci. 1999;40(9):1891–8.

64. Potentia pharmaceuticals' POT-4 drug candidate for age-related macular degeneration successfully completes phase I clinical trial. http://www.medicalnewstoday.com/articles/148725.php. Accessed 24 Dec 2009.

65. Safety of intravitreal POT-4 therapy for patients with neovascular age-related macular degeneration (AMD) (ASaP). ClinicalTrials.gov identifier: NCT00473928. http://www.clinicaltrials.gov/ct2/show/NCT00473928. Accessed 24 Dec 2009.

66. ARC1905 (ANTI-C5 APTAMER) given either in combination therapy with Lucentis® 0.5 mg/eye in subjects with neovascular age-related macular degeneration. ClinicalTrials.gov identifier: NCT00709527. ClinicalTrials.gov online. http://www.clinicaltrials.gov/ct2/show/NCT00709527. Accessed 25 Dec 2009.

67. A Study of ARC1905 (Anti-C5 Aptamer) in subjects with dry age-related macular degeneration. ClinicalTrials.gov identifier: NCT00950638. ClinicalTrials.gov online. http://www.clinicaltrials.gov/ct2/show/NCT00950638. Accessed 25 Dec 2009.

68. Olson JL, Courtney RJ, Mandava N. Intravitreal infliximab and choroidal neovascularization in an animal model. Arch Ophthalmol. 2007;125(9):1221–4.

69. Theodossiadis PG, Liarakos VS, Sfikakis PP, et al. Intravitreal administration of the anti-TNF monoclonal antibody infliximab in the rabbit. Graefes Arch Clin Exp Ophthalmol. 2009;247(2):273–81.

70. Theodossiadis PG, Liarakos VS, Sfikakis PP, et al. Intravitreal administration of the anti-tumor necrosis factor agent infliximab for neovascular age-related macular degeneration. Am J Ophthalmol. 2009;147(5):825–30, 30.e1.

71. Intravitreal infliximab for diabetic macular edema (DME) and choroidal neovascularization (CNV) (ITVR). ClinicalTrials.gov identifier: NCT00695682. ClinicalTrials.gov online. http://www.clinicaltrials.gov/ct2/show/NCT00695682. Accessed 24 Dec 2009.

72. Hay N, Sonenberg N. Upstream and downstream of mTOR. Genes Dev. 2004;18(16):1926–45.

73. Guba M, von Breitenbuch P, Steinbauer M, et al. Rapamycin inhibits primary and metastatic tumor growth by antiangiogenesis: involvement of vascular endothelial growth factor. Nat Med. 2002;8(2):128–35.

74. Wang W, Jia WD, Xu GL, et al. Antitumoral activity of rapamycin mediated through inhibition of HIF-1alpha and VEGF in hepatocellular carcinoma. Dig Dis Sci. 2009;54(10):2128–36.

75. Dejneka NS, Kuroki AM, Fosnot J, et al. Systemic rapamycin inhibits retinal and choroidal neovascularization in mice. Mol Vis. 2004;10:964–72.

76. Phase 1/2 Study of an ocular sirolimus (Rapamycin) formulation in patients with age-related macular degeneration. ClinicalTrials.gov identifier: NCT00712491. ClinicalTrials.gov online. http://www.clinicaltrials.gov/ct2/show/NCT00712491. Accessed 26 Dec 2009.

77. MacuSight (TM) announces positive preliminary results from phase 1 study of Sirolimus in wet age-related macular degeneration. http://www.medicalnewstoday.com/articles/98491.php. Accessed 26 Dec 2009.

78. Phase 2 study of an ocular sirolimus (Rapamycin) formulation in combination with Lucentis® in Patients with age-related macular degeneration (EMERALD). ClinicalTrials.gov identifier: NCT00766337. ClinicalTrials.gov online. http://www.clinicaltrials.gov/ct2/show/NCT00766337. Accessed 26 Dec 2009.

79. Campochiaro PA. Gene therapy for ocular neovascularization. Curr Gene Ther. 2007;7(1):25–33.
80. Steele FR, Chader GJ, Johnson LV, Tombran-Tink J. Pigment epithelium-derived factor: neurotrophic activity and identification as a member of the serine protease inhibitor gene family. Proc Natl Acad Sci USA. 1993;90(4):1526–30.
81. Duh EJ, Yang HS, Suzuma I, et al. Pigment epithelium-derived factor suppresses ischemia-induced retinal neovascularization and VEGF-induced migration and growth. Invest Ophthalmol Vis Sci. 2002;43(3):821–9.
82. Mori K, Gehlbach P, Ando A, et al. Regression of ocular neovascularization in response to increased expression of pigment epithelium-derived factor. Invest Ophthalmol Vis Sci. 2002;43(7):2428–34.
83. Gehlbach P, Demetriades AM, Yamamoto S, et al. Periocular injection of an adenoviral vector encoding pigment epithelium-derived factor inhibits choroidal neovascularization. Gene Ther. 2003;10(8):637–46.
84. Campochiaro PA, Nguyen QD, Shah SM, et al. Adenoviral vector-delivered pigment epithelium-derived factor for neovascular age-related macular degeneration: results of a phase I clinical trial. Hum Gene Ther. 2006;17(2):167–76.
85. Study of AdGVPEDF.11D in neovascular age-related macular degeneration (AMD). ClinicalTrials.gov identifier: NCT00109499. ClinicalTrials.gov online. http://www.clinicaltrials.gov/ct2/show/NCT00109499. Accessed 26 Dec 2009.
86. Rasmussen H, Chu KW, Campochiaro P, et al. Clinical protocol. An open-label, phase I, single administration, dose-escalation study of ADGVPEDF.11D (ADPEDF) in neovascular age-related macular degeneration (AMD). Hum Gene Ther. 2001;12(16):2029–32.
87. Hamilton MM, Brough DE, McVey D, et al. Repeated administration of adenovector in the eye results in efficient gene delivery. Invest Ophthalmol Vis Sci. 2006;47(1):299–305.
88. Pechan P, Rubin H, Lukason M, et al. Novel anti-VEGF chimeric molecules delivered by AAV vectors for inhibition of retinal neovascularization. Gene Ther. 2009;16(1):10–6.
89. Safety and tolerability study of AAV2-sFLT01 in patients with neovascular age-related macular degeneration (AMD). ClinicalTrials.gov identifier: NCT01024998. ClinicalTrials.gov online. http://www.clinicaltrials.gov/ct2/show/NCT01024998. Accessed 26 Dec 2009.
90. Kiuchi K, Matsuoka M, Wu JC, et al. Mecamylamine suppresses Basal and nicotine-stimulated choroidal neovascularization. Invest Ophthalmol Vis Sci. 2008;49(4):1705–11.
91. Safety and efficacy of ATG003 in patients with wet age-related macular degeneration (AMD). ClinicalTrials.gov identifier: NCT00414206. ClinicalTrials.gov online. http://www.clinicaltrials.gov/ct2/show/NCT00414206. Accessed 26 Dec 2009.
92. Safety and efficacy of ATG003 in patients with AMD receiving anti-VEGF. ClinicalTrials.gov identifier: NCT00607750. ClinicalTrials.gov online. http://www.clinicaltrials.gov/ct2/show/NCT00607750. Accessed 26 Dec 2009.
93. Connolly B, Desai A, Garcia CA, et al. Squalamine lactate for exudative age-related macular degeneration. Ophthalmol Clin North Am. 2006;19(3):381–91, vi.
94. Ciulla TA, Criswell MH, Danis RP, et al. Squalamine lactate reduces choroidal neovascularization in a laser-injury model in the rat. Retina. 2003;23(6):808–14.
95. A safety and efficacy study of MSI-1256F (Squalamine Lactate) to treat "wet" age-related macular degeneration. ClinicalTrials.gov identifier: NCT00593450. ClinicalTrials.gov online. http://www.clinicaltrials.gov/ct2/show/NCT00089830. Accessed 26 Dec 2009.
96. A study of MSI-1256 F (Squalamine Lactate) to treat "wet" age-related macular degeneration. ClinicalTrials.gov identifier: NCT00333476. ClinicalTrials.gov online. http://www.clinicaltrials.gov/ct2/show/NCT00333476. Accessed 26 Dec 2009.
97. MSI-1256 F (Squalamine Lactate) in combination with verteporfin in patients with "wet" age-related macular degeneration (AMD). ClinicalTrials.gov identifier: NCT00094120. ClinicalTrials.gov online. http://www.clinicaltrials.gov/ct2/show/NCT00094120. Accessed 26 Dec 2009.
98. A Safety and Efficacy Study of Squalamine Lactate for Injection (MSI-1256F) for "wet" age-related macular degeneration. ClinicalTrials.gov identifier: NCT00139282. ClinicalTrials.gov online. http://www.clinicaltrials.gov/ct2/show/NCT00139282. Accessed 26 Dec 2009.
99. Tozer GM, Prise VE, Wilson J, et al. Mechanisms associated with tumor vascular shut-down induced by combretastatin A-4 phosphate: intravital microscopy and measurement of vascular permeability. Cancer Res. 2001;61(17):6413–22.
100. Vincent L, Kermani P, Young LM, et al. Combretastatin A4 phosphate induces rapid regression of tumor neovessels and growth through interference with vascular endothelial-cadherin signaling. J Clin Invest. 2005;115(11):2992–3006.
101. Kador PF, Blessing K, Randazzo J, et al. Evaluation of the vascular targeting agent combretastatin a-4 prodrug on retinal neovascularization in the galactose-fed dog. J Ocul Pharmacol Ther. 2007;23(2):132–42.
102. OXiGENE announces interim results of wet age-related macular degeneration trial of Combretastatin A4 prodrug. http://www.thefreelibrary.com/OXiGENE+Announces+Interim+Results+of+Wet+Age-Related+Macular . . . -a0116742838. Accessed 9 Jan 2010.
103. Wong TP BD, Benz MS. Phase II clinical trial of intravenous combretastatin a4 phosphate in patients with subfoveal choroidal neovascular membranes (CNV) in pathologic myopia. Presented at ARVO, Ft. Lauderdale, 2007.

104. OXiGENE announces positive results from its phase II CA4P clinical trial in myopic macular degeneration (MMD-213). http://www.thefreelibrary.com/OXiGENE+Announces+Positive+Results+from+its+Phase+II+CA4P+Clinical+ . . . -a0159340756. Accessed 9 Jan 2010.

105. OXiGENE reports positive preclinical ocular penetration data with topical formulation of ZYBRESTAT(TM) for Ophthalmology. http://www.highbeam.com/doc/1G1-172903545.html. Accessed 27 Dec 2009.

106. Ramakrishnan V, Bhaskar V, Law DA, et al. Preclinical evaluation of an anti-alpha5beta1 integrin antibody as a novel anti-angiogenic agent. J Exp Ther Oncol. 2006;5(4):273–86.

107. Maier AK, Kociok N, Zahn G, et al. Modulation of hypoxia-induced neovascularization by JSM6427, an integrin alpha5beta1 inhibiting molecule. Curr Eye Res. 2007;32(9):801–12.

108. Zahn G, Vossmeyer D, Stragies R, et al. Preclinical evaluation of the novel small-molecule integrin alpha5beta1 inhibitor JSM6427 in monkey and rabbit models of choroidal neovascularization. Arch Ophthalmol. 2009;127(10):1329–35.

109. Li R, Maminishkis A, Zahn G, et al. Integrin alpha-5beta1 mediates attachment, migration, and proliferation in human retinal pigment epithelium: relevance for proliferative retinal disease. Invest Ophthalmol Vis Sci. 2009;50(12):5988–96.

110. A phase 1 safety study of single and repeated doses of JSM6427 (intravitreal injection) to treat AMD. ClinicalTrials.gov identifier: NCT00536016. ClinicalTrials.gov online. http://www.clinicaltrials.gov/ct2/show/NCT00536016. Accessed 26 Dec 2009.

111. A phase 1 ascending and parallel group trial to establish the safety, tolerability and pharmacokinetics profile of volociximab (alpha 5 beta 1 integrin antagonist) in subjects with neovascular age-related macular degeneration. ClinicalTrials.gov identifier: NCT00782093. ClinicalTrials.gov online. http://www.clinicaltrials.gov/ct2/show/NCT00782093. Accessed 27 Dec 2009.

112. Mones J. combined inhibition of $\alpha5\beta1$ integrin and vascular endothelial growth factor for neovascular age-related macular degeneration – phase 1 study. Retina Congress, NYC, NY, 2009.

113. Tao W, Wen R, Goddard MB, et al. Encapsulated cell-based delivery of CNTF reduces photoreceptor degeneration in animal models of retinitis pigmentosa. Invest Ophthalmol Vis Sci. 2002;43(10):3292–8.

114. Emerich DF, Thanos CG. NT-501: an ophthalmic implant of polymer-encapsulated ciliary neurotrophic factor-producing cells. Curr Opin Mol Ther. 2008;10(5):506–15.

115. Wen R, Song Y, Kjellstrom S, et al. Regulation of rod phototransduction machinery by ciliary neurotrophic factor. J Neurosci. 2006;26(52):13523–30.

116. A study of an encapsulated cell technology (ECT) implant for patients with atrophic macular degeneration. ClinicalTrials.gov identifier: NCT00447954. ClinicalTrials.gov online. http://www.clinicaltrials.gov/ct2/show/NCT00447954. Accessed 16 Dec 2009.

117. Jaffe G. CNTF-secreting implant for dry AMD. Retina Today. 2009;4(7):52–3.

118. Xie B, Shen J, Dong A, et al. Blockade of sphingosine-1-phosphate reduces macrophage influx and retinal and choroidal neovascularization. J Cell Physiol. 2009;218(1):192–8.

119. Caballero S, Swaney J, Moreno K, et al. Anti-sphingosine-1-phosphate monoclonal antibodies inhibit angiogenesis and sub-retinal fibrosis in a murine model of laser-induced choroidal neovascularization. Exp Eye Res. 2009;88(3):367–77.

120. Safety study of iSONEP (Sonepcizumab/LT1009) to treat neovascular age-related macular degeneration. ClinicalTrials.gov identifier: NCT00767949. ClinicalTrials.gov online. http://www.clinicaltrials.gov/ct2/show/NCT00767949. Accessed 21 Feb 2010.

121. Lpath's ISONEP is well tolerated at all dose levels in a phase 1 trial in wet-AMD patients. http://www.medicalnewstoday.com/articles/166897.php. Accessed 21 Feb 2010.

The Economics of Age-Related Macular Degeneration

10

Gary C. Brown, Melissa M. Brown, Heidi B. Lieske, Philip A. Lieske, and Kathryn Brown

Key Points

- The Patient Protection and Affordable Care Act of 2010 funded the Patient-Centered Outcomes Research Institute to promote the use of comparative effectiveness analysis and cost-effectiveness analysis in the Unites States.
- There are four healthcare economic analysis variants: (1) cost-minimization analysis, (2) cost-benefit analysis, (3) cost-effectiveness analysis, and (4) cost-utility analysis. Cost-utility analysis, which uses the outcome $/QALY (dollars expended per QALY gained) is the most sophisticated.
- The comparative effectiveness, or *human value gain* conferred by an intervention can be objectively measured using the QALY (quality-adjusted life year).
- Most commonly, only the direct ophthalmic medical costs of therapy for neovascular age-related macular degeneration (AMD) are addressed in the literature. Societal costs are more desirable.
- Intravitreal ranibizumab therapy versus no therapy for subfoveal neovascular AMD confers

a 15.9–28.2% value gain (improvement in the quality of life), intravitreal bevacizumab with intraocular brachytherapy a 22.4% value gain, photodynamic therapy an 8.1% value gain, intravitreal pegaptanib a 5.9% value gain, and laser therapy a 4.4% value gain. Extrafoveal laser photocoagulation confers an 8.1% value gain over no therapy.

- US interventions costing <$100,000/QALY are usually considered cost-effective, and those costing <$50,000/QALY very cost-effective.
- The direct nonophthalmic medical costs (depression, trauma), direct nonmedical costs (caregiver, shelter, transportation), and indirect costs (decreased salary, decreased incidence of employment) associated with neovascular AMD exceed the direct ophthalmic costs associated with treating neovascular AMD by several hundred percent.
- Untreated atrophic AMD causes an estimated annual wage loss of $26.1 billion (2010 real US dollars) and untreated neovascular AMD results in an annual wage loss of $5.8 billion, for a total wage loss of $31.9 billion (2010 real US dollars). This is essentially a loss to the GDP, since consumer spending is the most important component of the GDP.

G.C. Brown (✉)
Department of Ophthalmology, Jefferson Medical College, 910 E. Willow Grove Ave., Wyndmoore, PA 19038, USA

Center for Value-Based Medicine, 6010 Mill Road, Flourtown, PA 19031, USA
e-mail: gary0514@gmail.com

Introduction

The economics of age-related macular degeneration (AMD) is typically discussed with regard to the direct ophthalmic medical costs associated with management of the neovascular entity [1–15]. These costs are considerable, especially since there are approximately 1,65,000 new cases of neovascular ("wet") AMD in the USA annually. Nonetheless, the costs associated with the 1.7 million annual new cases of atrophic ("dry") AMD are even more substantial [14, 15].

The direct ophthalmic medical costs associated with the management of neovascular AMD are the most visible, especially to those who allocate healthcare resources. Numerous papers have dealt with the subject of therapies for the neovascular variant, including laser photocoagulation [1, 2], intravitreal pegaptanib injections [3, 4], photodynamic therapy with verteporfin [3, 5, 6] and intravitreal VEGF-A inhibitors [7–13].

The costs associated with a disease, however, include not only the very apparent direct medical costs, but also the direct nonmedical costs and the indirect medical costs [13]. It appears that these direct nonmedical costs and indirect costs for neovascular AMD actually exceed the direct medical costs several times over [13].

Background information on healthcare economic analysis is helpful in understanding the current economics associated with AMD. Included herein are the four major variants of healthcare economic analysis, as well as a more extensive discussion on the most sophisticated form, cost-utility analysis, which integrates clinical outcomes with their associated costs. Value-Based Medicine®, the standardization of input variables and outcomes associated with cost-utility analysis, is also discussed in detail [15–23]. Lastly, the macroeconomic aspects (economics on a national level) associated with AMD are addressed.

There are essentially four major variants of healthcare economic analysis [23–25]. No matter the variant, however, a healthcare economic analysis is more robust if it is based upon the highest level of evidence-based medicine, a discussion of which follows.

Evidence-Based Medicine

In 1972, Archie Cochrane advocated the randomized clinical trial to promote the highest quality, most reproducible, medical evidence [26]. But, it was not until the last decade of the twentieth century that the term "evidence-based medicine" was popularized [27, 28].

Interventional Evidence

There are basically five levels of medical interventional evidence [29]. The higher the level of evidence (Levels 1 and 2), the greater confidence the clinician can have that the data from a study are reproducible (reliable). A summary of the levels of interventional evidence is shown in Table 10.1 [29].

Level 1 interventional evidence is typically provided by a randomized clinical trial with low type 1 and type 2 errors.
- *Type I error.* The type 1 error, or "false positive" error, in a Level 1 clinical trial is typically associated with a probability, the p-value, designated by the letter α(alpha), of <0.05 for detecting significantly different outcomes. This indicates that a false positive result will occur in <5% of instances. The α(alpha) is analogous to the probability of a jury finding an innocent person guilty.
- *Type II error.* The type II error, or "false negative" error, is typically associated with a probability, designated by the letter β(beta), <0.20, meaning that the chance of missing a significant outcome is less than or equal to 20%. The β(beta) is the probability of failing to detect a significant association, analogous to the probability of a jury finding a guilty person innocent.
- *Power.* The power of a clinical trial is calculated by subtracting the type II error, or β(beta), from 1.0. For level 1 interventional evidence, a power of (1.0–0.20 =) *80%* or greater is generally required to detect a predetermined outcome [29].

Table 10.1 Levels of interventional evidence [29]

Level 1 – randomized clinical trial with type 1 error <0.05 and type 2 error <0.20
Level 2 – randomized clinical trial with higher type 1 and/or type 2 error
Level 3 – nonrandomized clinical trial
Level 4 – case series
Level 5 – case report

- *The negative study.* Knowing the type 2 error is not as relevant for a clinical trial that has a significant outcome ($p < 0.05$) as it is when no significant difference is found. With a negative clinical trial, one that does not demonstrate a significant difference, it is important to know whether sufficient numbers of participants participated in the study to effectively assess a given outcome. For example, a 70% beneficial outcome when $n = 10$ is not nearly as relevant as a 70% beneficial outcome when $n = 1,000$. Knowing the power is most important to assess whether there are sufficient participants in a study to make it clinically relevant.
- *Meta-analysis.* In instances in which Level 1 interventional evidence is not available, a good meta-analysis can provide Level 1 evidence by combining two or more clinical trials, which may be underpowered. While much less costly than a clinical trial, this type of analysis can suffer from the reality that participating cohorts, treatments, and treatment outcomes in different trials may not be exactly the same.

Level 2 interventional evidence is supplied by the randomized clinical trial with a type 1 error >0.05 and/or a type 2 error >0.20.

Level 3 interventional evidence occurs with a nonrandomized clinical trial.

Level 4 interventional evidence is supplied by a case series.

Level 5 interventional evidence or anecdotal evidence is gleaned from a case report.

Of course, Level 1 clinical evidence is not available for all interventions. It is very expensive to obtain, and often requires long time periods to ideally assess an outcome. The other levels of interventional evidence, however, can provide important information as well, especially concerning the demographic features of a cohort, life expectancy, and the incidence of adverse events.

Masking

The clinician should also be aware of whether a study is appropriately masked [23, 28]. Masking can occur in the form of a *single-blind study,* in which a participant typically does not know which treatment is given, a *double-blind study,* in which neither the researcher nor the participant knows which treatment is administered, or a *triple-blind study,* in which neither the researcher, the participant nor the person evaluating the treatment response knows who is receiving which treatment. A triple- or double-blind study is preferable, but may not always be possible. Masking greatly reduces the possibility of bias. An *open-label* clinical trial is one in which there is no masking; it is commonly encountered with drug trials following an initial period of masking.

Dropout Rate

A dropout rate of <5% is considered excellent, while a rate of 5–15% is still acceptable. A rate greater than 20%, however, casts suspicion upon the validity of a study [28]. For example, a 10% event rate can be misleading if there is a 30% dropout rate and half of those who dropped out (15% of all participants) also had the event. Consequently, the true event rate might have been 25%, or 250% higher than the 10% event rate reported in the study with the 30% dropout rate. An *intent to treat* study keeps in data from all patients who are randomized, thereby allowing a clinician know the dropout rate.

> **Pearl**
> A dropout rate of >20% makes the results of a clinical trial suspect.

Validity

There are two basic types of validity: criterion validity and construct validity.

Criterion validity measures how well an intervention measures up to the *criterion,* or "gold standard" in the field. For the treatment of neovascular AMD, one might assess how well a new drug measures up to the current criterion of the VEGF-A inhibitor ranibizumab [1–3, 5–7].

Construct validity assesses how effectively something measures what it is supposed to measure. For example, how well does the quality-of-life instrument NEI-VFQ-25 [30] for ocular diseases actually measure the quality of life associated with neovascular macular degeneration?

Risk Reduction

The two variants of risk reduction are absolute risk reduction and relative risk reduction [24]. They produce very different outcomes and are often confused.

Absolute risk reduction (ARR) is defined as [(Control event rate)—(treatment event rate)]. For example, if an intervention reduces the incidence of blindness in a cohort of 100 treated people from 10% to 5%, the ARR = 10% − 5% = 5%, or a 5% reduction in blindness among the entire cohort.

Number needed to treat. The ratio of 1.0/ARR is the number of patients needed to treat to obtain a therapeutic benefit in one person. For the blindness intervention, the ARR = 1.0/5% = 20, meaning that 20 people must be treated with the intervention to prevent one outcome of blindness.

Relative risk reduction. Relative risk reduction (RRR) is defined as the [Control Event Rate (CER) − Treatment Event Rate (TER)]/Control Event Rate (CER). Thus, the RRR for the above blindness intervention is (10 − 5%)/10% = 50%. The RRR essentially illustrates the reduction in an event that occurs among the people who would have definitely become blind without therapy.

The type of risk reduction is critically important for patient counseling. Some clinicians present the RRR, suggesting that treatment reduces the incidence of blindness by 50%, which is true for those who would have otherwise become blind. Patients should know, however, that among *all* patients treated, the intervention reduces the incidence of blindness from 10% to 5%.

Pharmacoeconomic Analysis

Healthcare economic instruments, or pharmacoeconomic instruments for purposes herein, occur in four basic variants. In the order of increasing complexity, these include: (1) cost-minimization analysis, (2) cost-benefit analysis, (3) cost-effectiveness analysis, and (4) cost-utility analysis [23]. An understanding of the different forms of analysis is important for clinicians, especially since H.R.3590, the Patient Protection and Affordable Care Act [31] of 2010 funded the Patient-Centered Outcomes Research Institute. While established primarily for promoting comparative effectiveness standards, the center will most assuredly promote and regulate the cost-effectiveness arena as well.

A description of each of the healthcare economic instruments follows.

Cost-Minimization Analysis

A cost-minimization analysis assesses the cost of two identical interventions to ascertain which is less expensive. Unfortunately, cost-minimization analysis often suffers from the dilemma that it compares two different interventions that may seem similar, but are not. For example, while two VEGF inhibitors for the treatment of neovascular, age-related macular degeneration (AMD) may have similar visual outcomes, the associated adverse events, and the incidences of these events, may be very different. This form of analysis is therefore used infrequently today.

An example of a simplistic cost-minimization analysis is one that compares cataract surgery in a hospital outpatient setting versus an ambulatory surgical center setting, using the same technique in each location. Here, the same intervention is undertaken in a different setting and the cost is compared to ascertain which is least expensive.

Cost-Benefit Analysis

A cost-benefit analysis assesses the dollars expended for an intervention with those gained from that intervention. As an example, let us assume that ranibizumab therapy for neovascular AMD has direct medical cost of $10,000/year. The treatment may considerably decrease the human burden of disease, but the primary factor here is the overall cost expended versus the cost saved. Therapeutically, the MARINA Study [32] demonstrated that intravitreal ranibizumab results in 42% of treated individuals reaching a vision of 20/40, thereby allowing many who would otherwise be disabled to obviate caregiver costs. Thus, the weighted caregiver saving gain per patient might be $600/month, or $7,200 accrued per year. If half of the 42% of patients who achieve >20/40 vision now work at least part time as well, the weighted gain to the economy accrued per treated person might be approximately $8,000 annually.

Using a societal cost perspective, the caregiver costs saved and wages gained ($7,200 + $8,000 = *$15,200/year*) exceed the cost of therapy ($10,000/year) by $5,200 a year, indicating a positive cost-benefit for ranibizumab therapy. Cost-benefit analysis, however, typically fails to account for the quality-of-life and/or length-of-life gain associated with an intervention [23].

Cost-Effectiveness Analysis

A cost-effectiveness analysis quantifies the resources expended for an intervention for a given outcome. The outcome can be years of healthy life gained, years of normal vision gained, disability-free years gained, lines of vision gained, or virtually any other endpoint [23].

It is important to appreciate the confusion that has arisen around cost-effectiveness analysis. Authors in the USA often use the term *cost-effectiveness analysis* synonymously with *cost-utility analysis* [24, 33, 34]. In these instances, cost-utility analysis has been considered a subgroup of cost-effectiveness analysis.

Others [23, 25], including the current authors, reserve the term *cost-utility analysis* for those studies which specifically use the QALY (quality-adjusted life-year) in a cost-utility ratio ($/QALY), or dollars expended per QALY gained from an intervention. Nonetheless, the outcome of a cost-utility analysis is still considered to be more or less cost-effective, rather than more or less cost-utilitarian.

Tengs et al. [35] produced a superb treatise on 500 life-saving treatments published in the form of cost-effectiveness analysis. In each of these instances, the analysis was performed using cost per year of life saved. Adjusting the 1993 U. S. dollars from the Tengs et al. study [35] to year 2010 dollars reveals the median cost to save a year of life with a *medical intervention* is approximately $28,000, while that for an *injury reduction intervention* is 72,000, and that for a toxin *control intervention* is $4.1 million. Injury reduction entities include setting speed limits and the mandatory use of seatbelts, while toxin control interventions include regulation of benzene emission levels in tire plants or maximum arsenic levels permissible in water. Needless to say, the average medical intervention is far more cost-effective than the average injury reduction and toxin control interventions.

> **Pearl**
> Medical interventions which save lives are far more cost-effective than injury reduction interventions or toxin control interventions.

Cost-Utility Analysis

A cost-utility analysis is the most sophisticated form of pharmacoeconomic analysis since it integrates: (1) the improvement in quality of life conferred by an intervention, (2) the gain in length of life conferred by an intervention, and (3) the costs associated with that intervention [23]. The increase in longevity conferred by an intervention can generally be ascertained from evidence-based data in the literature, but the measurement of quality of life is more difficult. That said, it should be noted there is no universally accepted criterion of what exactly defines the quality of life, or wellbeing, of an individual.

> **Pearl**
> Cost-utility analysis is the most sophisticated method of the healthcare economic analysis.

Quality-of-Life Instruments, Function-Based

Many instruments have been utilized to assess the quality of life associated with a health state (one disease alone or with comorbidities). *Generic* instruments, including the Medical Outcomes Short-Form-36 (SF-36) [36], the Sickness Impact Profile (SIP) [37], and the Quality of Well-Being Scale [38], are theoretically applicable to interventions across multiple specialties. Among the *specialty-specific* instruments are the VF-14 [39] and the NEI-25 [30], both used to assess ophthalmic quality of life. In general, the generic medical instruments are not applicable to ophthalmic diseases and the ophthalmic instruments are not applicable across medical health states [23]. All of these tests primarily measure the function (physical, social, psychological, pain-associated, and so forth) associated with a given health state [23].

Quality-of-Life Instruments, Preference-Based

Preference-based quality-of-life instruments are essentially synonymous with utility instruments. Utilities, the outcomes, quantify the quality of life associated with a health state. Utility analysis is believed to be more all-encompassing than function-based quality-of-life measures in that it integrates all functions, psychological overlay, caregiver availability, socioeconomic conditions, occupational aspects and virtually every other aspect that comprises quality of life [23, 40]. The time tradeoff methodology has been demonstrated to have good ophthalmic construct validity [41], and correlates most closely with visual acuity in the better seeing eye [41–45].

> **Pearl**
> Utility analysis is a preference-based, all-encompassing instrument that allows a measure of the quality of life associated with any health state.

Utilities generally vary from 0.00 (death) to 1.00 (normal health, or normal vision, permanently).

The closer a utility is to 1.00, the better the quality of life associated with the health state, while the closer a utility is to 0.00, the poorer the quality of life associated with the health state. As examples, the utility associated with treated systemic arterial hypertension is 0.98, while that associated with a severe stroke is 0.34 [23]. A great advantage of utilities is that they compare health states across all of medicine using the same outcome.

> **Pearl**
> Utilities typically vary from 0.00 (death) to 1.00 (normal health, or normal vision in each eye permanently).

A time tradeoff utility is calculated by asking a study participant two questions:
- How long do you expect to live?
- What is the maximum percentage of your remaining time, if any, you would be willing to trade for an intervention that immediately returns your health problem to normal on a permanent basis?

The utility is calculated by subtracting the proportion of time traded from 1.0. For example, if a person with 20/200 vision in the better seeing eye believes they will live for another 30 years, and is willing to trade 10 of the 30 years in return for a normal vision permanently, their resultant ocular utility is $1.0 - 10/30 = 0.67$ [41]. Because patients can prefer to trade time for better health or prefer to trade no time and remain in the same health state, utility analysis is referred to as a *preference-based* quality-of-life instrument [23].

Utility Acquisition

It is important to note that the researcher who obtains utilities by interview will likely have different results for the same health state compared to the investigator who obtains utilities via mail or some other noninterview format. Participants reveal very personal information when they answer the above questions and, unless the researcher has a good rapport, are often hesitant to disclose their true preferences to strangers [23].

Utilities associated with visual acuity in the better-seeing eye are shown in Table 10.2 [16, 41, 44], while utilities associated with general medical conditions are shown in Table 10.3 [16]. The ocular utilities are directly comparable with the general medical utilities. Ocular utilities appear to correlate closely with the vision in the better-seeing eye, rather than the underlying cause of visual loss [16, 17, 41–46].

Pearl
Utilities can compare health states across all of medicine. For example, if 20/40 vision in the better-seeing eye is associated with a utility of 0.80 and American College of Rheumatology Global Functional Status Class III osteoarthritis of the hip also is associated with a utility of 0.80, the two entities are associated with similar quality of life.

Utility Gain

The improvement in quality of life conferred by an intervention can be analytically quantified with utility analysis. For example, if the vision in the better-seeing eye improves from 20/800 (utility of 0.52) to 20/25 (utility of 0.87), the gain in utility is (0.87 − 0.52 =) 0.35 [42].

Decision Analysis

Decision analysis is a mathematical instrument that utilizes the weighted averages of utilities to arrive at the most probable utility outcome associated with an intervention (Fig. 10.1). It is often helpful in amalgamating the benefits of a drug with its 40 or 50 adverse events, as well as the incidences of those adverse events, to more effectively demonstrate the overall utility associated with use of the drug (Fig. 10.1). Markov modeling is a useful tool within decision analysis in assessing the risk of a recurrent event, such as the yearly incidence of the occurrence of neovascular AMD in an eye contralateral to one

Table 10.2 Time tradeoff utilities associated with vision in the better-seeing eye [16, 42, 45]

Vision	Utility
20/20 OU permanently	1.00
20/20–20/25 OU	.97
20/20	.92
20/25	.87
20/30	.84
20/40	.80
20/50	.77
20/70	.74
20/100	.67
20/200	.66
20/400	.54
20/800	.52
HM-LP	.35
NLP	.26

OU both eyes, *HM* hands motions, *LP* light perception, *NLP* no light perception

Table 10.3 Time tradeoff utilities for general medical health states [16]

Health state	Utility
AIDS, CD4 count 0–50	0.94
AIDS, CD4 count 201–300	0.79
Mild angina	*0.88*
Moderate angina	0.83
Severe angina	0.53
Cancer, breast, early	0.94
Cancer, breast, radiotherapy	0.89
Cancer, breast, chemotherapy	0.74
Diabetes mellitus	0.88
Myocardial infarction, mild	0.91
Myocardial infarction, moderate	0.80
Myocardial infarction, severe	0.30
Osteoarthritis, hip, mild	0.69
Osteoarthritis, S/P hip replacement	0.82
Renal transplant	0.74
Hemodialysis	0.49
Stroke, minor	0.89
Stroke, major	0.30
Ulcerative colitis, severe	0.58
Ulcerative colitis, 1 yr post-op	0.98

1 yr post-op 1 year after bowel resection

that has already developed neovascular AMD. The TreeAge program (TreeAge Software, Inc. @ www.treeage.com) is a well-supported, widely used decision analysis program utilized by the current authors.

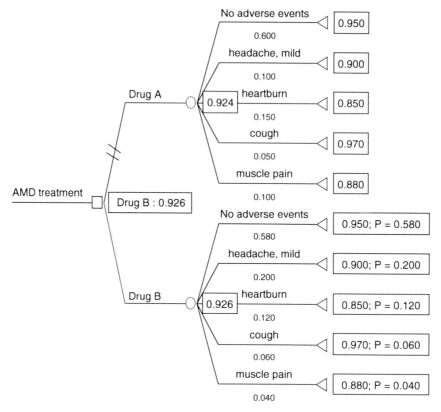

Fig. 10.1 Decision analysis tree comparing Drug A and Drug B for the treatment of AMD (age-related macular degeneration). The tree is read from left to right. The preferred strategy is the use of Drug B because it has a final utility (0.926) greater than the final utility of Drug A (0.924). The □ indicates a decision node, the *o* indicates a chance node and the Δ indicates a terminal node. The incidence of each health state is shown beneath its respective branch furthest to the right. The utility associated with no adverse events (0.950) is shown at the right of each respective terminal node, while the utility associated with mild headache is 0.900, that associated with heartburn is 0.850, that for cough is 0.97 and that for muscle pain is 0.880 (*P* probability). The // through the line going from the decision node to the chance node for Drug A indicates this drug is not the preferred intervention

Pearl

Decision analysis quantifies the most probable outcome associated with an intervention. It integrates all benefits and adverse events conferred by an intervention to ascertain the most probable quality-of-life outcome associated with use of that intervention.

Comparative Effectiveness (Human Value Gain)

Human value gain, the most sophisticated measure of comparative effectiveness, is objectively assessed in quality-adjusted life-years (QALYs), an entity first described by Klarman et al. [47] in 1968. The (improvement in utility) × (years of duration of treatment benefit) quantifies the total *human value* gain conferred by an intervention [5–7, 13]. As used in Value-Based Medicine® [13, 23], a standardized variant of cost-utility analysis, *(human) value gain* does not refer to money, but rather signifies the quantifiable improvement in quality of life and/or length of life conferred by an intervention.

Thus, an interventional utility gain of (0.87 − 0.52 =) *0.35* for 10 years results in a QALY gain of (0.35 × 10 years =) *3.5 QALYs*. For most ophthalmologic interventions, value gain equates to the improvement in the quality of life, rather than a gain in length of life.

If the improvement in vision also results in a change in life expectancy from 10–12 years, the total QALY gain is [(0.87 − 0.52) × 10 years] + (0.87 × 2 years), or 3.5 QALYs + 1.74 QALYs, a total gain of *5.24* QALYs.

Value gain can also be measured in *percent gain in value.* As people go through life, they accrue QALYs. People should theoretically try to maximize their value gain (QALYs accrued) during their lifetimes. If an intervention adds 10 QALYs to the life of a patient who would otherwise accrue 20 QALYs during their remaining lifetime, the *value gain* is (10/20 =) *50%.*

> **Pearl**
>
> The quality-adjusted life-year quantifies the *comparative effectiveness* or *human value gain* conferred by any intervention. It is calculated by multiplying (utility gain) × (years of benefit). If length of life is also gained, the (years of gain) × (the person's utility) is also added.

> **Pearl**
>
> The *percent gain in human value,* similar to the QALY, is a measure of comparative effectiveness that can be utilized to compare interventions across all specialties, no matter how disparate.

Value Trumps Cost

All patients should want and deserve the intervention, which confers the greatest human value [23]. Only when the human value conferred by interventions is the same should cost be a consideration. In the event of equal value gain, the intervention which is least expensive becomes the preferred interventional strategy. At the current time, the VEGF inhibitor ranibizumab

Table 10.4 Human value gain conferred by healthcare interventions

Intervention	Value gain (%)
Laser, subfoveal choroidal neovascularization [1]	4.4
AREDS supplements for atrophic AMD [17]	4.8
Pegaptanib therapy, subfoveal choroidal neovascularization [3]	5.9
β(beta)-blockers for arterial hypertension[a]	6.3–9.1
Photodynamic therapy for classic, subfoveal, neovascular AMD [3, 5]	8.1
Cataract surgery, second eye [48]	12.7
Cataract surgery, first eye [49]	20.8
Brachytherapy/bevacizumab therapy for subfoveal neovascular AMD	22.4
Antidepressants (SSRIs)[a]	20–24
Ranibizumab, intravitreal, subfoveal neovascular AMD, minimally classic and occult choroidal neovascularization [8][a]	15.8–28.2
Proton pump inhibitors, Zollinger–Ellison syndrome[a]	28.9–38.2

AREDS age-related eye disease study, *AMD* age-related macular degeneration, *SSRI* selective serotonin reuptake inhibitor
[a]Data from Center for Value-Based Medicine Pharmaceutical Value Index® internal files

appears to deliver the greatest value among interventions for neovascular AMD (Table 10.4) [2, 3, 5, 7].

> **Pearl**
>
> A Value-Based Medicine® pillar is the paradigm that *all patients deserve* the intervention, which confers the greatest *(human) value.* Only when interventional value is the same does cost become a factor; in this instance the intervention which is the least costly is the *preferred strategy.*

An example of the comparative effectiveness potential the QALY allows in cost-utility, pharmacoeconomic analyses is demonstrated by the head-to-head comparison of intravitreal pegaptanib and photodynamic therapy with verteporfin

Table 10.5 Value-based medicine®, cost-utility analysis standards

a. Cost-utility
   • *Average* cost-utility: intervention under study vs. no treatment
   • *Incremental* cost-utility: intervention under study vs. other interventions available
b. Cost perspective– Third Party Insurer (using direct medical costs) and Societal (direct medical, direct nonmedical and indirect medical costs)
c. Population analysis– base case (average case)
d. Utilities
   • Methodology: time tradeoff utility analysis
   • Respondents: patients with the health state under study
e. Cost basis

Direct healthcare costs	Cost reference source
Providers	Average national Medicare payment
Hospital, acute	Average national Medicare payment
Ambulatory surgical center	Average national Medicare payment
Skilled nursing facility	Average national Medicare payment
Rehabilitation	Average national Medicare payment
Home health care	Average national Medicare payment
Clinical tests	Average national Medicare payment
Durable goods	Average national Medicare payment
Nursing home care	Average national *Medicaid* payment
Pharmaceuticals	Average Medicare Sales Price (ASP)

f. *Annual discount rate* – 3% for quality-adjusted life-years (QALYs) and costs
g. Sensitivity analysis – should perform at least one-way. Those input variables in which there is the least confidence should be analyzed.

(PDT) for the treatment of classic, neovascular, subfoveal AMD. The final two-year vision in the pegaptanib VEGF IS trial [50] was 20/126–1 in the treatment cohort versus 20/200+1 in the control group, while in the PDT TAP trial [51] the two-year vision was 20/160+1 in the treatment cohort versus 20/320+1 in the control group. Comparing these vision outcomes, much less the accompanying adverse events and the incidences of these adverse events, is virtually impossible without using QALYs. Value-Based Medicine® comparative effectiveness analysis clearly demonstrates PDT to confer the greatest value gain, an 8.1% improvement in the quality of life, compared to a 5.9% improvement in the quality of life conferred by pegaptanib (Table 10.4) [3].

Costs

The costs used in cost-utility analysis are major determinants of the cost-utility ratio [23, 52]. There are three major cost categories: (1) *direct medical costs,* which include physician and other provider costs, facility costs (acute hospital, ambulatory sur-

gical center, subacute nursing facility, nursing home), pharmaceutical costs, and durable goods; (2) *direct nonmedical costs,* such as caregiver costs, transportation costs, costs of shelter, and babysitting costs; and (3) *indirect costs,* including employment costs, and costs related to volunteering.

Cost Basis

The average Medicare Fee Schedule is the most standardized reimbursement schedule in the United States [53]. Virtually all healthcare insurers in the USA adhere to the Medicare Fee Schedule in some form. Suggested standardized costs in the USA are shown in Table 10.5 [2, 6–8, 17].

Cost Perspective

The *third party* insurer cost perspective utilizes the direct medical costs, or those relevant for a healthcare insurer. The *societal cost perspective,* that recommended by NICE (National Institute for Health and Clinical Excellence in the UK) [54] and the Panel for Cost-Effectiveness in Health and Medicine in the USA [24, 33, 34], utilizes direct medical costs, direct nonmedical costs, and the indirect costs. Other cost perspectives include the governmental cost perspective and the patient cost perspective [52].

The societal cost perspective typically results in a more favorable cost-utility ratio than the third party insurer cost perspective [13]. Costs that result in more favorable cost-effectiveness with the societal cost perspective include those related to increased patient employment, decreased caregiver costs, decreased transportation costs, and the diminution of shelter (nursing home, assisted living, and so forth) costs.

Cost-Utility Ratio

When the total number of QALYs gained from an intervention is amalgamated with the associated costs, the cost-utility ratio, or $/QALY, is the result. The cost-utility of an intervention can be compared with that of any other intervention in healthcare, whether pharmacologic, surgical, or medical.

The cost-utilities of various nonophthalmic healthcare interventions and interventions for atrophic and neovascular ARMD are shown in Table 10.6 [5–8, 16, 55–58]. While laser photocoagulation is more cost-effective in treating neovascular AMD than intravitreal pegaptanib therapy, photodynamic therapy with verteporfin and intravitreal ranibizumab therapy, it confers the least human value among the interventions, and is thus the least desirable among neovascular AMD interventions. This case illustrates the fact that cost-utility (cost-effectiveness) analysis should never be used in a vacuum without knowing the human value gain. In this instance, ranibizumab, while not the most cost-effective, confers the greatest patient *value*.

Pearl

Cost-utility ratios should never be used in a vacuum. The conferred human value gain for an intervention should also be known, since the most cost-effective intervention may not be the one which confers the greatest patient value (improvement in quality of life and/or length of life).

Table 10.6 Cost-utility of neovascular AMD and other healthcare interventions *(in year 2010 real US dollars)*

Intervention	Cost-utility ($/QALY)
Laser, threshold ROP [55]	$932
SSRIs, depression*	$1,124–$11,342
PPV, diabetic vitreous hemorrhage [56]	$2,488
B(BETA) – blockers for systemic arterial hypertension	$2,544–$26,924
Cataract extraction, first eye [48]	$2,591
AREDS supplements for atrophic AMD [17]	$2,978
Cataract surgery, second eye [49]	$3,440
Laser, DME [57]	$4,039
Laser, subfoveal CNVM [2]	$8,670
Cochlear implant, children [16]	$12,318
Photodynamic therapy with verteporfin for subfoveal neovascular AMD [3, 5]	$33,427
Rx, occupational HIV exposure [16]	$51,580
Ranibizumab, intravitreal, subfoveal neovascular AMD, minimally classic & occult choroidal neovascularization [7]	53,732
Surgery for PVR, C3F8 gas, no previous Vitrectomy [58]	$60,187
Pegaptanib therapy, classic, minimally classic and occult subfoveal choroidal neovascularization [7]	$70,806
Simultaneous kidney and pancreas transplant [16]	$152,274
Acute CRAO treatment with AC tap and 95% O_2:5% CO_2 inhalation [16]	$4.93 million

ROP retinopathy of prematurity, *SSRI* selective serotonin reuptake inhibitor, *PPV* pars plana vitrectomy, *DME* diabetic macular edema, *ME* macular edema, *BVO* branch retinal vein obstruction, *Rx* treatment, *HIV* human immunodeficiency virus, *PVR* proliferative vitreoretinopathy, *C3F8* perfluoropropane, *PDT* photodynamic therapy, *Va* visual acuity, *CRAO* central retinal artery obstruction, *AC* anterior chamber, CO_2 carbon dioxide, O_2 oxygen
* = internal data   from the Center for Value-Based Medicine®

It is very likely that combination therapies for neovascular AMD will be more commonly undertaken in the near future. In this instance, Value-Based Medicine® cost-utility analysis objectively assesses the value and cost-utility (cost-effectiveness) of these interventions in the same fashion as for monotherapies [13]. The Patient-Centered Outcomes Research Institute will likely play a major role in the

Table 10.7 Summary of upper limits of cost-effectiveness in resources/QALY (quality-adjusted life-year)

Organization	Very cost effective	Cost effective
United States	$50,000	$100,000
NICE (UK)	£20,000 (~US $28,700)	£30,000 (~US $43,100)
WHO	1 × GDP per capita	3 × GDP per capita
WHO (US GDP)	$46,400	$139,200

NICE (UK) National Institute for Health and Clinical Excellence in the United Kingdom, *WHO* World Health Organization, *GDP* Gross Domestic Product, or the sum of all final goods and services produced within the national borders of a country in a 1-year period

comparative effectiveness and cost-effectiveness arenas within five years, and hopefully set a number of standards to better allow the comparability of cost-utility analyses [31]. It is likely that this institute will resemble NICE55 (National Institute for Health and Clinical Excellence) in the UK, an entity formed in 1999 to assess comparative effectiveness and cost-effectiveness.

Cost-Effectiveness Standards

An intervention is typically thought to be cost-effective in the USA if its costs <$100,000/QALY [59], and very cost-effective if it costs <$50,000/QALY [60, 61]. Nonetheless, there is no formal body that sets cost-effectiveness standards in the United States. World Health Organization standards suggest interventions costing <1× GDP per capita (~2010 US $47,000/QALY) are very cost-effective and those costing <3× GDP per capita (~2010 US $141,000/QALY) are cost-effective [62]. NICE in the UK typically considers interventions cost-effective if they cost <£20,000/QALY, on occasion, going as high as £30,000/QALY [54]. NICE recommends to the National Health Service whether interventions are cost-effective or not, and thus whether they should be covered for payment or not. A summary of cost-effectiveness standards is shown in Table 10.7.

> **Pearl**
> Interventions associated with a cost-utility ratio <$50,000/QALY are generally considered to be very cost-effective in the USA, while those associated with a cost-utility <$100,000/QALY are thought to be cost-effective.

> **Pearl**
> NICE (National Institute for Health and Clinical Excellence) in the UK evaluates healthcare interventions to ascertain if they are cost-effective and should be recommended to the National Health Service for coverage.

Discounting

Both costs and value outcomes (QALYs gained) are discounted [23] using net present value (NPV) analysis to account for the time value of money and of good health. Essentially, a dollar now is worth more than a dollar in 20 years since that dollar now can be invested to yield more dollars over time. Good health now can also be viewed to create more dollars and other resources that can be invested for a greater yield over time.

Value-Based Medicine®

Value-Based Medicine® is the practice of medicine based upon the value (improvement in quality of life and/or length of life) conferred by healthcare interventions [23]. It utilizes cost-utility analysis with standardized input parameters and outcomes to allow comparisons of all interventions within and across medical specialties, no matter how disparate [14–23, 63].

Standardization

Unfortunately, most of the cost-utility studies in the current literature are not comparable since they use different utilities, diverse utility respondents, unlike cost perspectives, different costs and cost bases, and so forth [23]. Value-Based Medicine® cost-utility analyses use the standards listed in Table 10.5, therefore permitting comparisons of virtually all cost-utility ratios.

> **Pearl**
> Most cost-utility analyses in the current literature are not comparable due to different inputs: type of utility analysis, utility respondents, costs, costs basis, discounting, year of publication, and so forth.

> **Pearl**
> Value-Based Medicine® cost-utility ratios use standardized inputs and outcomes, and are therefore generally comparable.

Patient Respondents

Value-Based Medicine® cost-utility analyses specifically use patient utilities, since community and expert (physician) surrogate respondent utilities often differ considerably from those of patients. With regard to AMD, physicians who treated the disease underestimated its diminution upon quality of life compared to patients with the condition by a range of 96–750% (Table 10.8) [14, 15, 20]. The authors herein adamantly believe that, while more difficult to acquire than utilities from the general community or professionals, utilities obtained from patients who have experienced a health state firsthand should be the criterion (gold standard).

> **Pearl**
> Utilities from patients who have experienced a health state can differ dramatically from those of physicians and other respondents. Patient utilities are the criterion for Value-Based Medicine® cost-utility analysis.

Cost Perspective

The *third party insurer cost perspective* includes only those costs the insurer has to pay, or the direct medical costs. The *societal cost perspective* includes third party insurer costs, as well as *direct nonmedical costs,* such as caregiver costs, shelter costs, and travel costs, and *indirect costs,* such as loss of employment and disability payments avoided. Both the third party insurer and societal cost perspectives performed together allow for much great comparability of cost-utility analyses.

The third party insurer cost perspective and societal cost perspective are often very different and not comparable. A cost-utility analysis is therefore more complete if it offers outcomes utilizing both cost perspectives. Generally, the societal cost perspective results in a more favorable cost-utility ratio compared to the third party insurer cost perspective. One note of caution, however, is the fact that societal costs are not as standardized or as available as direct medical costs [23].

A summary of Value-Based Medicine® comparative effectiveness value gains and cost-utility ratios for AMD interventions is shown in Table 10.9. Because of the standardization of the input variables, Value-Based Medicine® cost-utility analyses are typically comparable.

Table 10.8 Utilities from AMD patients and ophthalmologists who treat AMD

Vision (better eye)	AMD patients (n=82)	General public (n=142)	Ophthalmologists (n=46)	p-value
20/20–20/40	0.83	0.96	0.98	<.001
20/50–20/100	0.68	0.92	0.89	<.001
<20/200	0.47	0.86	0.73	<.001
<20/800	0.37	NA	0.69	<.001

AMD age-related macular degeneration, *NA* not available

Table 10.9 Comparative effectiveness and cost-utility ratios (2010 real US dollars) associated with interventions for age-related macular degeneration

Disease	Intervention	Value gain (%)	Cost-utility ratio ($/QALY)
Neovascular AMD, subfoveal	Laser photocoagulation	4.4	$8,670
Atrophic AMD	AREDS supplements	4.8	$2,978
Neovascular AMD, subfoveal	Intravitreal pegaptanib	5.9	$70,806
Neovascular AMD, subfoveal	PDT with verteporfin	8.1	$33,427
Neovascular AMD, extrafoveal	PDT with verteporfin	8.1	$28,832
Neovascular AMD	Brachytherapy + bevacizumab	22.4	$11,344
Neovascular AMD, subfoveal	Intravitreal ranibizumab	15.8–28.2	$30,289–$53,732

Atrophic AMD = dry age-related macular degeneration, $/QALY = dollars expended per quality-adjusted life-year gained, AREDS supplements = Age-Related Eye Disease Study oral supplements, or beta carotene, vitamin C, vitamin E, zinc and copper

Value-Based Medicine® pharmacoeconomics, as applied to AMD interventions and those across all of medicine, signals a *new era of quality in the healthcare arena*. The information is important to patients, physicians, Pharmacy & Therapeutic Committees [63], insurers, Pharmacy Benefit Managers, and those in public positions who allocate healthcare resources.

The advantages of Value-Based Medicine® pharmacoeconomic analyses for AMD and other interventions include the facts they:

- Integrate all benefits and adverse events associated with a drug to demonstrate its overall conferred value.
- Integrate patient quality-of-life preferences (utilities) often ignored in clinical trial primary outcomes.
- Allow physicians to better understand what patients consider most relevant so higher quality care can be provided.
- Identify drugs with superior value, as well as those with negligible value.
- Demonstrate the often underappreciated benefits of drugs, such as the facts that they prevent disability, decrease caregiver costs, and allow patients to continue to work.
- Allow a head-to-head comparison of the value conferred by drugs and other interventions.
- Assess the cost of comparator drugs of similar value so the least expensive can be identified.

In essence, Value-Based Medicine® pharmacoeconomics provides an information system which allows all stakeholders the ability to appreciate the human value conferred by AMD drugs and other interventions [48, 4955–58, 62], as well as the costs expended for that value [23]. It ushers in a new era of superior care for medicine as it takes evidence-based medicine outcomes to a higher level of quality by integrating patient preferences, at the same time it facilitates the most efficient use of healthcare resources.

The Future

Pharmacoeconomics has already had an impact on the use of retinal pharmacologic agents [1–23], a phenomenon that will only become more pronounced in the near future as the USA adopts cost-utility principles with the creation of the Patient Centered Outcomes Research Institute [31]. Pharmacoeconomic cost-utility principles are currently used in public policy in the UK, Canada, and Australia, and will be adopted in other countries as well. Why? Because there is no other instrument available that can integrate quality of life, length of life, costs, and the ability to objectively assess interventions across all of healthcare.

Macroeconomic Costs and AMD

Extrapolation of data from the Beaver Dam Eye Study [64] and the Eye Diseases Prevalence Research Group [65] suggests that 1.7 million new cases of atrophic macular degeneration and 1,65,000 new cases of neovascular AMD develop in the United States annually. Prevalence data show there are approximately 7.5 million cases of atrophic AMD and 1.2 million cases of neovascular AMD in the USA any time [64, 65].

Employment and Wage Loss

Data on disability and employment from the Bureau of Labor and Statistics demonstrate those with mild visual loss (<20/40 in the better eye) are employed at a rate 56% that of people with normal vision and those with severe visual loss (<20/200 in better eye) are employed only 39% as often as those with normal vision [66]. Furthermore, people with mild visual loss earn 30% less than those with normal vision, and those with severe visual loss earn 38% less than those with normal vision [66]. Consequently, the average person with mild visual loss earns 39% that of a person with normal vision, while the average person with severe visual loss earns only 24% that of a person with normal vision.

> **Pearl**
> The average person with mild vision loss (<20/40) earns 39% as much as their counterpart with normal vision, while the average person with severe vision loss (≤20/200) earns 24% that of their counterparts with normal vision.

Gross Domestic Product (GDP)

The GDP, or Gross Domestic Product [67], is the sum of all final goods and services produced within the national borders annually. Brown and colleagues [15] calculated that atrophic AMD in the USA, diminishes salaries, employment, and consumption, and therefore the GDP of the country, by approximately $26.1 billion annually (adjusted to year 2010 real dollars). Neovascular AMD in the USA decreases the GDP by approximately $5.8 billion annually. The total annual cost (in 2010 real dollars) to the GDP, the latter which is often considered a measure of the overall wealth of the country, is therefore ($26.1 + $5.8 =) $31.9 billion [15]. The financial loss due to wage loss from untreated AMD comprises approximately 0.22% of the entire 2010 US GDP of $14.75 trillion [67].

> **Pearl**
> Untreated, atrophic AMD causes wage loss of $26.1 billion annually, while neovascular AMD cause a $5.1 billion annual wage loss. Thus, AMD costs the economy, and therefore the GDP (Gross Domestic Product), $31.8 billion annually in real 2010 US dollars.

Other Costs

In addition to direct ophthalmologic medical costs, there are other direct costs associated with AMD and visual loss. Among the *direct, nonophthalmologic medical costs* are those associated with: (1) increased depression, (2) increased injury, (3) increased subacute nursing facility (SNF) costs, (4) increased nursing home costs, and (5) as yet unidentified costs associated with visual loss [68]. As per the work of Javitt and colleagues [68], the annual sum of these costs is greater than $12,700 (2010 US real dollars) for people with <20/400 vision in the better eye (World Health Organization definition of blindness), more than $8,200 for those with <20/200 in the better seeing eye (US definition of legal blindness) and more than $4,300 for those with vision <20/40 in the better eye.

The *direct nonmedical costs* include primarily transportation costs, the cost of shelter and caregiver costs, with the latter the greatest cost. Schmier and colleagues [69] have shown that caregiver costs for people with AMD increase as vision in the better-seeing eye decreases. The costs (adjusted to year 2010 real dollars) from the Schmier study [69] are shown in Table 10.10. Remarkably, caregiver costs exceed $58,000 per year for AMD patients whose vision in the better-seeing eye is 20/250 or worse.

Table 10.10 Caregiver costs associated with age-related macular degeneration (adjusted TO 2010 real US dollars)

Vision	Annual caregiver cost
>20/32	$278
20/32 to >20/50	$1,685
20/80 to >20/150	$14,280
20/150 to >20/250	$20,797
20/250 or worse	$58,214

Adapted from data in Schmier et al. [69]

> **Pearl**
> Among AMD patients with 20/250 or less vision, the annual caregiver costs exceed $58,000per year.

Among the *indirect costs* encountered in AMD patients with visual loss are those associated with lack of employment and decreased salary, as discussed above. The costs associated with volunteering should also be theoretically included, preferably at the average national wage per hour, but data in this arena are sparse. Disability costs are relevant for the patient and governmental perspectives, although some believe they are transfer costs, and thus should not be used in a societal cost perspective, cost-utility analysis [24].

Financial Return on Investment (ROI)

Brown and colleagues [13] demonstrated that brachytherapy/VEGF-A inhibitor therapy for neovascular AMD accrues a 16.2% annual financial return on investment (ROI) for the direct ophthalmic medical costs expended. Furthermore, this therapy adds $76,000 per capita to the GDP above the direct ophthalmic medical costs expended over the 13-year life expectancy of the average patient.

Data from the Center for Value-Based Medicine® suggest that ranibizumab therapy for neovascular AMD accrues four times over and above the direct, ophthalmic medical costs of approximately $51,000 expended over the 12-year life expectancy of the average patient in the MARINA [*M*inimally classic/occult trial of

the *A*nti-VEGF antibody *R*anibizumab *I*n the treatment of *N*eovascular Age-Related Macular Degeneration (*A*MD)] Study [32, 70].

> **Pearl**
> Intravitreal ranibizumab therapy for neovascular AMD returns approximately $4 to society for every $1 it consumes in direct ophthalmic medical cost.

Approximately, 1,65,000 people each year develop neovascular AMD in the USA. Assuming each is treated with ranibizumab as per the MARINA trial [32], the total cost would be $8.4 billion. Nonetheless, an economic analysis suggests that ranibizumab therapy returns a net $25 billion in wages generated and costs saved above the direct costs of ranibizumab therapy over the 12-year model [70]. This is an extraordinary ROI that creates considerable wealth for the country at the same time it greatly enhances human value [70]. It is safe to say that very few interventions in the last decade have conferred human value gain and financial value gain close to that of ranibizumab for neovascular AMD. The impact of the intervention is extraordinary.

Financial Disclosure Supported in part by the Center for Value-Based Medicine®, Flourtown, PA, the sponsor played no role in performance of the study, writing of the manuscript, or requiring direction of the study.

References

1. Brown GC, Brown MM, Sharma S. Incremental cost-effectiveness of laser photocoagulation for subfoveal choroidal neovascularization. Ophthalmology. 2000;107:1374–80.
2. Busbee B, Brown MM, Brown GC, Sharma S. A cost-utility analysis of laser photocoagulation for extrafoveal choroidal neovascularization. Retina. 2003;23:279–87.
3. Brown GC, Brown MM, Brown HC, Kindermann S, Sharma S. A value-based medicine comparison of interventions for subfoveal neovascular macular degeneration. Ophthalmology. 2007;114:1170–8.
4. Colquitt JL, Jones J, Tan SC, Takeda A, Clegg AJ, Price A. Ranibizumab and pegaptanib for the

treatment of age-related macular degeneration: a systematic review and economic evaluation. Health Technol Assess. 2008;12:iii–iv, ix–201.

5. Brown GC, Brown MM, Campanella J, Beauchamp GR. The cost-utility of photodynamic therapy in eyes with neovascular age-related macular degeneration. A reappraisal with 5-year data. Am J Ophthalmol. 2005;140:679–87.

6. Sharma S, Brown GC, Brown MM, Hollands H, Shah GK. The cost-effectiveness of photodynamic therapy for fellow eyes with subfoveal choroidal neovascularization secondary to age-related macular degeneration. Ophthalmology. 2001;108:2051–9.

7. Brown GC, Brown MM, Brown H, Peet JS. A value-based medicine analysis of ranibizumab (MARINA Study) for the treatment of subfoveal neovascular macular degeneration. Ophthalmology. 2008;115:1039–45.

8. Cohen SY, Bremond-Gignac D, Quentel G, Mimoun G, Citterio T, Bisot-Locard S, et al. Cost-effectiveness sequential modeling of ranibizumab versus usual care in age-related macular degeneration. Graefes Arch Clin Exp Ophthalmol. 2008;246:1527–34. Epub 2008 Jul 19.

9. Hurley SF, Matthews JP, Guymer RH. Cost-effectiveness of ranibizumab for neovascular age-related macular degeneration. Cost Eff Resour Alloc. 2008;6:12.

10. Neubauer AS, Holz FG, Schrader W, Back EI, Kühn T, Hirneiss C, et al. Cost-utility analysis of ranibizumab (Lucentis) in neovascular macular degeneration. Klin Monatsbl Augenheilkd. 2007;224:727–32.

11. Raftery J, Clegg A, Jones J, Tan SC, Lotery A. Ranibizumab (Lucentis) versus bevacizumab (Avastin): modeling cost effectiveness. Br J Ophthalmol. 2007;91:1244–6. Epub 2007 Apr 12.

12. Fletcher EC, Lade RJ, Adewoyin T, Chong HV. Computerized model of cost-utility analysis for treatment of age-related macular degeneration *corrected proof*. 2008. DOI: 10.1016/j.ophtha.2008.07.018, from the internet @http://download.journals.elsevierhealth.com/pdfs/journals/0161–6420/PIIS0161642008007677.pdf. Accessed 25 Oct 2008.

13. Brown MM, Brown GC, Brown HC, Irwin B, Roth Z. Comparative effectiveness and cost-effectiveness analyses of VEGF-A inhibitor and ^{90}Sr brachytherapy for neovascular macular degeneration. Evid Based Ophthalmol. 2009;10:107–22.

14. Brown MM, Brown GC, Sharma S, Stein J, Roth Z, Campanella J, et al. Age-related macular degeneration. Its burden and a value-based medicine analysis. Can J Ophthalmol. 2005;40:177–87.

15. Brown GC, Brown MM, Sharma S, Stein J, Roth Z, Campanella J, et al. The burden of age-related macular degeneration: a value-based analysis. Trans Am Ophthalmol Soc. 2005;103:180–93.

16. Brown MM, Brown GC, Sharma S, Landy J. Health care economic analyses and value-based medicine. Surv Ophthalmol. 2003;48:204–23.

17. Sharma S, Bakal J. The value component of evidence-based medicine. The cost-utility of high dose vitamin supplementation for macular degeneration. Evid Based Ophthalmol. 2002;3:105–9.

18. Brown GC, Brown MM, Sharma S, Brown H, Smithen L, Leeser D, et al. Value-based medicine and ophthalmology: an appraisal of cost-utility analyses. Trans Am Ophthalmol Soc. 2004;102:177–85.

19. Brown GC, Brown MM, Sharma S. Value-based medicine: evidence-based medicine and beyond. Ocul Immunol Inflamm. 2003;11:157–70.

20. Stein JD, Brown MM, Brown GC, Sharma S, Hollands H. Quality of life with macular degeneration: perceptions of patients, clinicians and community members. Br J Ophthalmol. 2003;87:8–12.

21. Brown GC. Value-based medicine: the new paradigm. Curr Opin Ophthalmol. 2005;16:139–40.

22. Brown MM, Brown GC, Sharma S. Value-based medicine: a paradigm for quality pharmaceutical care. Drug Benefit Trends. 2006;18:285–9.

23. Brown MM, Brown GC, Sharma S. Evidence-based to value-based medicine. Chicago: AMA Press; 2005. p. 151–265.

24. Gold MR, Patrick DL, Torrance GW, Fryback DG, Hadorn DC, Kamlet MS, et al. Identifying and valuing outcomes. In: Gold MR, Siegel JE, Russell LB, Weinstein MC, editors. Cost-effectiveness in health and medicine. New York: Oxford University Press; 1996. p. 82–134.

25. Drummond ME, O'Brien B, Stoddart GL, Torrance GW. Methods for the economic evaluation of health care programmes. 2nd ed. New York: Oxford University Press; 1999.

26. Cochrane AL. Effectiveness and efficiency: random reflections on health services. London: Nuffield Provincial Hospitals Trust; 1972 (Reprinted in 1989 in association with the BMJ, Reprinted in 1999 for Nuffield Trust by the Royal Society of Medicine Press, London).

27. Evidence-Based Medicine Working Group. A new approach to teaching the practice of medicine. JAMA. 1992;268:2420–5.

28. Sackett DL, Straus SE, Richardson WS, et al. Evidence-based medicine. How to practice and teach EBM. 2nd ed. Philadelphia: Churchill Livingstone; 2000.

29. Sharma S. Levels of evidence. Evid Based Eye Care. 2002;3:175–6.

30. National Eye Institute Visual Functioning Questionnaire-25 (VFQ-25). From the internet @ http://www.nei.nih.gov/resources/visionfunction/vfq_ia.pdf. Accessed 16 Apr 2010.

31. H.R.3590. Patient Protection and Affordable Care Act. From the internet @ http://thomas.loc.gov/cgi-bin/query/D?c111:7:./temp/~c111jCyAeo. Accessed 20 May 2010.

32. Rosenfeld PJ, Brown DM, Heier JS, MARINA Study Group, et al. Ranibizumab for neovascular age-related macular degeneration. N Engl J Med. 2006;355:1419–31.

33. Siegel JE, Weinstein MC, Russell LB, Gold MR. Panel on cost-effectiveness in health and medicine: recommendations for reporting cost-effectiveness analyses. JAMA. 1996;276:1339–41.

34. Weinstein MC, Siegel JE, Gold MR, et al. Recommendations of the panel on cost-effectiveness in health and medicine. JAMA. 1996;276:1253–8.

35. Tengs TO, Adams ME, Pliskin JS, Safran DG, Siegel JE, Weinstein MC, et al. Five-hundred life-saving interventions and their cost-effectiveness. Risk Anal. 1995;15:369–90.

36. Edelman D, Williams GR, Rothman M, Samsa GP. A comparison of three health status measures in primary care patients. J Gen Intern Med. 1999;14:759–62.

37. Bergner M, Bobbitt RA, Carter WB, Gilson BS. The sickness impact profile: development and final revision of a health status measure. Med Care. 1981;119:787–805.

38. Kaplan RM, Ganiats TG, Sieber WJ, Anderson JP. The quality of well-being scale: critical similarities and differences with the SF-36. Int J Qual Health Care. 1998;10:509–20.

39. Steinberg EP, Tielsch JM, Schein OD, et al. The VF-14. An index of functional impairment in patients with cataract. Arch Ophthalmol. 1994;112:630–8.

40. Redelmeier DA, Detsky A. A clinician's guide to utility measurement. Med Decis Making. 1995;22:271–81.

41. Sharma S, Brown GC, Brown MM, Hollands H, Robbins R, Shah G. Validity of the time trade-off and standard gamble methods of utility assessment in retinal patients. Br J Ophthalmol. 2002;86:493–6.

42. Brown GC. Vision and quality of life. Trans Am Ophthalmol Soc. 1999;97:473–512.

43. Brown MM, Brown GC, Sharma S, Shah G. Utility values and diabetic retinopathy. Am J Ophthalmol. 1999;128:324–30.

44. Brown GC, Brown MM, Sharma S, Kistler J. Utility values associated with age-related macular degeneration. Arch Ophthalmol. 2000;118:47–51.

45. Brown MM, Brown GC, Sharma S, et al. Utility values associated with blindness in an adult population. Br J Ophthalmol. 2001;85:327–31.

46. Brown MM, Brown GC, Sharma S, Landy J. Quality of life with visual acuity loss from diabetic retinopathy and age-related macular degeneration. Arch Ophthalmol. 2002;120:481–4.

47. Klarman H, Francis J, Rosenthal G. Cost-effectiveness applied to the treatment of chronic renal disease. Med Care. 1968;6:48–55.

48. Busbee B, Brown MM, Brown GC, Sharma S. Incremental cost-effectiveness of initial cataract surgery. Ophthalmology 2002;109:606–612.

49. Busbee B, Brown MM, Brown GC, Sharma S. A cost-utility analysis of cataract surgery in the second eye. Ophthalmology 2003;110:2310–2317

50. Gragoudas ES, Adamis AP, Cunningham Jr ET, VEGF Inhibition Study in Ocular Neovascularization Clinical Trial Group, et al. Pegaptanib for neovascular age-related macular degeneration. N Engl J Med. 2004;351:2805–16.

51. Bressler NM, Treatment of Age-Related Macular Degeneration with PhotodynamicTherapy (TAP) Study Group. Photodynamic therapy of subfoveal choroidal neovascularization in age-related macular degeneration with verteporfin: two-year results of 2 randomized clinical trials – TAP report 2. Arch Ophthalmol. 2001;119:198–207.

52. Smith A, Brown GC. Understanding cost-effectiveness: a detailed review. Br J Ophthalmol. 2000;54:794–8.

53. Centers for Medicare and Medicaid Services. Physician fee schedule. From the internet @ https://www.cms.gov/PhysicianFeeSched/. Accessed 20 May 2010.

54. National Institute for Health and Clinical Excellence (NICE). Incorporating health economics in guidelines and assessing resource impact. In: The Guidelines Manual. London: NICE, 2007, Chap. 8. Available on the internet @ http://www.nice.org.uk/page.aspx?o= 422950. Accessed 15 Mar 2008.

55. Brown GC, Brown MM, Sharma S, Tasman W, Brown HC. Cost-effectiveness of treatment for threshold retinopathy of prematurity. Pediatrics. 1999;104:e47.

56. Sharma S, Hollands H, Brown GC, Brown MM, Shah GK, Sharma SM. The cost-effectiveness of early vitrectomy for the treatment of vitreous hemorrhage in diabetic retinopathy. Curr Opin Ophthalmol. 2001;12:230–4.

57. Sharma S, Brown GC, Brown MM, Hollarnds H, Shah GK. The cost effectiveness of grid laser photocoagulation for the treatment of diabetic macular edema: results of a patient-based cost-utility analysis. Curr Opin Ophthalmol 2000;11(3): 175–9.

58. Brown GC, Brown MM, Sharma S, Busbee B. A Cost utility analysis of interventions for proliferative vitreoretinopathy. Am J Ophthalmol 2002;133:365–72.

59. Laupacis A, Feeny D, Detsky AS, Tugwell PX. How attractive does a new technology have to be to warrant adoption and utilization? Tentative guidelines for using clinical and economic evaluations. CMAJ. 1992;146:473–81.

60. Heudebert GR, Centor RM, Klapow JC, et al. What is heartburnworth? A cost-utility analysis of management strategies. J Gen Intern Med. 2000;15:175–82.

61. Kallmes DF, Kallmes MH. Cost-effectiveness of angiography performed during surgery for ruptured intracranial aneuryms. AJNR Am J Neuroradiol. 1997;18:1453–62.

62. World Health Organization. The World Health Report 2002. Reducing Risks, Promoting Healthy Life. Geneva, WHO, pp 101–144.

63. Brown MM, Brown GC. The Pharmacy & Therapeutics Committee and value-based medicine: A union whose time has come. Evidence-Based Ophthalmology 2006;7:8–9.

64. Klein R, Klein BEK, Tomany SC, et al. Ten-year incidence and progression of age-related maculopathy: the Beaver Dam Eye Study. Ophthalmology. 2002; 109:1767–79.

65. Friedman DS, O'Colmain BJ, Munoz B, Eye Diseases Prevalence Research Group, et al. Prevalence of age-related macular degeneration in the United States. Arch Ophthalmol. 2004;122:564–72.

66. Bureau of Labor and Statistics. Data on disability and unemployment. 1991/92, 1993/94, 1994/95, and 1997. From the survey of income and program participation. From the internet @ www.bls.census.gov. Accessed 4 Apr 2008.

67. The Financial Forecast Center. U.S. Gross Domestic Product GDP forecast. From the internet @http:// forecasts.org/gdp.htm. Accessed 20 May 2010.

68. Javitt JC, Zhou Z, Willke RJ. Association between visual loss and higher medical care costs in Medicare beneficiaries. Ophthalmology. 2007;114: 238–45.

69. Schmier JK, Halpern MT, Covert D, Delgado J, Sharma S. Impact of visual impairment on use of caregiving by individuals with age-related macular degeneration. Retina. 2006;26:1056–62.

70. Brown GC, Brown MM, Lieske HB, Cokman S, Tran I. A value-based medicine® analysis of ranibizumab for neovascular macular degeneration. The return-on-investment and wealth of the nation (in press).

Index

A.C. Ho and C.D. Regillo (eds.), *Age-related Macular Degeneration Diagnosis and Treatment*,
DOI 10.1007/978-1-4614-0125-4, © Springer Science+Business Media, LLC 2011